Color Handbook of

Dermatology

Color Handbook of

Dermatology

RJG Rycroft
MD FRCP FFOM DIH
Consultant Dermatologist
St John's Institute of Dermatology
St Thomas' Hospital
London, UK

SJ Robertson
BA FBIPP ARPS
Educational Technology Consultant
St John's Institute of Dermatology
St Thomas' Hospital
London, UK

APPLETON
& LANGE

First published in the United States of America in 1999 by
Appleton & Lange,
107 Elm Street,
PO Box 120041
Stamford CT 06912-0041, USA

ISBN: 0–8385–1622–X

Library of Congress Cataloging in Publication Data is available for this title
(Catalog Card Number 99–072077).

Project management: John Ormiston
Colour reproduction: Jade Reprographics, Braintree, UK
Printed by: Grafos SA, Barcelona, Spain

Contents

Preface

The purpose in compiling this little book is to combine excellence in pictorial quality with a concise but ordered text. Details of treatment have deliberately been omitted, to concentrate on dermatological diagnosis. The wide spectrum of skin disorders is covered by a loyal and industrious team of then-trainee dermatologists at St John's Institute of Dermatology – Daniel Creamer, David Fenton, Susan Handfield-Jones, Rachel Jenkins, Mary Judge, Sallie Neill, Bill Phillips, Charlotte Proby, Catherine Smith and Hywel Williams; Sarah Wakelin has been invaluable in assisting me with its subsequent editing.

We have aimed the book at all those who need some initial assistance in the recognition of disorders of the skin, from those starting out on formal dermatological training to experienced doctors in other disciplines who require some dermatological guidance, particular general practitioners. There are sure to be some errors and, as the dermatologist editor, I take full responsibility for these and look forward to being further educated. I thank my fellow-editor Stuart Robertson for his tireless pursuit of the illustrations that were required.

Richard J G Rycroft

Introduction

HISTORY

Diagnosis in dermatology follows the standard approach of history taking and physical examination. Questions relating to the presenting dermatosis should answer the following: time and site of onset; ensuing course; provoking and relieving factors (sunlight, temperature, occupation, etc.) and associated symptoms (itch, pain, etc.). It is important to elicit a history of any previous general medical or surgical problems as well as details of past dermatological conditions. A past history of eczema or psoriasis is of particular relevance. Enquiry into the occurrence of the common inherited dermatoses (such as atopic eczema, psoriasis or ichthyosis) in first-degree relatives is useful, as is a history of infectious illness in close personal contacts. Aspects of the patient's daily life are relevant to the diagnosis of many skin diseases: occupational or recreational contact with potentially sensitising substances may be pertinent as may a history of excess sun exposure. A detailed drug history is mandatory. A full list of medications taken for other conditions may reveal a possible culprit in iatrogenic skin disease, while knowledge of concomitant therapies may help to avoid drug interactions or polypharmacy. Current and past use of topical agents should be noted.

EXAMINATION

The diagnosis of skin disease is dependent on careful examination and the correct interpretation of cutaneous physical signs. In addition to an inspection of the area(s) of involvement, a dermatological examination should include visual assessment of the whole skin. Adequate illumination is imperative, while additional torch-light may be required to examine the oral cavity. At times, a light source positioned obliquely to the lesions can reveal important morphological information. Closer inspection of individual lesions is often helpful and is facilitated by the use of a hand lens. Palpation of the lesional skin should always be undertaken to provide information on temperature, consistency and level of tissue involvement. Examination of the regional lymph nodes is sometimes necessary.

In order to extract the maximum amount of information for diagnostic purposes, four aspects of the lesion(s) under scrutiny need to be recorded:

- Morphology.
- Shape.
- Distribution.
- Colour.

MORPHOLOGY

Most skin lesions have a characteristic morphology which, once defined, will narrow the differential diagnosis. The following list describes the features of the common primary lesions:

- Macule – a flat, non-palpable lesion (**1**) distinguished from adjacent, normal skin by a change in colour.
- Papule – a small, solid and raised lesion less than 5mm in diameter (**2**).
- Nodule – a larger, raised lesion greater than 5mm in diameter.
- Plaque – a flat-topped lesion with a diameter considerably greater than its height (**3**).
- Wheal – a transient swelling of the skin of any size, often associated with surrounding, localised erythema (the flare) (**4**).

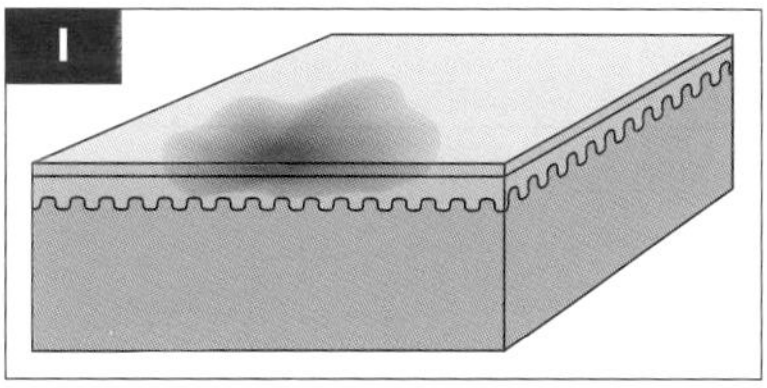

1 Macule.

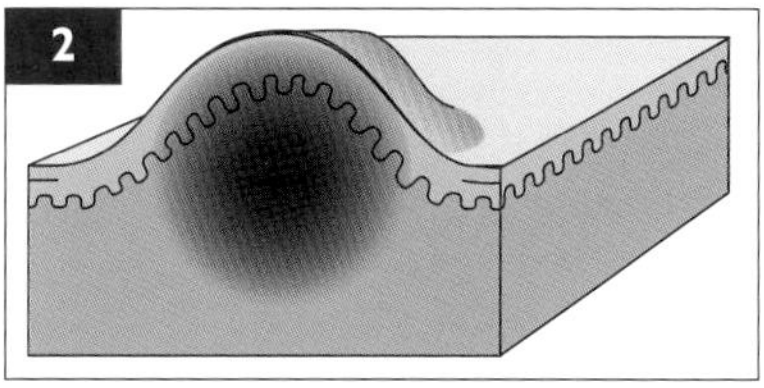

2 Papule.

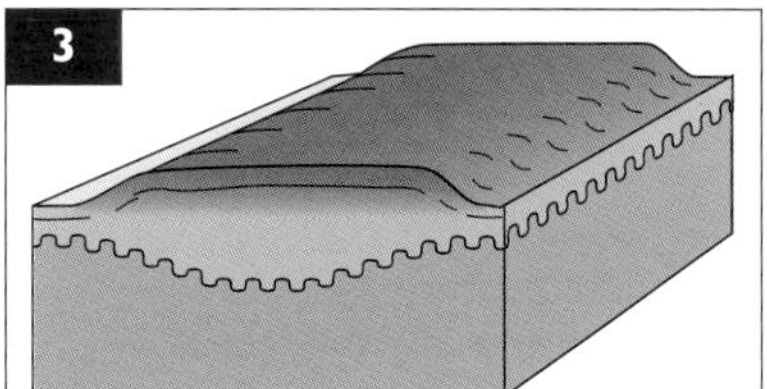

3 Plaque.

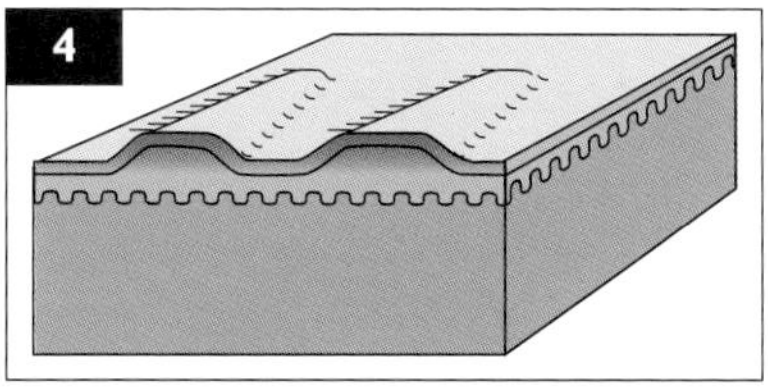

4 Weal.

Introduction

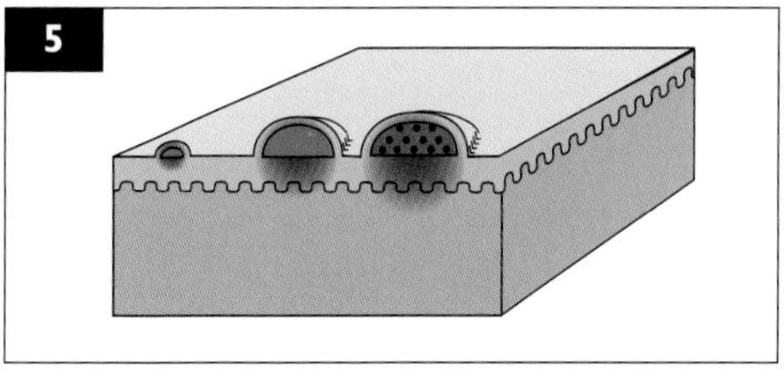

5 Vesicle.

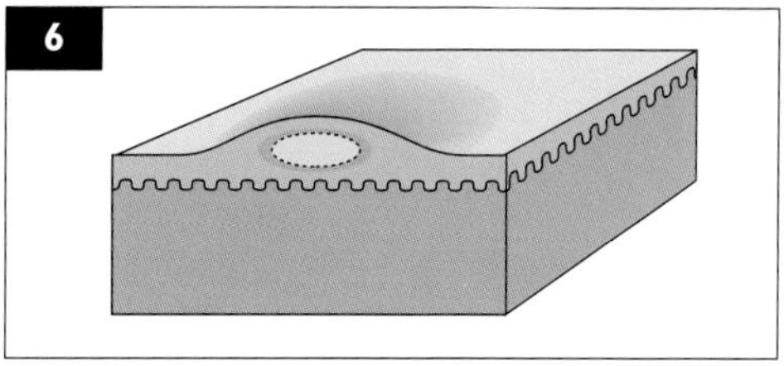

6 Pustule.

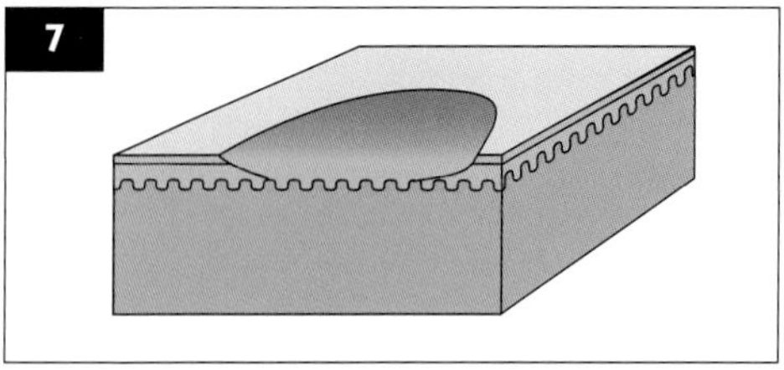

7 Erosion.

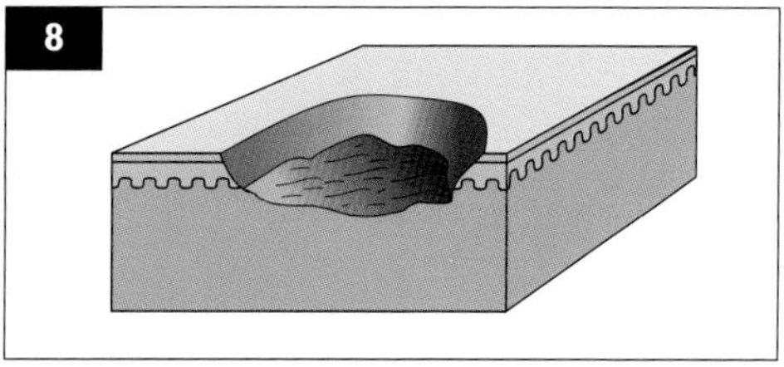

8 Ulcer.

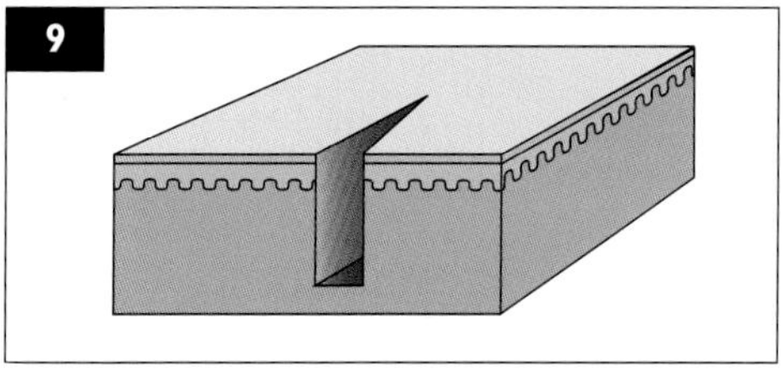

9 Fissure.

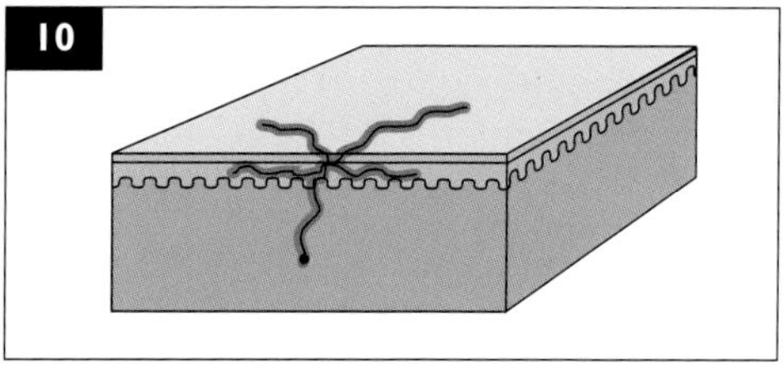

10 Telangiectasia.

- Vesicle – a blister less than 5mm in diameter (**5**).
- Bulla – a blister greater than 5mm in diameter.
- Pustule – a visible accumulation of pus, therefore white, yellow or green in colour (**6**).
- Erosion – an area of skin from which the epidermis alone has been lost (**7**).
- Ulcer – an area of skin from which the epidermis and part of the dermis has been lost (**8**).
- Fissure – a cleft-shaped ulcer (**9**).
- Telangiectasia – a visibly-dilated, small, dermal blood vessel (**10**).
- Comedone – accumulation of keratin and sebum lodged in dilated pilosebaceous orifice (**11**).

A primary lesion can be associated with additional, superimposed features:

- Scale – a flake of keratinised epidermal cells lying on the skin surface (**12**).
- Crust – dried serous or sanguineous exudate (**13**).
- Hyperkeratosis – an area of thickened stratum corneum (**14**).
- Atrophy – thinning of the skin due to the partial loss of one or more of the tissue layers of the skin (epidermis, dermis, subcutis) (**15**).
- Sclerosis – hardening of the skin due to dermal pathological change (often an expansion of collagenous elements) characterised by induration.
- Lichenification – thickened skin with increased markings usually due to prolonged scratching (**16**).
- Umbilicated – shaped like the umbilicus (**17**).
- Exudate – material escaped from blood vessels with a high content of protein, cells, cellular debris, etc. (**18**).
- Warty – horny excrescence (**19**).
- Excoriation – scratch or abrasion of the skin (**20**).

Introduction

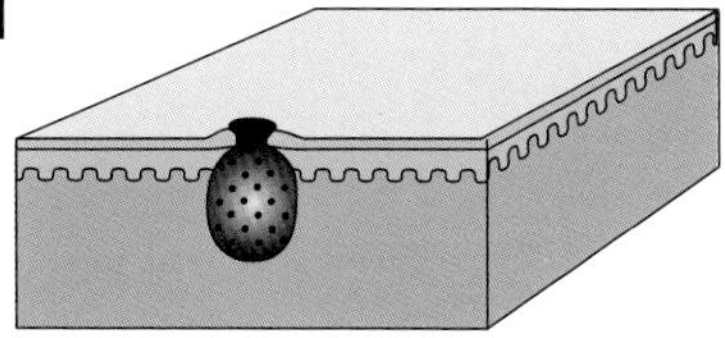

11 Comedone.

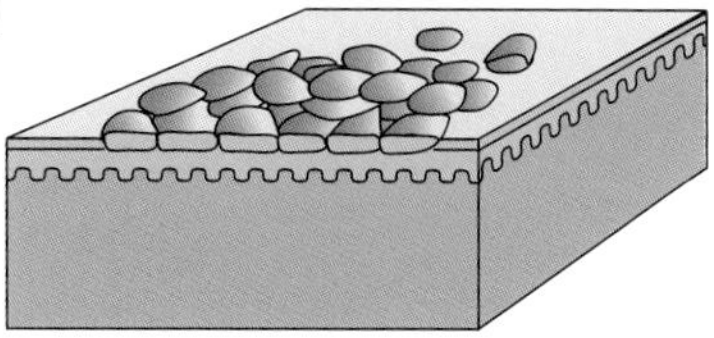

12 Scale.

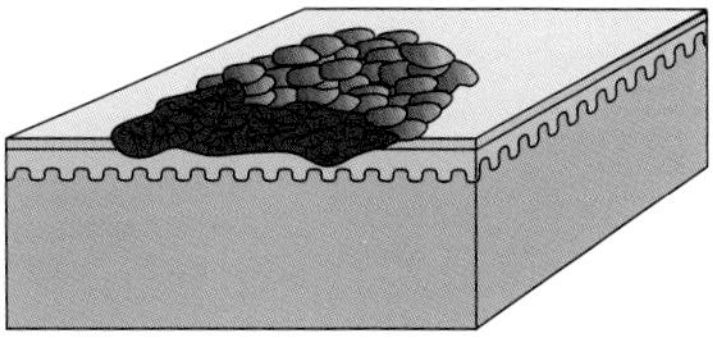

13 Crust.

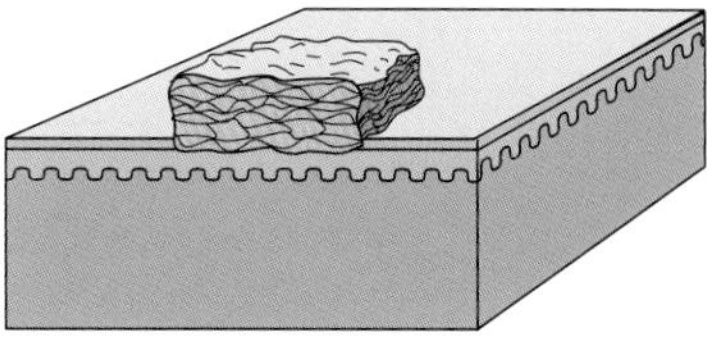

14 Hyperkeratosis.

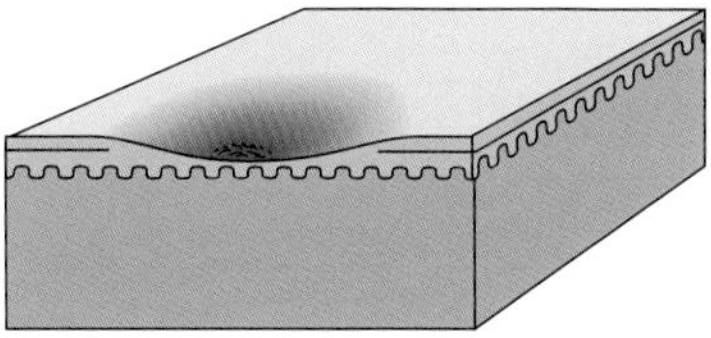

15 Atrophy.

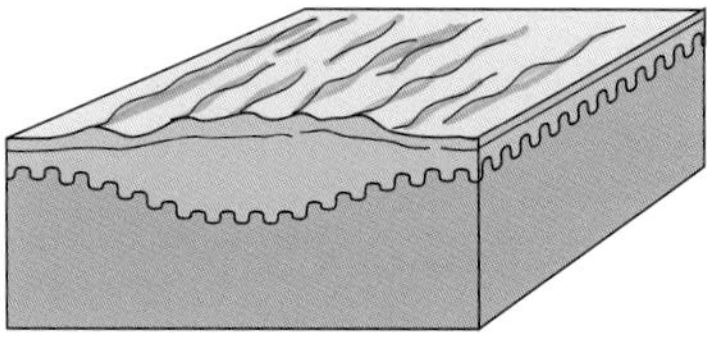

16 Lichenification.

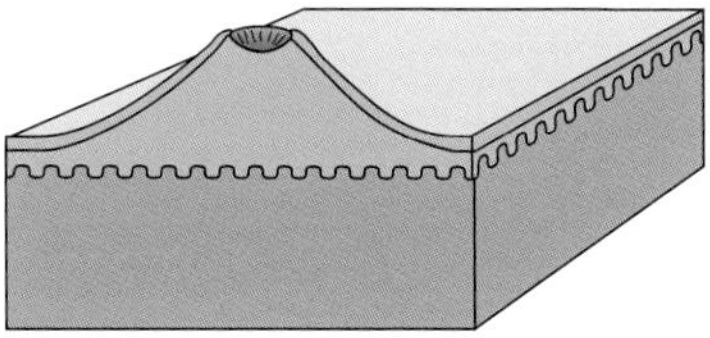

17 Umbilicated.

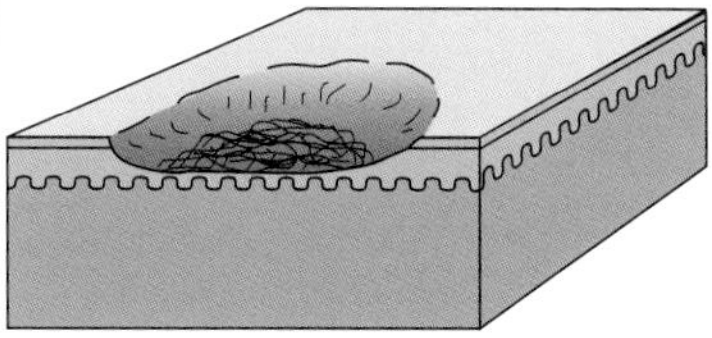

18 Exudate.

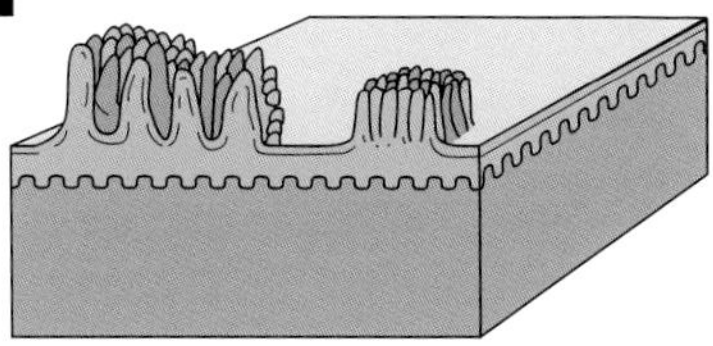

19 Warty.

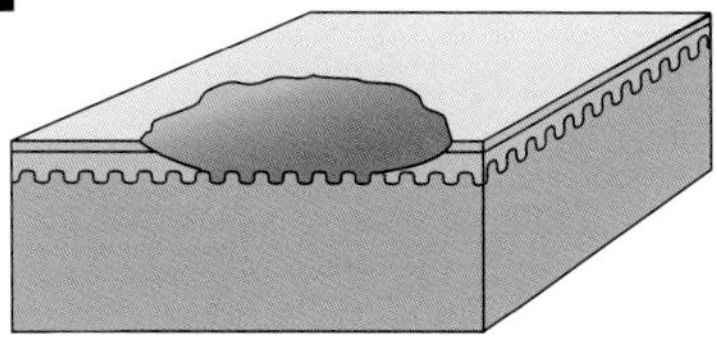

20 Excoriation.

Introduction

SHAPE

The shape of individual lesions has a clinical significance as certain dermatoses consist of lesions possessing a characteristic shape. The following list defines the nomenclature for the commonly observed shapes or patterns:

- Linear (**21**).
- Discoid refers to a coin-shaped lesion.
- Annular describes a ring-shaped lesion (**22**).
- Target describes a lesion consisting of concentric rings.
- Polycyclic describes a pattern of interlocking rings.
- Arcuate describes lesions that are arc shaped.
- Serpiginous describes a linear lesion which is wavy in shape (**23**).
- Whorled is used to describe lesions which follow the developmental lines of Blaschko and demonstrate a curved or spiral pattern.
- Digitate refers to lesions which are finger-like in shape.
- Zosteriform means resembling herpes zoster (see p. 76).

DISTRIBUTION

The majority of skin diseases have a characteristic distribution or a predilection for certain sites. Other dermatoses vary in extent of involvement according to their severity. The recognition of particular configurations is important diagnostically, while defining the extent of involvement is useful for prognostic and therapeutic reasons. Discrete lesions occurring in a localised area are called grouped (**24**) while multiple lesions distributed over a wide area of skin are called scattered (**25**). There are terms which define widespread distributions more exactly:

- Exanthem refers to a predominantly truncal eruption consisting of multiple, symmetrical, erythematous, maculopapular lesions. Such dermatoses (called exanthematous) can be further described as being either morbilliform (meaning measles-like, comprised of blotchy, pink, slightly elevated lesions) or scarlatiniform (meaning scarlet fever-like, comprised of tiny erythematous papules).
- Confluent describes the appearance of a coalescence of individual lesions to form a large area of involvement.
- Erythroderma implies that a particular dermatosis involves more than 90% of the body surface area and that the involvement is confluent.

The distribution of lesions can also be described according to regional involvement, the recognition of which can help pinpoint a diagnosis:

- Centrifugal – mostly affecting the extremities, e.g. granuloma annulare.
- Centripetal – mostly affecting the trunk, e.g. pemphigus vulgaris.
- Centrifacial – mostly involving the forehead, nose and chin, e.g. rosacea.
- Palmoplantar – affecting the palms and soles, e.g. palmoplantar pustulosis.
- Flexural – involving the flexural skin, e.g. erythrasma.
- Extensor – involving the extensor skin, e.g. plaque psoriasis.
- Dermatomal – affecting the skin of one or more dermatomes, e.g. shingles (herpes zoster).
- Periorbital – distributed around the eyes, e.g. syringomata.
- Perioral – distributed around the mouth, e.g. perioral dermatitis.
- Light-exposed – involving the skin routinely exposed to sunlight, e.g. chronic actinic dermatitis.

COLOUR

Cutaneous lesions can be flesh-coloured, demonstrate a change in pigmentation (hyper- or hypo-pigmentation) or be characterised by redness. Erythema is redness due to microvascular dilatation which can be blanched by pressure. Purpura is a darker cutaneous redness due to erythrocyte extravasation; purpura cannot be blanched by pressure.

Introduction

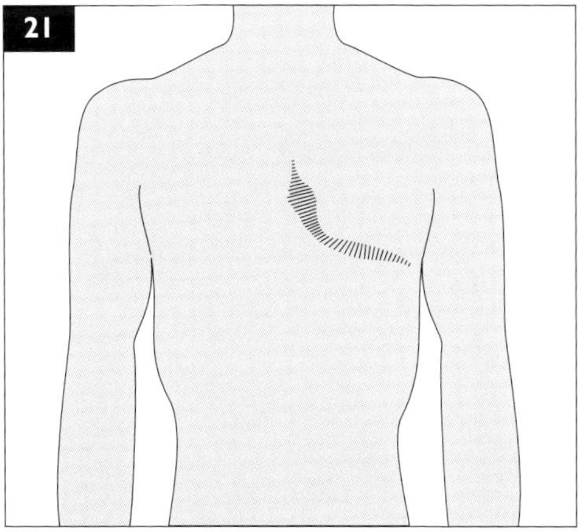

21 Linear lesion.

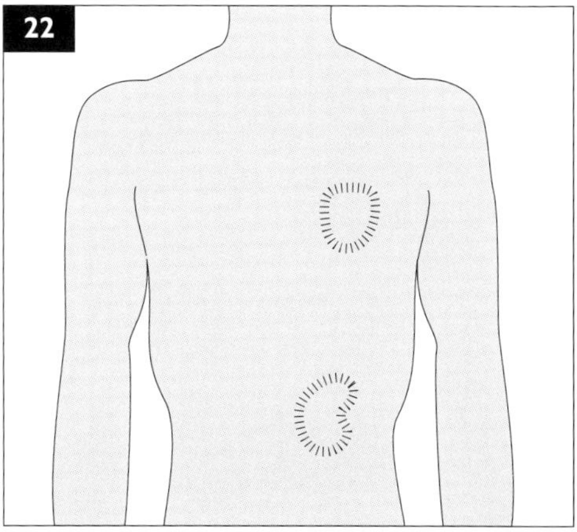

22 Annular lesion.

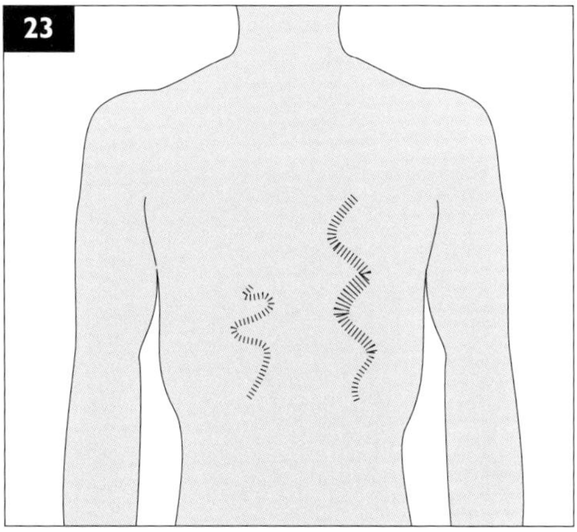

23 Serpiginous lesion.

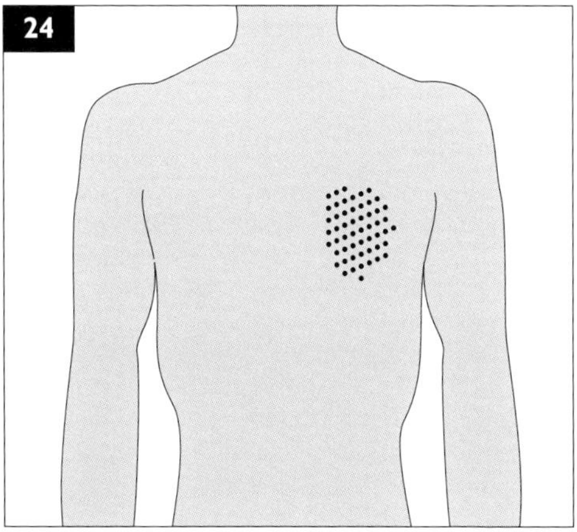

24 Grouped lesions.

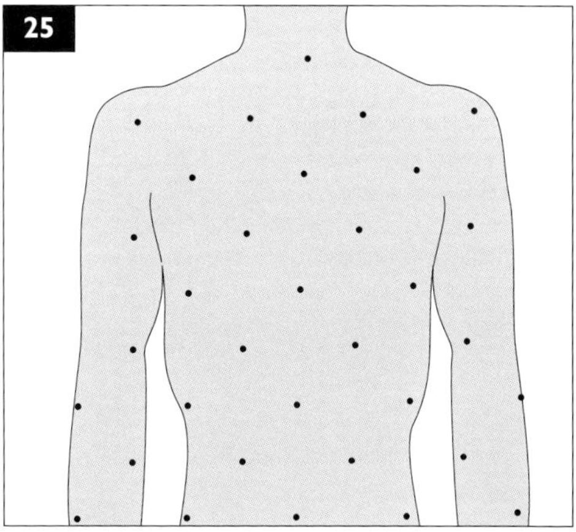

25 Scattered lesions.

The Eczemas

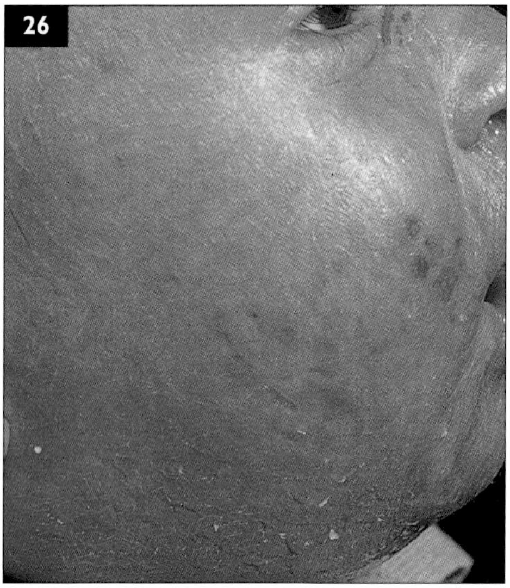

26 Infantile eczema.

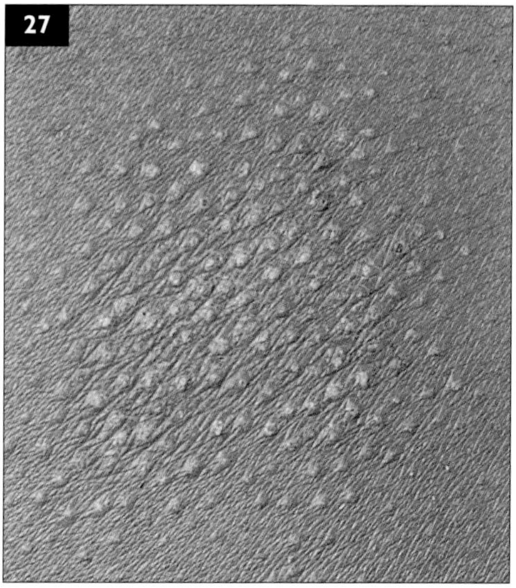

27 Follicular eczema.

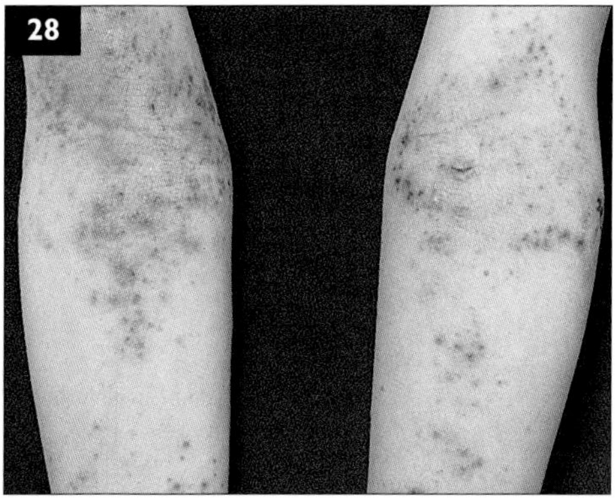

28 Flexural eczema.

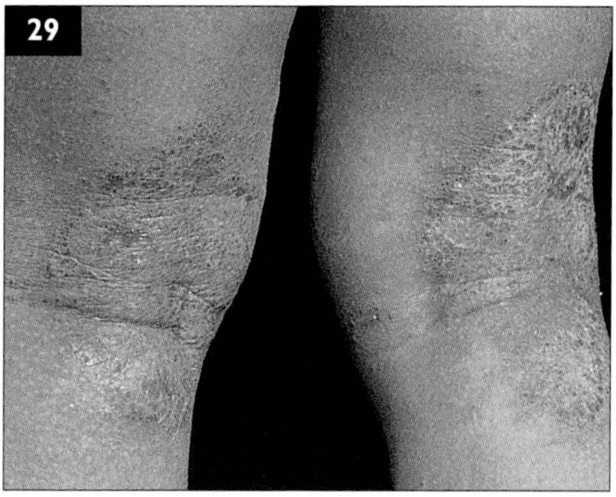

29 Flexural eczema.

Endogenous eczemas are a group of eczemas where the primary role of external factors is not established. Like anaemia the word eczema is not a diagnosis in itself and should prompt further enquiry to identify the subtype of eczema or a treatable cause.

ATOPIC ECZEMA (ATOPIC DERMATITIS)

Definition and clinical features

A chronic, pruritic skin condition which commonly affects skin flexures. In the first 2 years of life eczematous lesions are often present on exposed areas such as the cheeks (**26**) or outer aspects of the forearms or legs. The lesions are red, poorly defined and surface changes such as scaling, erosions, papules or vesicles are present. Follicular eczema may occur, especially in black skin (**27**). In the older child, eczema usually affects flexural sites such as the antecubital (**28**) and popliteal fossae (**29**), the fronts of the ankles (**30**) and around the neck (**31**) and face. Children are often miserable as a result of intractable itching. A generally dry skin is almost always present even in the absence of active eczema.

The Eczemas

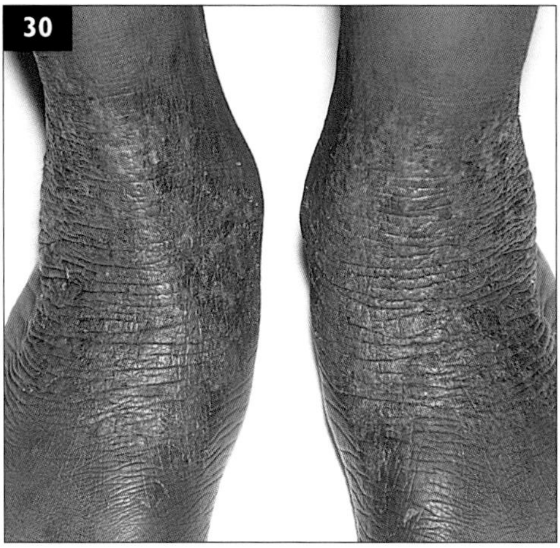

30 Ankle eczema.

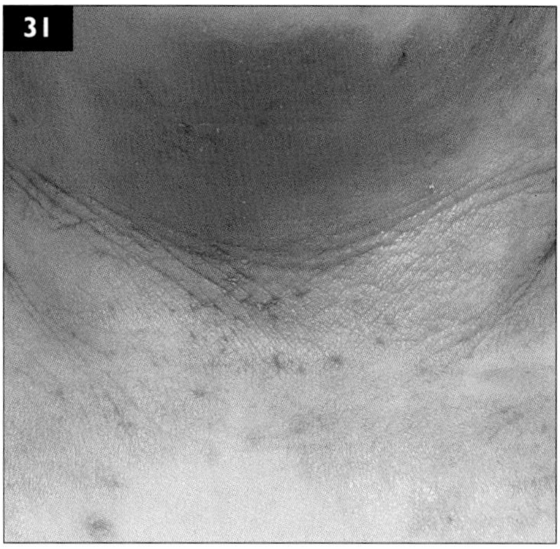

31 Neck eczema.

Epidemiology

Atopic eczema affects around 10% of children in developing countries and its prevalence is rising. Onset in the first year of life occurs in around 70% of cases. Around half of these children go on to develop asthma or hay fever or both. Two-thirds of children with atopic eczema are clear by the age of 16 but the condition may recur as hand eczema in adulthood (**32**). Genetic and environmental factors are probably equally important in the development of atopic eczema. Allergic factors such as house dust mite and food allergies play a role but physical factors such as microbial infection and irritation from soaps and textiles are also important.

Differential diagnosis

Irritant contact dermatitis of the hands in older patients and napkin dermatitis in infants. Scabies must be excluded in any widespread pruritic eruption of recent onset. Contact dermatitis is not usually flexural except in the case of clothing, wood dust dermatitis or autosensitisation eczema.

Investigations

These are not usually necessary to establish the diagnosis but a raised serum IgE level and multiple skin prick test positivity are useful supportive features in difficult cases. Skin swabs may be useful to determine the sensitivities of microbial secondary infection or the presence of the herpes simplex virus. Patch testing may occasionally be used to establish contact factors.

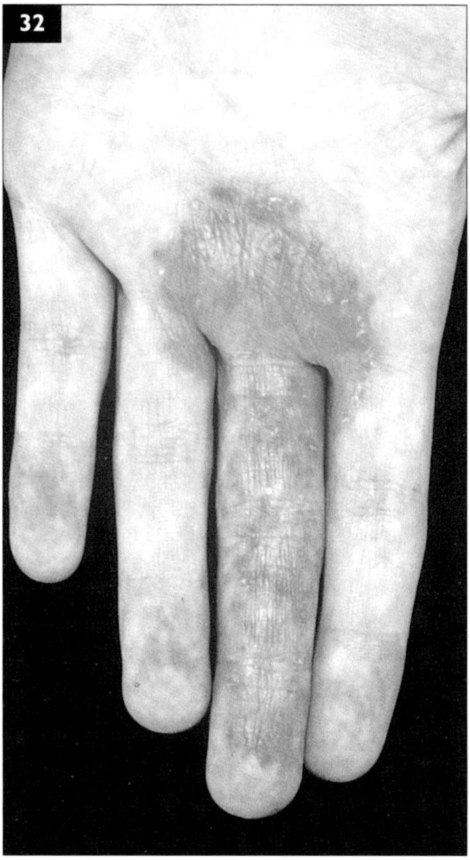

32 Hand eczema.

The Eczemas

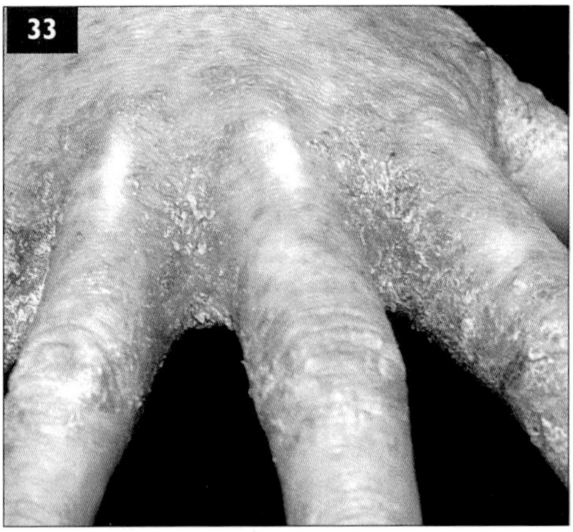

33 Secondary infection with *Staphylococcus aureus*.

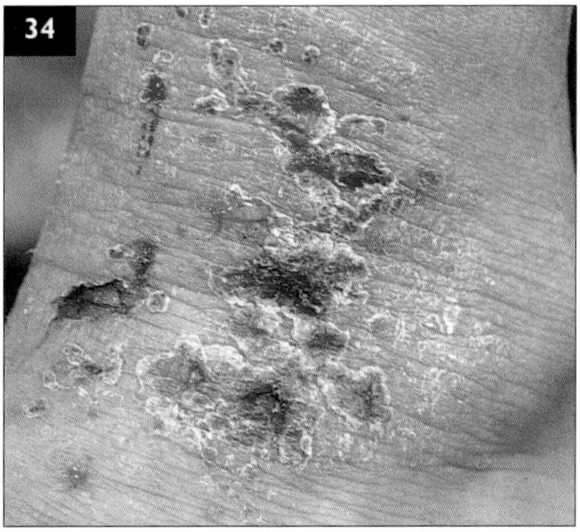

34 Secondary infection with *Staphylococcus aureus*.

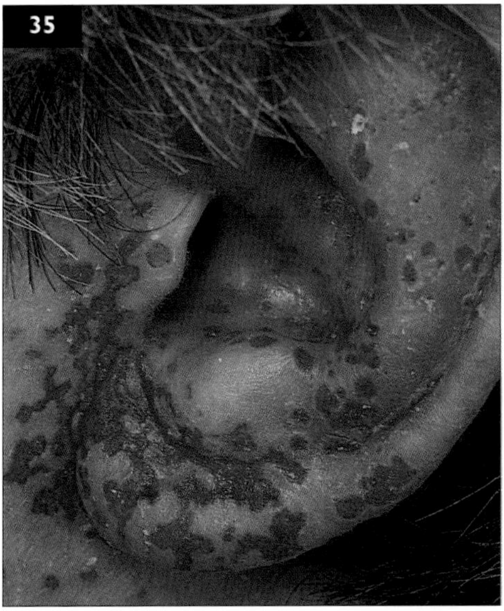

35 Eczema herpeticum.

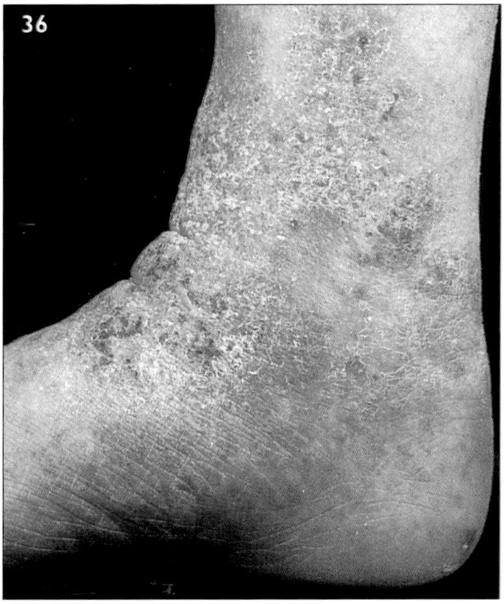

36 Venous eczema.

Special points

Secondary infection with *Staphylococcus aureus* is common where soreness, crusting and pustules may be present (**33**, **34**). Occasionally, the herpes simplex virus may grow very rapidly on an area of atopic eczema (eczema herpeticum) and may warrant treatment with systemic acyclovir (**35**). Allergic contact dermatitis may be superimposed on atopic eczema.

VENOUS ECZEMA (GRAVITATIONAL, VARICOSE OR STASIS ECZEMA)

Definition and clinical features

Eczema secondary to venous hypertension. Venous eczema typically occurs on the lower legs (**36**). The inner aspect of the lower leg is the first area to be affected; possibly also present are accompanying changes such as pigmentation from haemosiderin deposition, small white areas

The Eczemas

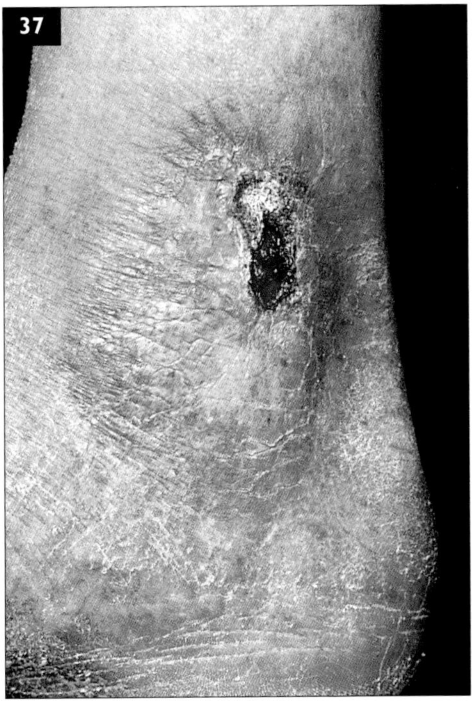

37 Venous ulcer.

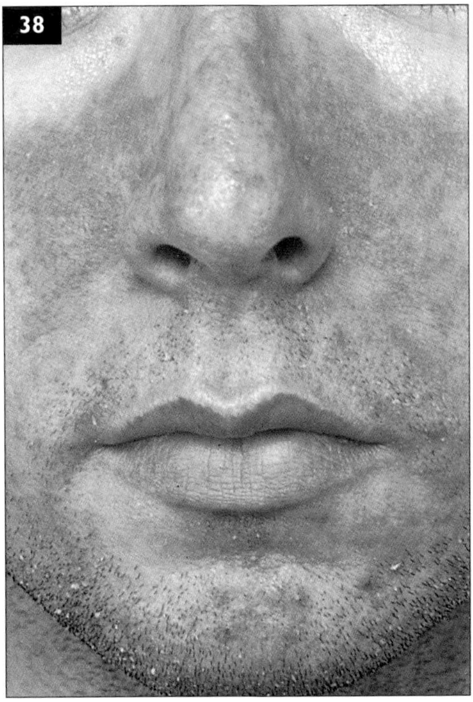

38 Seborrhoeic eczema.

of atrophy (atrophie blanche), oedema, purpura and venous varicosities. Trivial injury can often lead to the development of a venous ulcer (**37**).

Epidemiology

The exact mechanism of venous eczema is still unknown, but venous hypertension secondary to a previous deep vein thrombosis is the most common cause. The condition is commonest in middle and old age; and females outnumber males.

Differential diagnosis

Contact dermatitis secondary to rubber hosiery or impregnated bandages usually involves the whole of the lower leg and shows a sharp cut-off point. Cellulitis is very tender, red and hot, and the patient usually feels unwell. Eczematous changes are not seen in erythromelalgia, a syndrome of intense burning and heat of the lower legs and feet.

Investigations

Doppler studies will help to identify the source of any perforating veins amenable to surgery and will test the adequacy of the distal arterial circulation. Swabs may be indicated if secondary infection is suspected. Patch testing is needed to detect medicament sensitivity.

Special points

Contact dermatitis from medicaments is a common problem at this site, for which treatment should be kept as simple as possible.

SEBORRHOEIC ECZEMA (SEBORRHOEIC DERMATITIS)

Definition and clinical features

A relapsing eczema affecting seborrhoeic areas such as the scalp, face and upper trunk. Patients usually complain of the cosmetic effects of scaling and redness rather than itching. Lesions of seborrhoeic eczema are covered with a fine scale and are often quite well demarcated. The scalp may be diffusely involved or lesions may be localised to the scalp margins. On the face, the paranasal areas (**38**), eyebrows and external ears are commonly affected.

The Eczemas

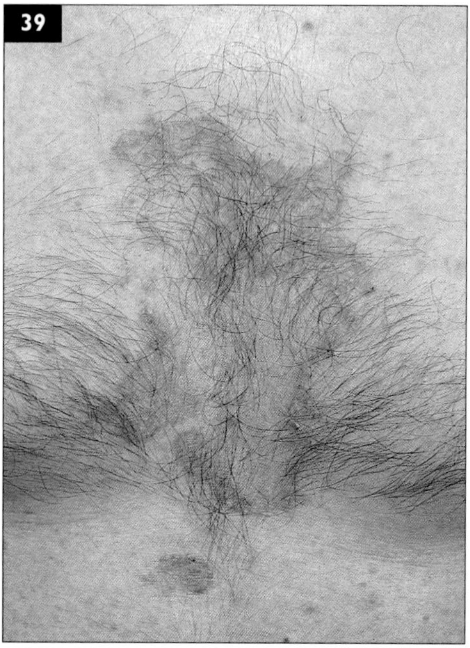

39 Seborrhoeic eczema.

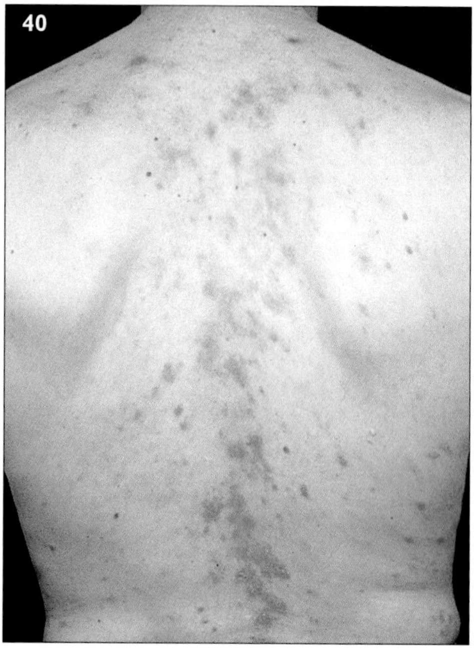

40 Seborrhoeic eczema.

Elsewhere the presternal area (**39**), interscapular area (**40**), axillae and groins may be involved.

Epidemiology
Although the exact aetiology is unknown, there is strong evidence to link seborrhoeic eczema with the presence of the yeast *Pityrosporum ovale*. Adults are affected and the condition may indicate underlying debilitation if very extensive.

Differential diagnosis
Mild facial and scalp psoriasis can be very difficult to distinguish from seborrhoeic eczema. However, the lesions of the latter are usually less well demarcated and less scaly than those of psoriasis. Systemic lupus erythematosus usually affects the malar as opposed to the paranasal areas and such patients are systemically unwell.

Investigations
None are usually necessary. Any facial dermatitis which does not fit the above clinical description should be investigated for possible contact factors.

Special points
Whilst most seborrhoeic eczema occurs in healthy adults, the sudden appearance of widespread involvement in a sexually active person should raise the possibility of underlying immunosuppression such as HIV infection.

Seborrhoeic eczema of infancy is a non-pruritic, well-demarcated eczema of the napkin area which presents in the first 6 weeks of life and has an excellent prognosis (**41**). Its precise relationship to adult seborrhoeic eczema is unclear.

DISCOID ECZEMA (NUMMULAR ECZEMA)
Definition and clinical features
This is an eczema of unknown cause characterised by multiple coin-shaped lesions over the limbs and trunk. It is very pruritic and consists of multiple coin-shaped lesions measuring 2–6 cm in diameter (**42**). They are quite well demarcated (**43**).

The Eczemas

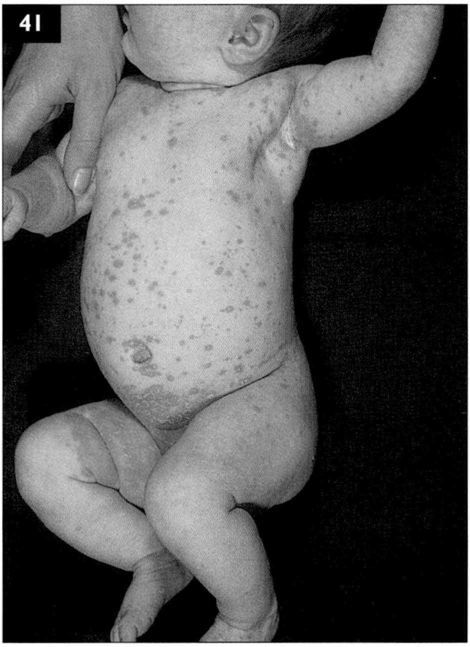

41 Seborrhoeic eczema of infancy.

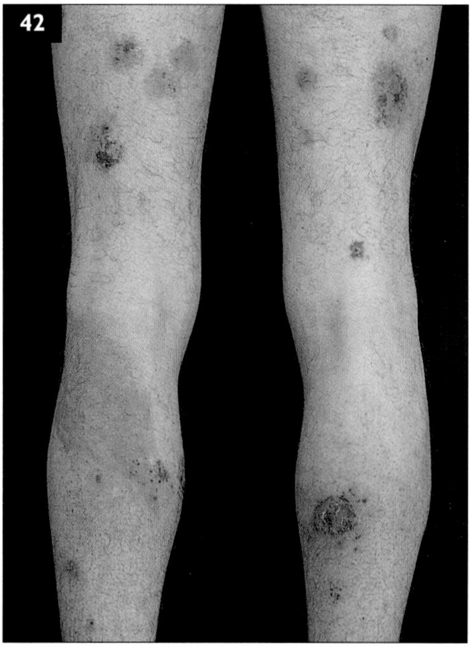

42 Discoid eczema.

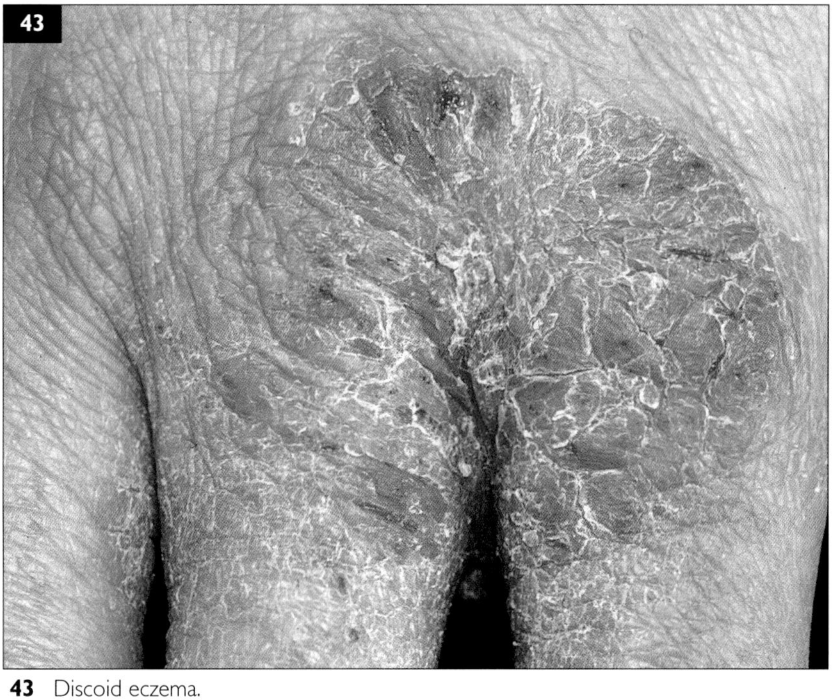

43 Discoid eczema.

The Eczemas

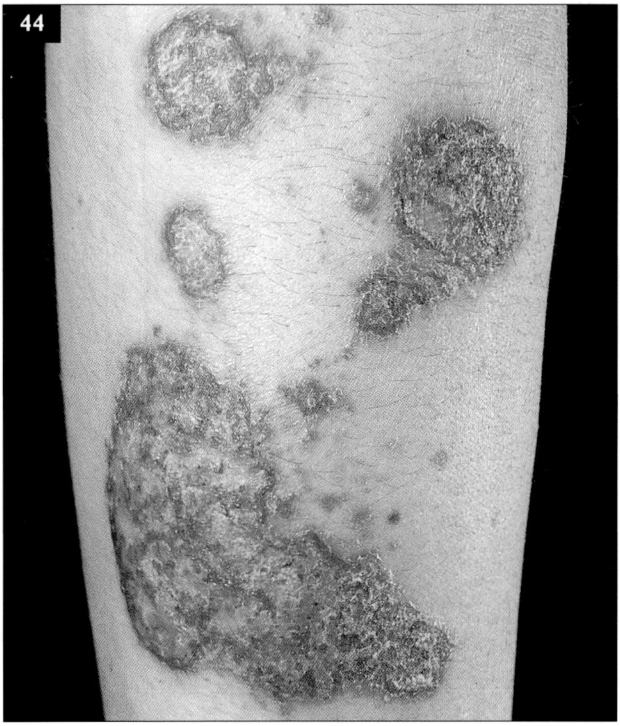

44 Discoid eczema.

The centres of the lesions could possibly contain vesicles, oozing, crusts and scaling (**44**). The limbs are usually the first areas to be affected (**45**) but the trunk may be involved in more extensive cases. A general dryness of the skin is often evident.

Epidemiology

Discoid eczema may be seen at any age but is most common in middle-aged adults. Its precise relationship to atopic eczema is unknown. Emotional stress, excessive drying of the skin and secondary infection may be important factors in the dissemination of lesions.

Differential diagnosis

The lesions of guttate psoriasis are usually smaller (1–2 cm) than in discoid eczema and are not especially pruritic. Tinea corporis exhibits a distinct border and vesicles are not usually present.

Investigations

None are usually required. Swabs for microbial culture may reveal secondary infection. Scrapings must be taken from solitary lesions to exclude infection with tinea. Atypical cases should be patch tested.

Special points

The condition often responds dramatically to treatment with potent topical corticosteroids but relapses are common.

ASTEATOTIC ECZEMA

Definition and clinical features

Eczema caused by the excessive loss of skin lipids. This eczema may occur at any age but elderly people are particularly prone with the lower limbs commonly affected. The skin is generally dry (**46**) and in some areas cracks appear which become red (eczéma craquelé) (**47**). A generalised eczema or discoid pattern may eventually develop.

Epidemiology

The exact prevalence of this condition is unknown but it is one of the commonest reasons for a dermatologist to be called to see a hospital inpatient. Lesions develop when natural skin

The Eczemas

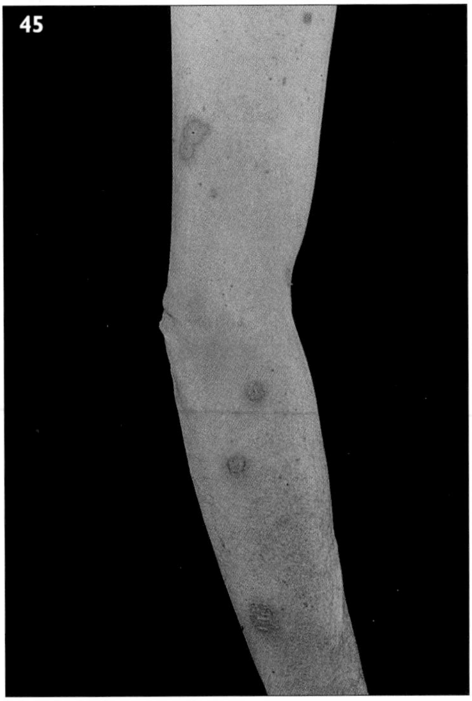
45 Discoid eczema.

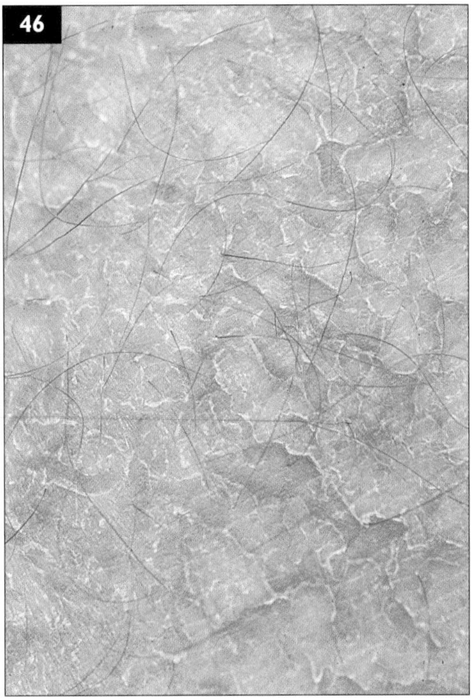
46 Asteatotic eczema.

lipid production can no longer keep up with its removal by frequent washing with soaps. This commonly occurs in elderly inpatients in whom lipid production may be reduced. High ambient temperatures of wards also play a role.

Differential diagnosis

Drug eruptions are usually more proximal and symmetrical, inflamed cracks in the skin surface being unusual. Atopic eczema sufferers also have a tendency to a generally dry skin which may develop features of eczéma craquelé if excessive washing occurs. Congenital ichthyosis, as the name implies, is present from birth. Lymphoma or treatment with clofazimine may occasionally give rise to a generalised dryness of the skin.

Investigations

No investigations are usually necessary.

Special points

The use of soap substitutes and emollients is all that is usually required to treat and prevent this condition.

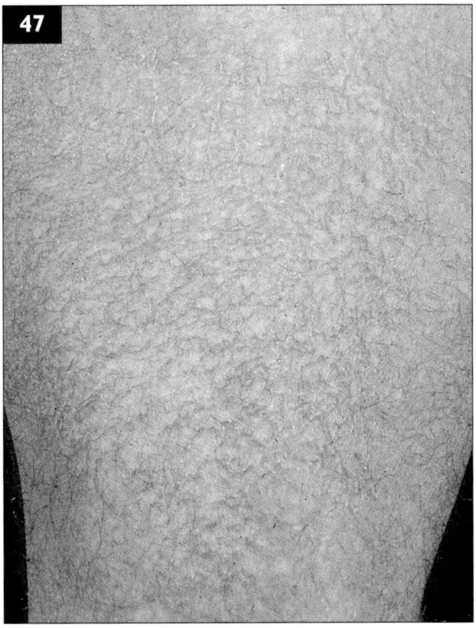
47 Asteatotic eczema (eczéma craquelé).

The Eczemas

48

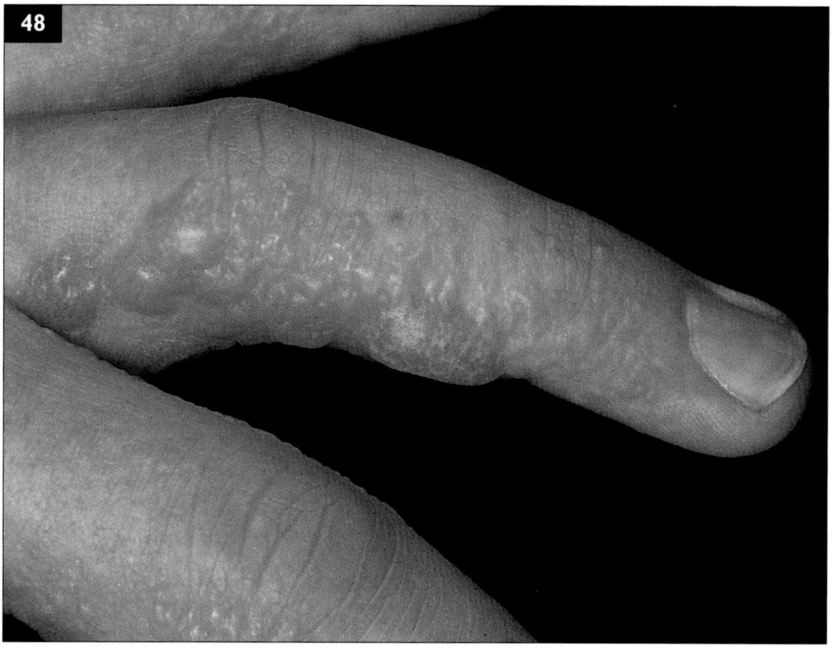

48 Pompholyx.

POMPHOLYX

Definition and clinical features

A severe form of eczema of the palms and/or soles in which there are vesicles up to 10 mm in diameter, becoming confluent. Sudden crops of clear vesicles that appear deep-seated and sago-like. Confluence produces large bullae (**48**). Itching may be severe. Secondary bacterial infection may complicate the condition.

Epidemiology

Pompholyx may occur at any age but its onset is usually between the ages of 10 and 40 years. Recurrence is often over long periods, especially in the summer.

Differential diagnosis

While many cases are forms of endogenous eczema, both irritant and allergic contact dermatitis may at times confuse, as may pustular psoriasis, tinea and sometimes even pemphigoid.

Investigations

Mycological and/or bacterial examination, as well as patch testing, may be indicated.

Special points

There is possibly a case for dropping the term pompholyx in favour of severe vesicular eczema.

Lichen Simplex

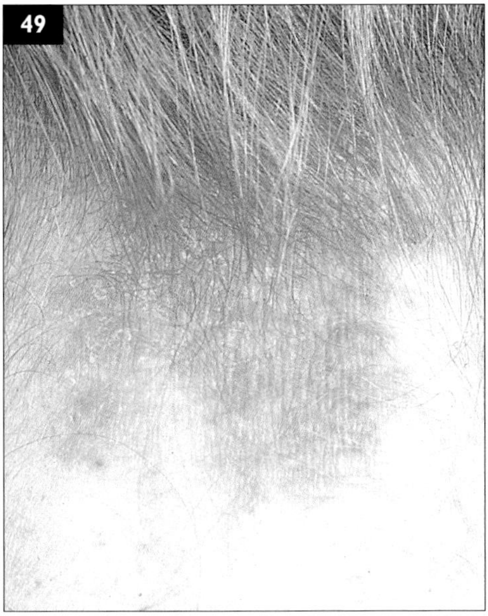

49 Lichen simplex.

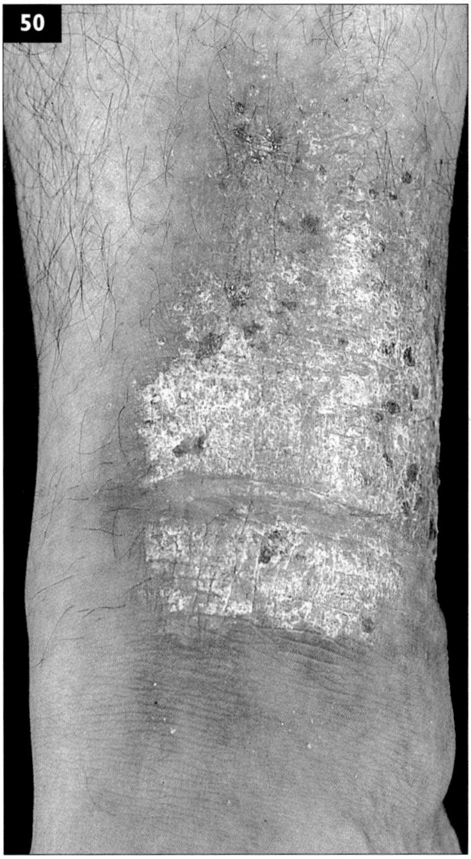

50 Lichen simplex.

Definition and clinical features
Lichenification where there is no known predisposing skin disorder. Circumscribed patches of intensely itchy lichenification which may be surrounded by closely set lichenoid papules and peripheral hyperpigmentation. Common sites are the nape (**49**) and sides of the neck, scalp, backs of the forearms, lower legs and ankles (**50**), upper inner thighs, pubis, vulva and scrotum. Chronicity is common.

Epidemiology
Peak incidence is between the ages of 30 and 50 years but it can be seen at any time after puberty.

Differential diagnosis
Lichen planus, psoriasis, tinea and contact dermatitis (e.g. nail varnish).

Investigations
Biopsy, mycological examination or patch testing may be required.

Special points
Underlying emotional tension may benefit from exploration and assistance in reduction. Topical corticosteroids under occlusion are otherwise useful in treatment.

Contact Dermatitis

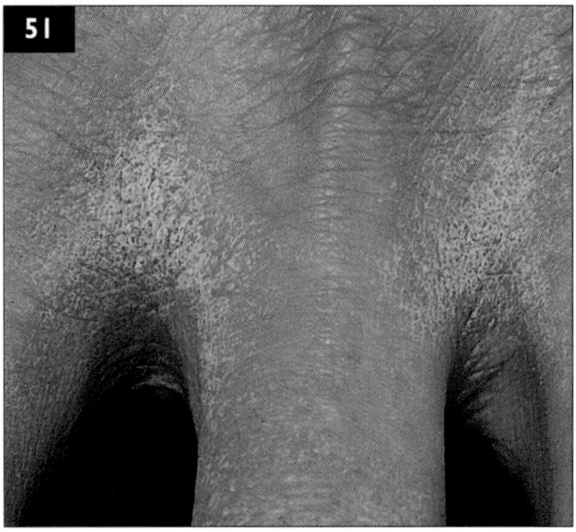

51 Irritant contact dermatitis.

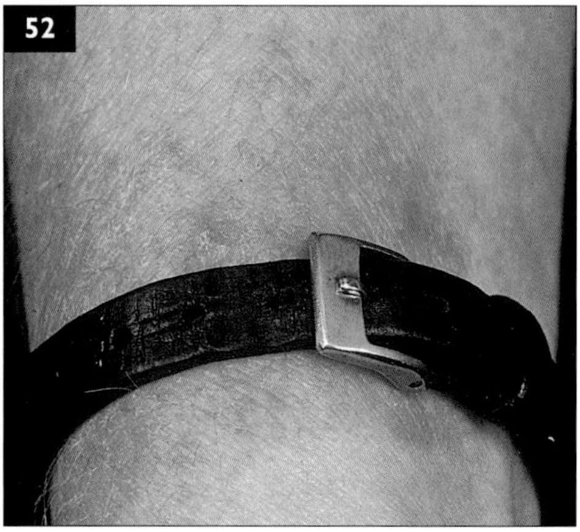

52 Allergic contact dermatitis from nickel.

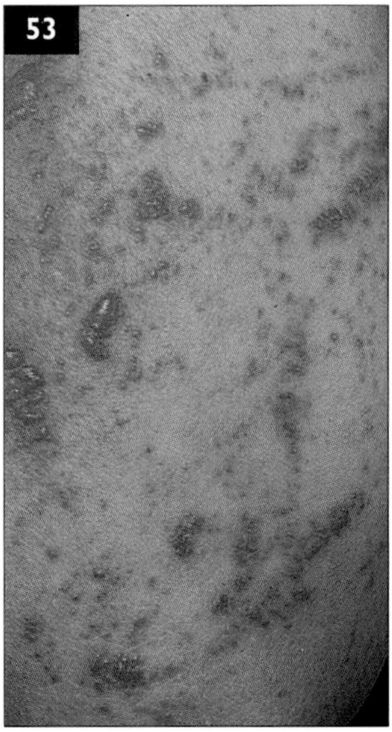

53 Allergic contact dermatitis from primula.

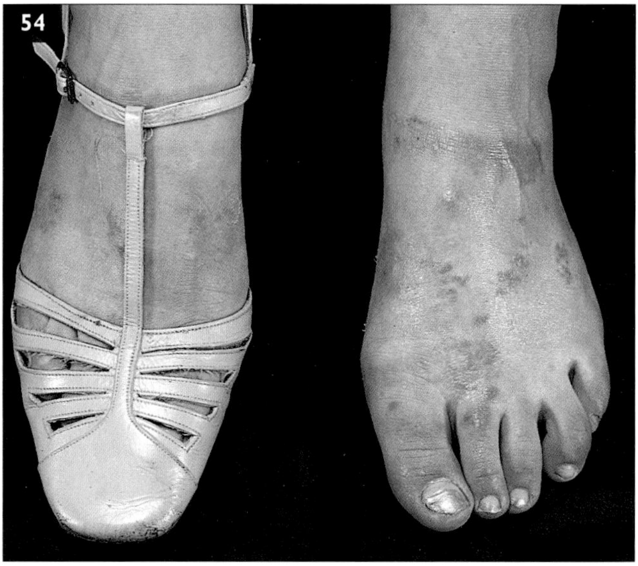

54 Allergic contact dermatitis from a shoe.

Definition and clinical features

This is a dermatitis (i.e. an eczema) caused by contact with external substances (contact factors). It may be allergic (immunological) or irritant (non-immunological) (**51**). Morphologically indistinguishable from endogenous eczema (see above). Certain patterns are characteristic of some contact factors, e.g. nickel (**52**), primula (**53**), shoe dermatitis (**54**) and hat bands (**55**).

Contact Dermatitis

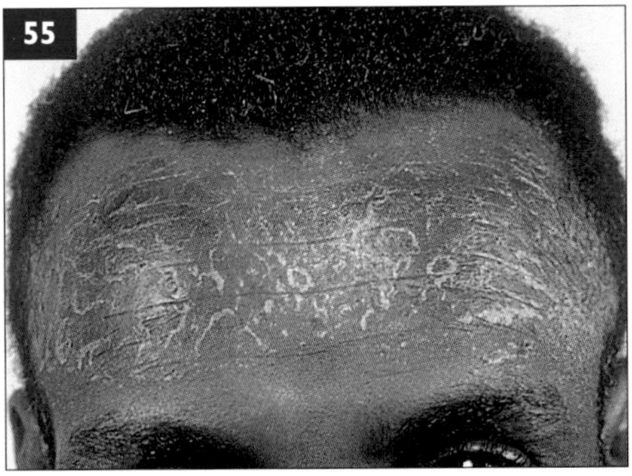

55 Allergic contact dermatitis from a hat band.

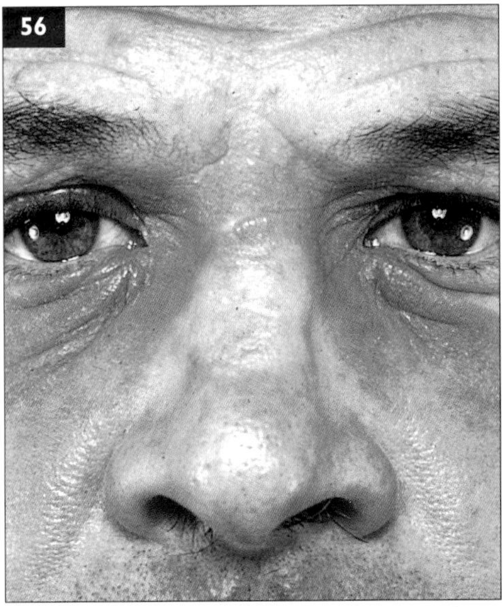

56 Occupational allergic contact dermatitis from airborne epoxy resin.

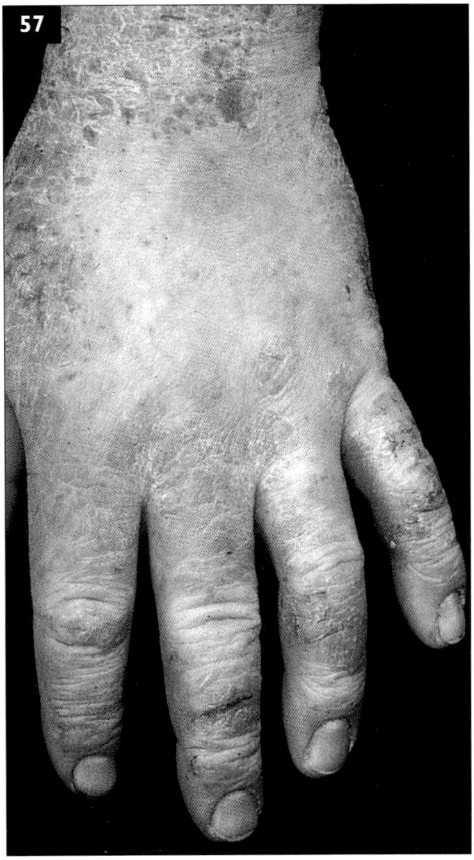

57 Occupational allergic contact dermatitis from chromate in wet cement.

Epidemiology

Point prevalences of contact dermatitis in the general population higher than 5% have been found, and higher than 10% in high-risk occupations.

Differential diagnosis

Due to its clinical identity with endogenous eczema a high level of suspicion is required, particularly in chronic eczema, eczema subject to rapid and recurrent relapse, eczema of an unusual clinical pattern (**56**) and hand eczema (**57**). Psoriasis and tinea are the main non-eczematous causes of confusion, particularly on the hands.

Investigations

Patch testing is essential to distinguish allergic (cell-mediated, Type IV) from irritant (non-immunological) contact dermatitis and endogenous eczema.

Special points

Occupational contact dermatitis is among the commonest of all occupational diseases.

Non-Dermatitic Occupational Dermatoses

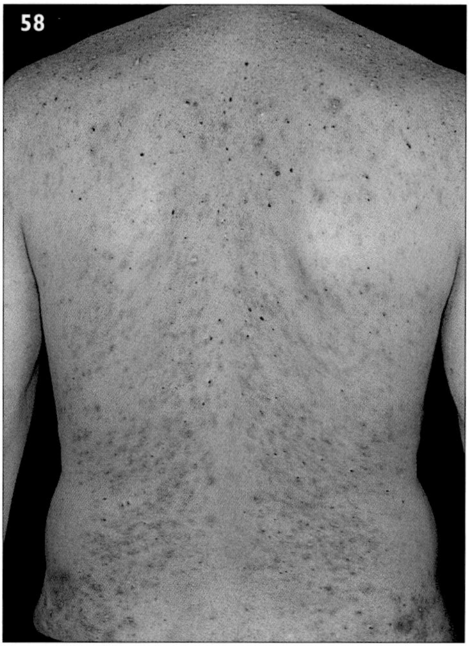

58 Chloracne.

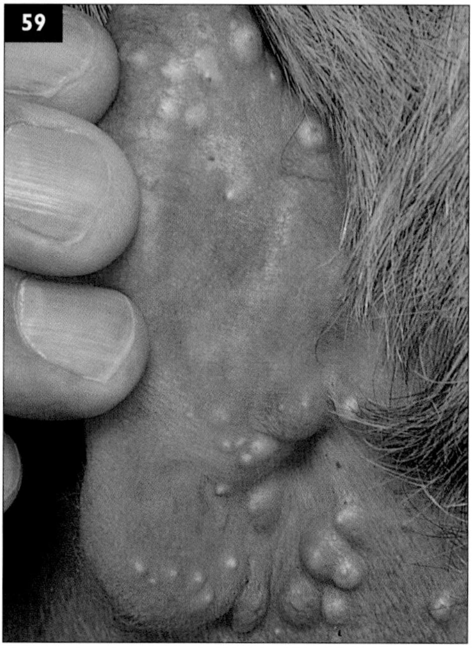

59 Chloracne cysts.

CHLORACNE

Definition and clinical features

A refractory follicular dermatosis caused by occupational or environmental exposure to halogenated aromatic compounds of a specific molecular shape (e.g. dioxins) which may be accompanied by systemic toxicity. Open comedones (blackheads) (**58**) with small, pale-yellow cysts (**59**) predominate in milder cases. In more severe cases, inflammatory pustules and even cold abscesses develop. The skin just below and to the outer side of the eye and behind the ear (**59**) is the most sensitive, next the cheeks, forehead (but not the nose) and male genitalia, followed in severe cases by the shoulders, chest and back (**58**), buttocks and abdomen. Lesions may continue to appear after exposure ceases and tend to persist in spite of treatment.

Epidemiology

Epidemics have occurred from accidental ingestion or inhalation as well as from external skin contact in chemical plants (and surrounding populations after plant explosions) and chemical waste disposal plants. All ages are susceptible.

Differential diagnosis

Acne vulgaris in younger patients, senile comedones in older patients, cystic acne in severe cases.

Investigations

Occupational or community clustering of similar cases and appropriate exposure should be enquired for. Biopsy shows characteristic keratinous cysts replacing sebaceous glands. The patient's weight, peripheral nervous system, lung function, liver function, blood lipids and urinary porphyrins should be checked.

Special points

Chloracne is generally the most sensitive indicator of toxic exposure to such chemicals. Mild cases are easily missed.

OTHER OCCUPATIONAL DERMATOSES

Definition and clinical features

Non-dermatitic skin conditions primarily caused by the patient's work. A wide variation, e.g. glass-fibre dermatitis (**60**), contact urticaria, oil acne (**61**), chrome ulceration (**62**), cement burns (**63**),

Non-Dermatitic Occupational Dermatoses

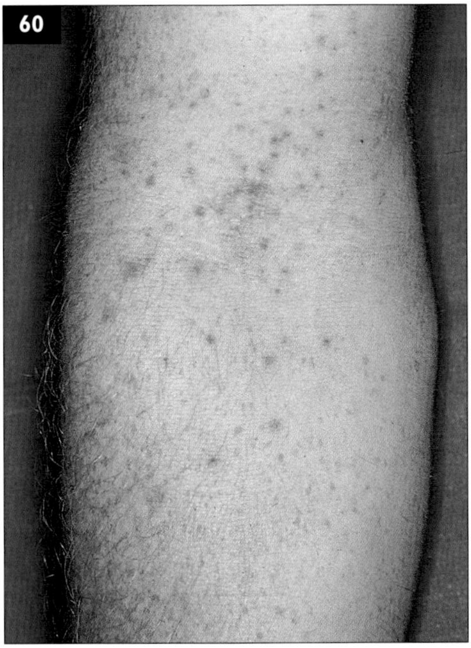

60 Glass-fibre dermatitis.

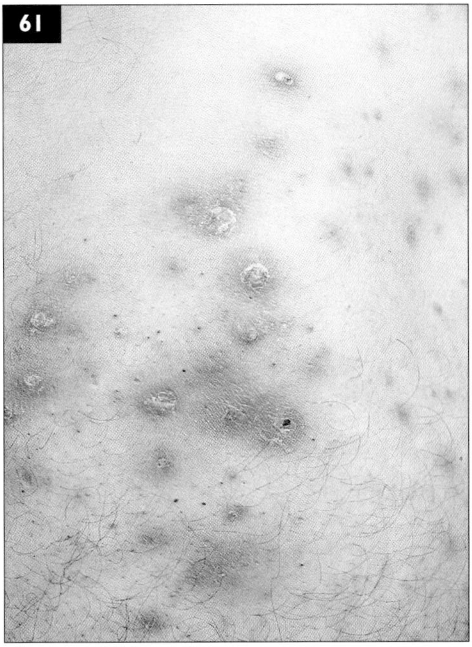

61 Oil acne.

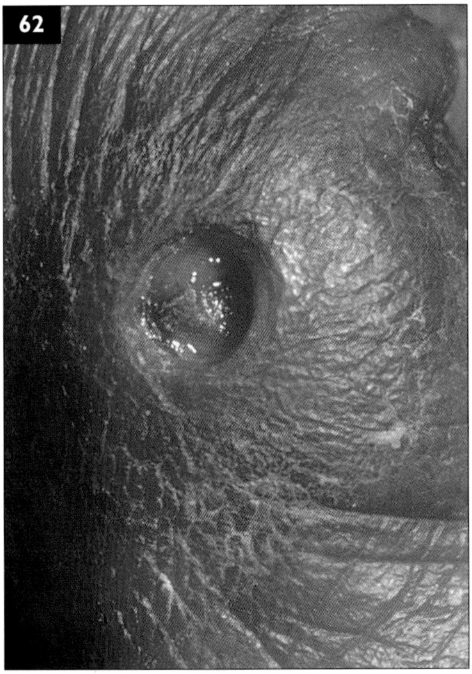

62 Chrome ulceration.

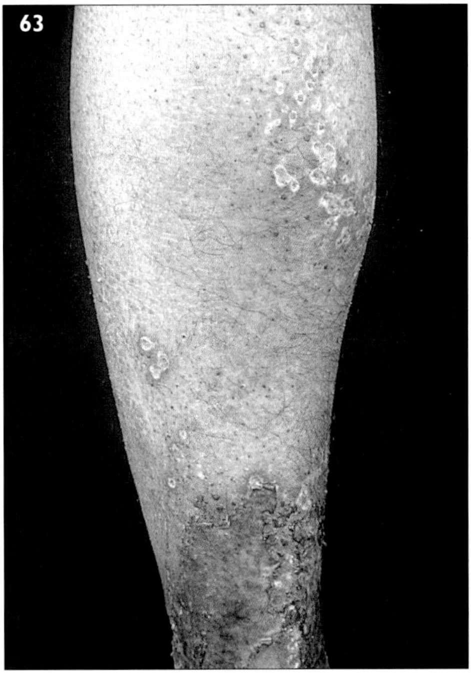

63 Cement burns.

Non-Dermatitic Occupational Dermatoses

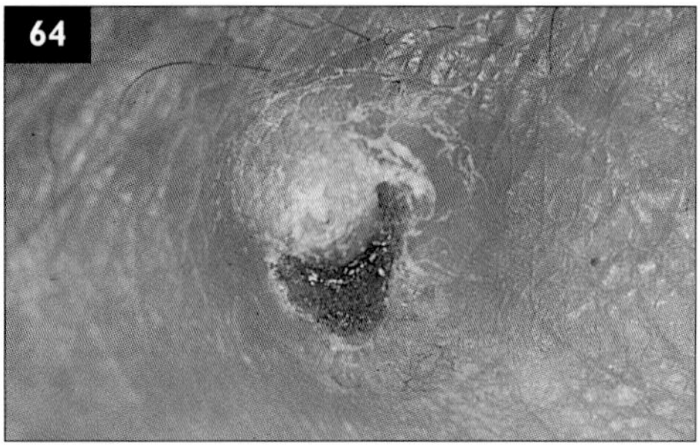

64 Epithelioma.

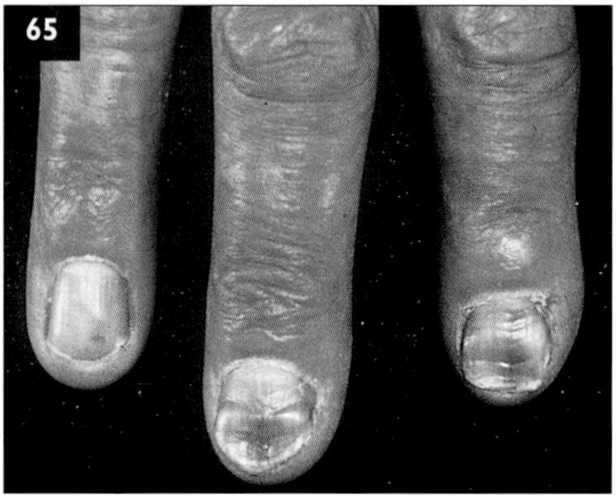

65 Koilonychia.

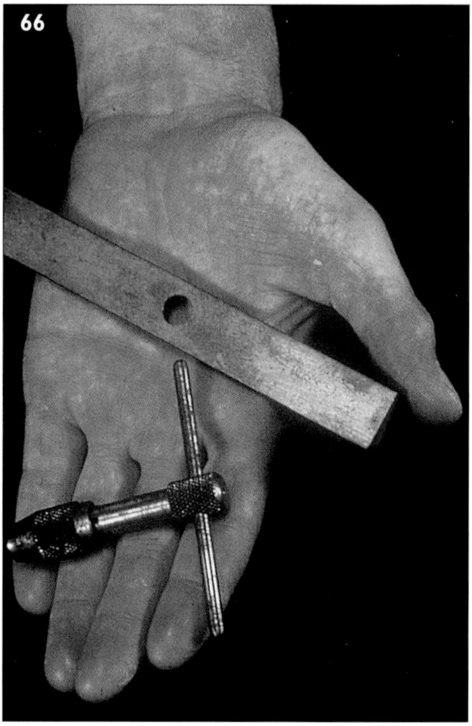

66 Rusty ferrous metal after handling by a 'ruster'.

leukoderma, scleroderma-like disease (see p. 101), epithelioma (**64**) and koilonychia (**65**).

Epidemiology
These account for 10% or less of occupational dermatoses, the remainder being contact dermatitis (see above).

Differential diagnosis
Non-occupational forms of, for example, contact urticaria and epithelioma, and idiopathic forms of such conditions as leukoderma, scleroderma and koilonychia.

Investigations
As indicated by the condition in question, e.g. prick testing in contact urticaria.

Special points
Always know your patient's occupation!

RUSTERS

Definition and clinical features
Rusters are those people whose touch is capable of rusting ferrous metals (with a delay dependent on the ambient relative humidity). Ferrous metal handled by rusters in engineering work later becomes rusty (**66**). Problems arise especially when this occurs on finished metal products in transit to the customer. It used to be thought that rusters were persons with some special quality of sweat but palmar hyperhidrosis is now thought to be the reason.

Special points
Adequate control of the hyperhidrosis may be achieved by tap water iontophoresis or, in severe cases, sympathectomy.

Dermatitis Artefacta

67 Excoriated dermatitis artefacta.

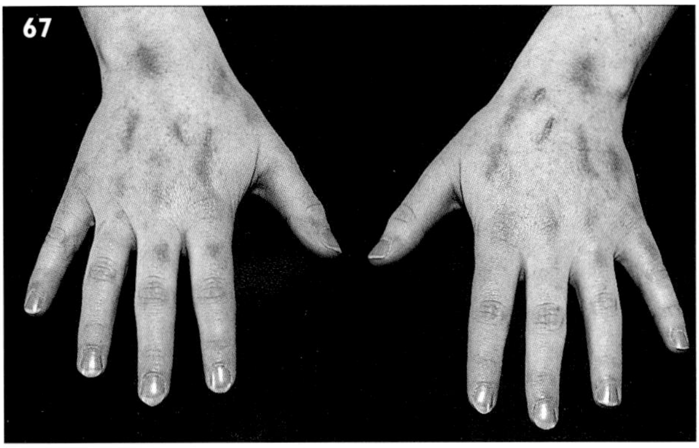

68 Dermatitis artefacta on thigh from chemical applied on glove.

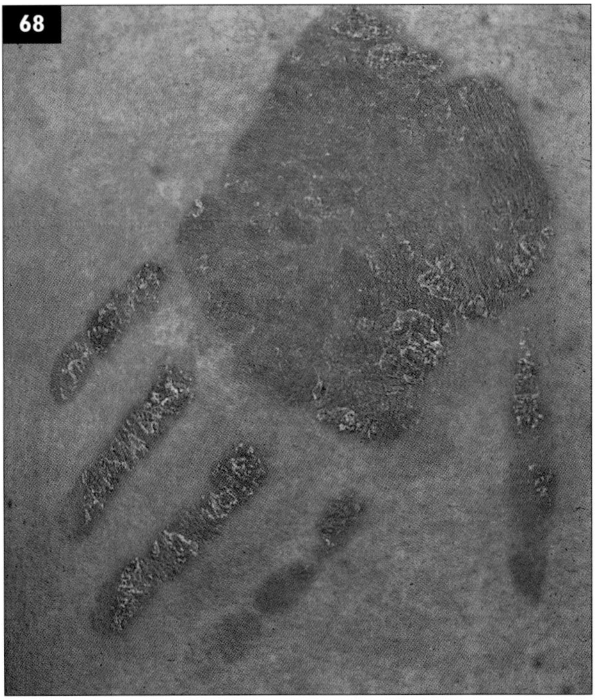

Definition and clinical features

Dermatitis artefacta are self-inflicted skin lesions. Lesions with sharp edges and sharp angulation in accessible sites (**67**, **68**).

Epidemiology

More common in women than in men, and commoner in younger people.

Investigations

Other possible causes of skin lesions need to be excluded.

Special points

Care is required in the management of dermatitis artefacta to prevent symptom conversion into depressive, even suicidal, reactions.

Contact Urticaria

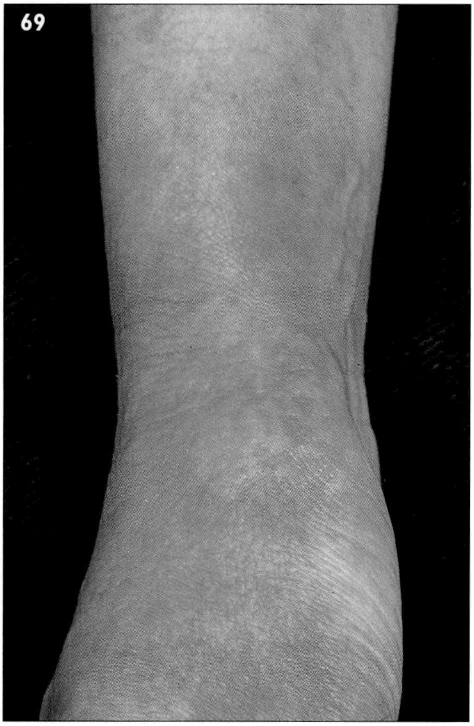

69 Immunological contact urticaria from rubber latex glove.

Definition and clinical features
Contact urticaria is the localised wheal-and-flare reaction to contact with external substances; it may be immunological or non-immunological. It is morphologically indistinguishable from idiopathic urticaria, and history and site are characteristic.

Epidemiology
Increasing diagnostic awareness indicates a higher frequency than formerly thought.

Differential diagnosis
Idiopathic urticaria, contact dermatitis.

Investigations
Use test, RAST or prick test (take care!).

Special points
Immunological contact urticaria from rubber latex (**69**) is currently important to diagnose because of the risk of anaphylaxis from surgical interventions.

Urticaria

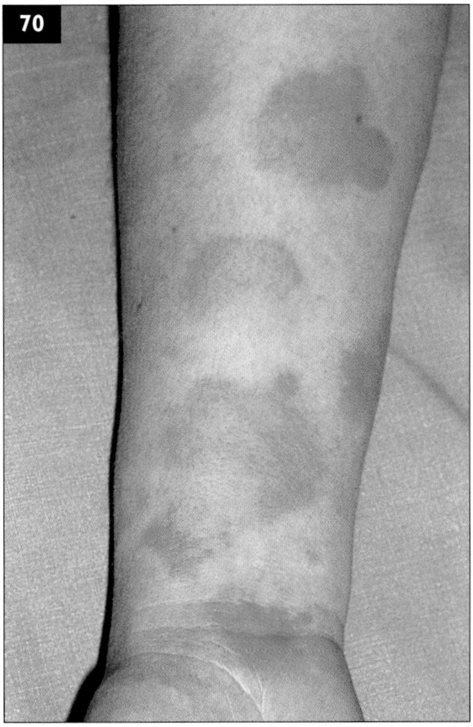

70 Urticaria.

Definition and clinical features

Urticaria commonly known as hives consists of transient pruritic areas of erythema and dermal oedema which resolve within 24 hours without leaving residual cutaneous signs. The lesions consist of focal papules, plaques or annular areas of palpable dermal oedema with or without erythema (**70**). The distribution and morphology of the lesions is influenced by the precipitating cause, especially in the physical urticarias. Dermographism the most common physical urticaria consists of urticated weals developing at sites where the skin is firmly stroked. Other precipitants of physical urticaria include pressure, vibration, cold, heat, sunlight and water. Some patients may have no physical signs at presentation because of the transient nature of the lesions.

Epidemiology

Idiopathic urticaria is common and usually mild and self-limiting. In addition to the physical urticarias, some patients have clear precipitating factors including drugs such as salicylates, opiates, angiotensin converting enzyme inhibitors and antibiotics. Other patients give a clear history of allergy to foods or food additives and, in a small proportion of cases, underlying infection or systemic illness such as lupus erythematosus or a lymphoproliferative disorder may be found.

Differential diagnosis

The diagnosis of urticaria is rarely a problem, although urticarial vasculitis should be considered in patients with lesions that persist for longer than 24 hours or that resolve leaving post-inflammatory changes. Efforts should be directed at identifying any precipitating cause.

Investigations

Patients with mild to moderate urticaria do not require investigation. In those with severe or persistent lesions, urinalysis, a full blood count, ESR, CH50 and ANF should be checked.

Angio-Oedema

71

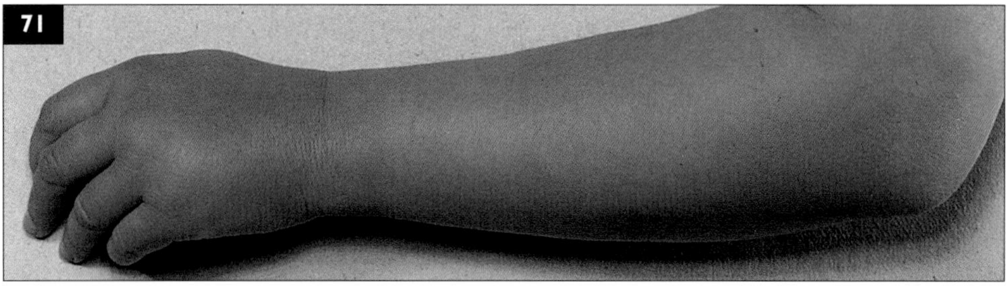

71 Angio-oedema.

72

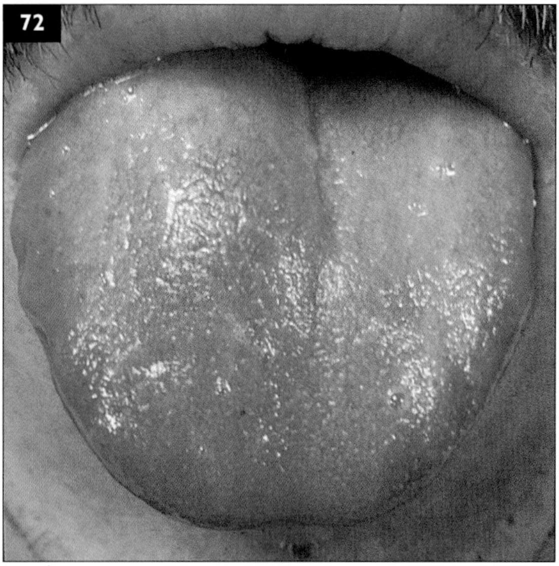

72 Glottal angio-oedema.

Definition and clinical features

Angio-oedema consists of transient episodes of focal subcutaneous and dermal oedema (**71**) which may affect any body site but which are most commonly seen in a perioral or periorbital distribution. Glottal (**72**) and laryngeal angio-oedema are of particular concern because, in rare instances, sudden severe episodes may cause fatal obstruction of the airway. Lesions which are usually non-pruritic frequently last 24 to 48 hours.

Epidemiology

Idiopathic angio-oedema is common and is frequently associated with urticaria. Hereditary angio-oedema is a rare autosomal dominant disorder in which patients suffer from symptoms related to subcutaneous and gastrointestinal angio-oedema. These patients are at risk of sudden death due to laryngeal oedema.

Investigations

Most patients with mild and occasional angio-oedema do not require investigation. Those with a persistent or severe condition should have their CH50, C2 and C4 checked, as well as C1 esterase inhibitor. A full blood count, ESR and ANF are also advisable.

Special points

Patients with a history of severe oral angio-oedema should carry an adrenaline injection device or inhaler with them at all times, to be used as emergency treatment for life-threatening laryngeal oedema.

Urticaria Pigmentosa

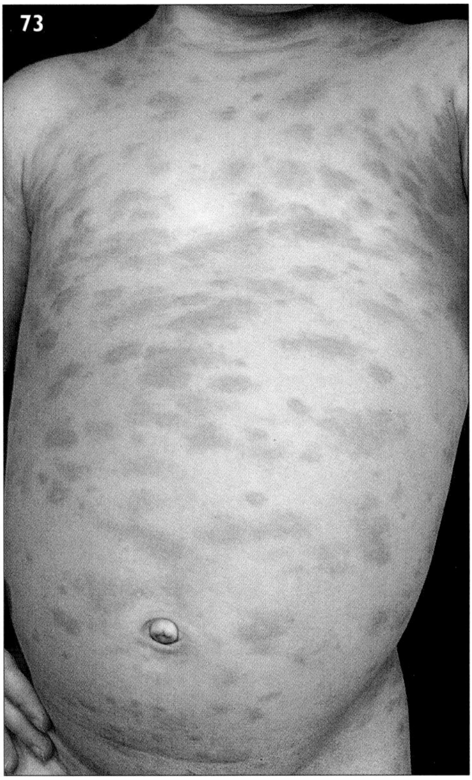

73 Childhood urticaria pigmentosa.

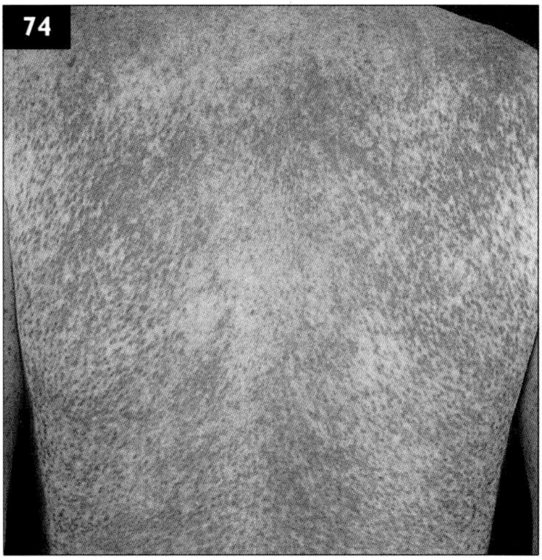

74 Adult urticaria pigmentosa.

Definition and clinical features

Urticaria pigmentosa is a skin disease in which symptoms and signs are due to a pathological increase in dermal mast cell numbers. Childhood and adult variants exist with a different natural history.

Childhood (paediatric) urticaria pigmentosa usually presents with a number of brownish dermal papules and plaques widely distributed over the body (**73**). When rubbed, these plaques become urticated (Darier's sign). Patients suffer from pruritus due to the release of mast cell products and, in severe cases with extensive involvement, may have systemic symptoms including wheezing, diarrhoea and syncope. Individual lesions may become bullous, especially in younger children. Clinical evidence of systemic involvement is uncommon in children and spontaneous resolution of the cutaneous manifestations is the rule.

Adult urticaria pigmentosa presents with an insidious onset of monomorphic pigmented maculopapular lesions, sometimes with prominent telangiectasia on the trunk and limbs (**74**). Systemic symptoms include weight loss, bone pain due to either osteoporosis or osteosclerosis, abdominal pain due to peptic ulceration and occasional neuropsychiatric symptoms.

Differential diagnosis

Paediatric urticaria pigmentosa is usually confirmed by the presence of Darier's sign but other infiltrative processes, such as Langerhans' cell histiocytosis and sarcoidosis, need to be considered if Darier's sign is negative. The differential diagnosis is similar for adult urticaria pigmentosa.

Investigations

Paediatric urticaria pigmentosa usually requires no investigation although a skin biopsy can be helpful in cases of diagnostic difficulty. Symptoms suggesting systemic involvement should be investigated. Patients with possible adult urticaria pigmentosa should have a skin biopsy to confirm the diagnosis. A full blood count should be monitored for evidence of significant bone marrow involvement; other symptoms should be investigated on merit.

Special points

It is important to consider the diagnosis of urticaria pigmentosa actively as skin biopsies may not be diagnostic unless special stains for mast cells are performed.

Urticarial Vasculitis

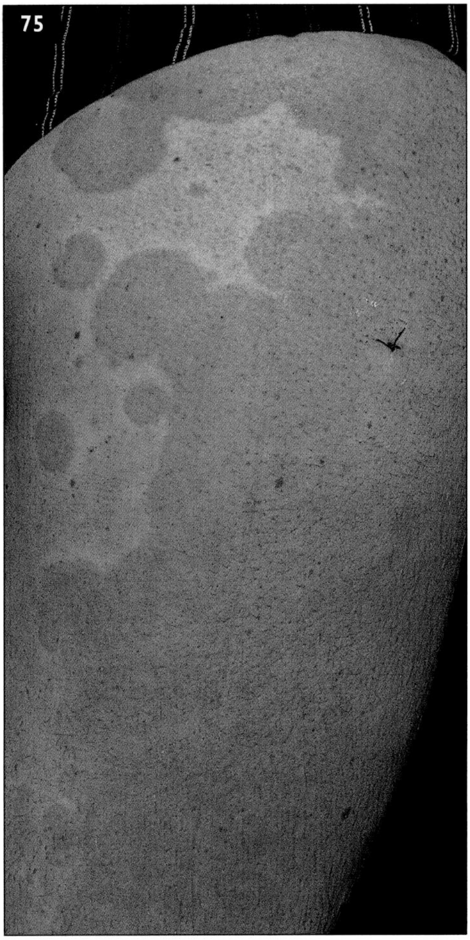

75 Urticarial vasculitis.

Definition and clinical features

Urticarial vasculitis may be defined as urticaria in which the individual lesions persist for more than 24 hours and resolve leaving post-inflammatory hyperpigmentation (**75**), though this may simply represent the more severe end of the spectrum of common urticaria. Such patients more frequently have arthralgias and reduced C2 and C4.

Epidemiology

Urticarial vasculitis is uncommon. The majority of cases are idiopathic, though in some patients it may be the presenting feature of underlying connective tissue disease.

Differential diagnosis

Urticarial vasculitis needs to be distinguished from a reactive erythema or exanthem, as well as from simple urticaria.

Investigations

A general physical examination of patients with urticarial vasculitis is important. Urine must be stick tested for proteinuria or haematuria and, if either is present, sent for microscopy and culture. Full blood count, ESR, urea and electrolytes, creatinine, liver function tests, C2, C4, CH50 and ANF should be done as baseline investigations, as well as a skin biopsy. Infective precipitants of the process, such as recent streptococcal infection, mycoplasma, hepatitis A, B or C, should also be sought.

Acute and Chronic Effects of Ultraviolet Irradiation

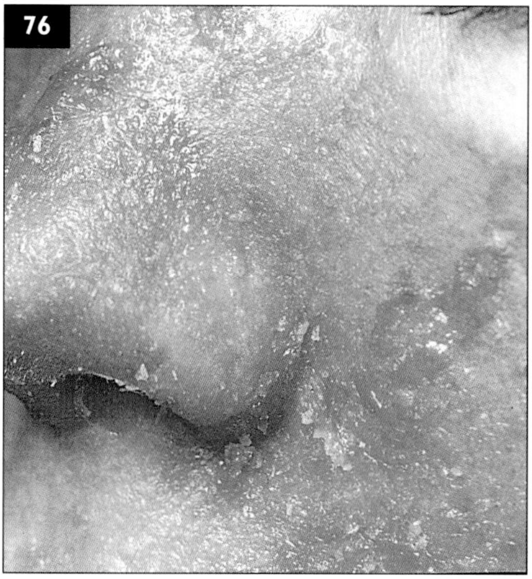

76 Sunburn.

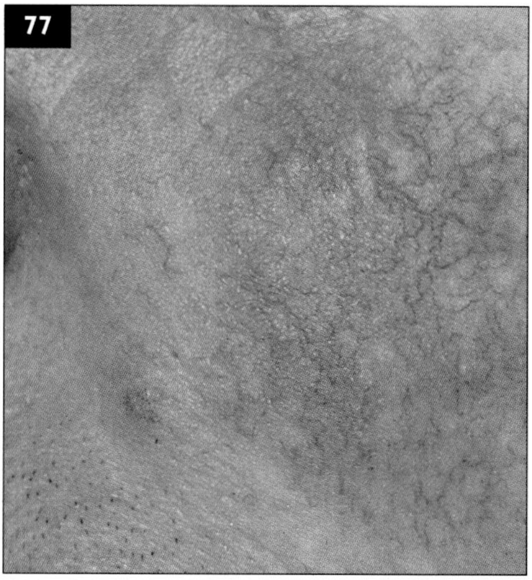

77 Telangiectasia.

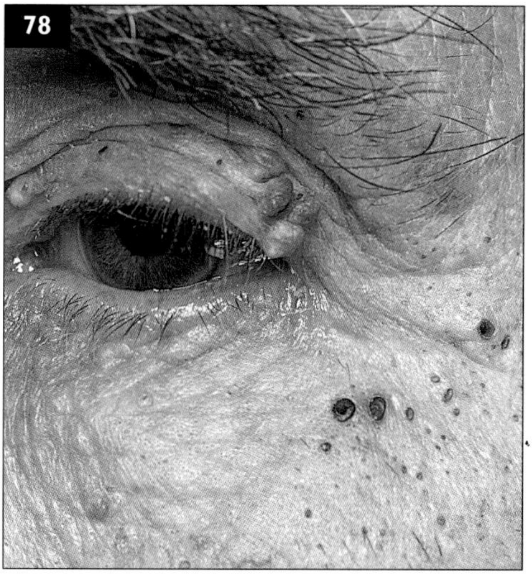

78 Comedones.

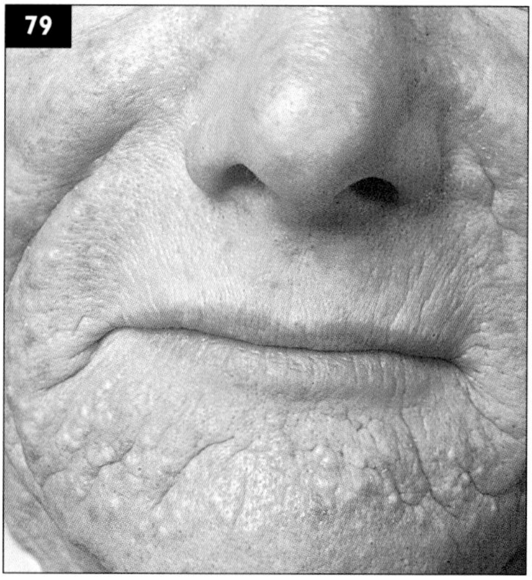

79 Colloid milium.

Ultraviolet irradiation (UVR) has early and late effects on the skin. Early effects include inflammation (sunburn), tanning, hyperplasia, vitamin D synthesis and immunological changes. Late effects include photoageing and photocarcinogenesis.

The erythema, pain, heat, swelling and, in severe cases, blistering of sunburn develops over hours (maximal effects 18–24 hours) and settles over days (**76**). Photoageing effects include wrinkling, dryness, coarseness, laxity, loss of tensile strength, telangiectasia (**77**), mottled pigmentation and comedones (**78**). Histologically, changes of solar elastosis are seen. Colloid milium is a degenerative change with yellowish, translucent papules on light-exposed skin (**79**).

Acquired Idiopathic Photodermatoses

80

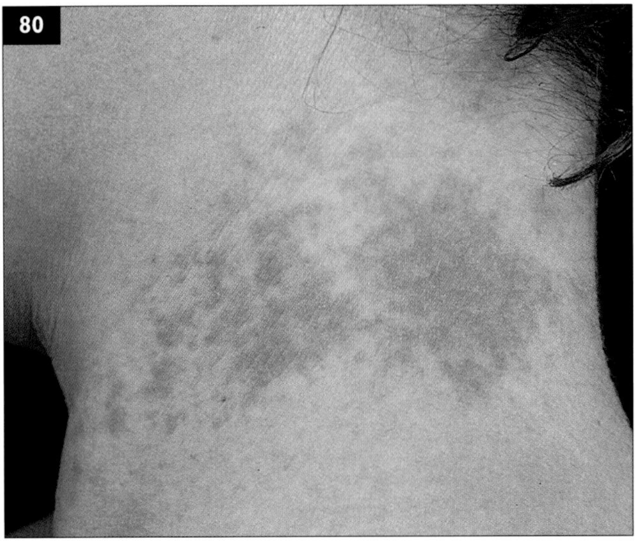

80 Polymorphic light eruption.

Acquired idiopathic photodermatoses include polymorphic light eruption (the commonest of all photodermatoses), actinic prurigo, chronic actinic dermatitis and solar urticaria. They all appear to be immunologically mediated. The history and examination are distinctive in each case.

POLYMORPHIC LIGHT ERUPTION (PLE)

Definition and clinical features

A common photodermatosis that may represent a delayed-type hypersensitivity response to UV-induced cutaneous antigens. PLE gives a delayed onset, itchy eruption in light-exposed sites, typically appearing within hours or days of significant sun exposure. PLE is transient, usually resolving within 7–14 days without scarring. The eruption is polymorphic and may give plaques of oedematous erythema or even blisters but most commonly consists of discrete pruritic papules in a symmetrical distribution on some, but not all, light-exposed sites (**80**). Chronically exposed sites such as the face are often spared. The eruption is restricted to the summer months and often improves (i.e. tolerance develops) as the summer progresses.

Epidemiology

PLE probably affects 10–15% of the population in temperate climates. It is significantly more common in females and onset is usually between the ages of 10 and 30 years.

Differential diagnosis and investigations

The temporal features of PLE will usually distinguish it from other photodermatoses on history alone. Early stages of subacute cutaneous lupus erythematosus (SCLE) may present identically so an extractable nuclear antigen (ENA) antibody test is mandatory to exclude a positive Ro autoantibody.

Special points

PLE is often provoked by longer wavelength UVA, or UVA and UVB, and so may be induced through window glass (e.g. when driving) or through thin clothing. It is generally adequately controlled by sensible sun avoidance and regular applications of highly protective combined UVA/UVB sunscreens. More severely affected patients may need treatment with low-dose photochemotherapy (PUVA).

ACTINIC PRURIGO

Definition and clinical features

Also known as Hutchinson's summer prurigo, this rare and chronic photodermatosis is likely to have an immunological basis. Actinic prurigo (AP) is regarded as a persistent variant of PLE by some investigators and as a distinct entity by others.

It is clinically separable from PLE, being a persistent, excoriated papular or nodular eruption on light-exposed and, to a lesser extent, non-exposed sites (**81**). There may be

Acquired Idiopathic Photodermatoses

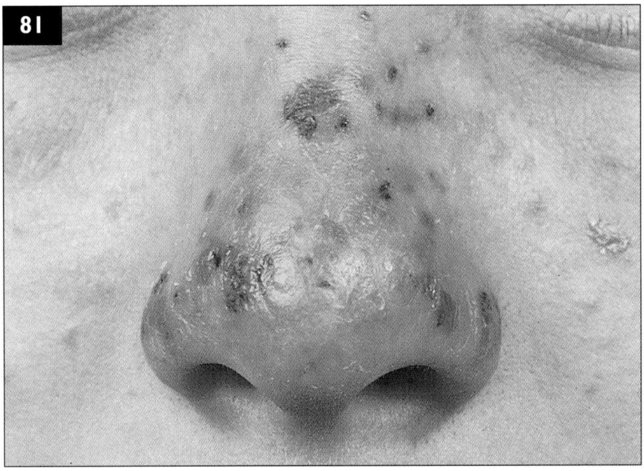

81 Actinic prurigo.

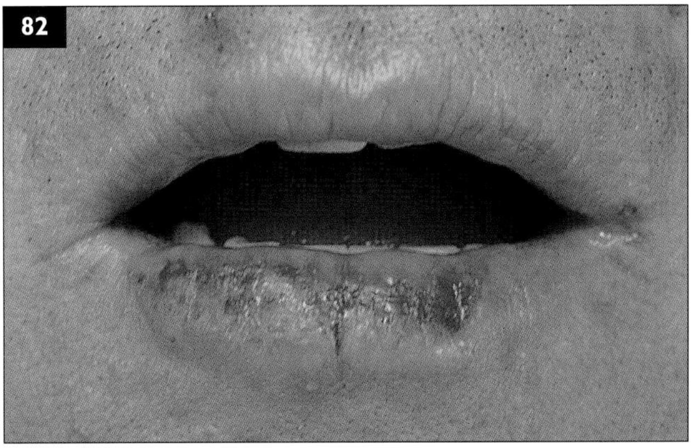

82 Associated cheilitis.

crusting and secondary infection. Unlike PLE the eruption usually starts in childhood and may improve following puberty. Lesions persist into winter, often failing to clear completely and, when severe, the eruption often extends to involve the covered skin of the limbs and buttocks. Characteristically all light-exposed sites are affected, the lesions leaving pitted scars on resolution. Cheilitis (**82**) and conjunctivitis are recognised associations.

Epidemiology

AP is more common in females and has an association with atopy and with HLA DR4 in Caucasoid populations. It has different HLA associations in the American Indians where it is a relatively common and frequently severe dermatosis.

Investigations

Two-thirds of patients are abnormally sensitive to monochromatic irradiation, most commonly within the UVA wavelengths.

Special points

Intermittent courses of low-dose thalidomide are effective in severe cases. PUVA or UVB phototherapy may be helpful (as for PLE).

CHRONIC ACTINIC DERMATITIS

Definition and clinical features

Chronic actinic dermatitis (CAD) also known as photosensitivity dermatitis (PD) or actinic reticuloid syndrome (AR) is a disabling eczematous photodermatosis mostly affecting light-exposed sites. It is probably immunologically based, possibly a delayed-type

Acquired Idiopathic Photodermatoses

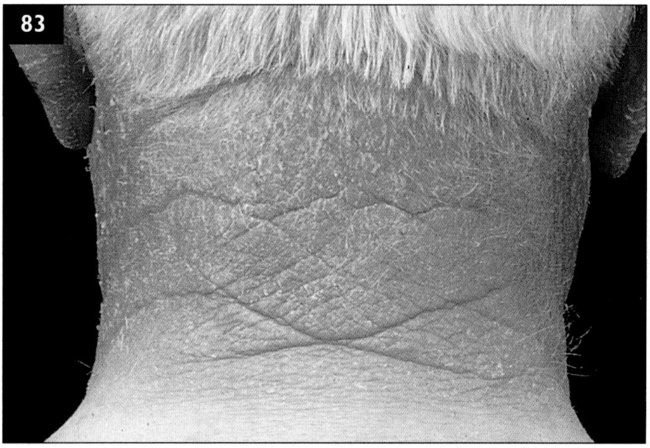

83 Chronic actinic dermatitis (CAD).

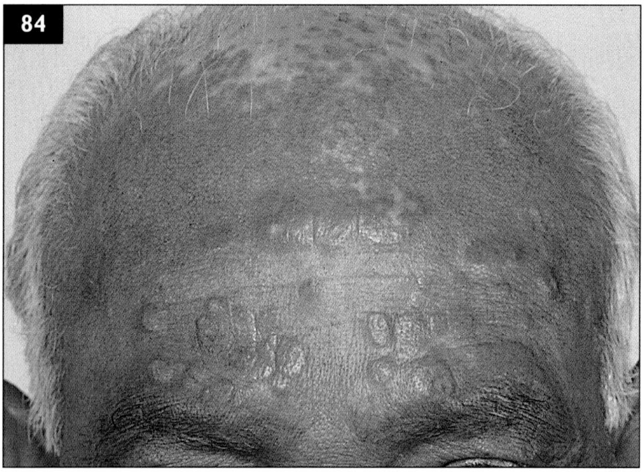

84 Severe CAD mimicking lymphomatous infiltration.

hypersensitivity reaction to an UV-induced neoantigen.

Older men are most commonly affected with persistent eczematous papules and plaques on photo-exposed sites (**83**). CAD may, when severe, mimic lymphomatous infiltration both clinically (**84**) and histologically. Some patients have had a preceding photoallergic contact dermatitis, others a history of endogenous or atopic eczema while many have associated, often multiple, contact allergies. Contact sensitivities to airborne allergens, especially to the Compositae family of plants, are characteristic. CAD is worse in summer and after sun exposure but patients may fail to recognise this, particularly if affected all year round.

Epidemiology

Middle-aged or elderly males represent 90% of most CAD populations. Any skin type may be affected although it is seen most commonly in fair-skinned individuals with an occupational or recreational history of many years of outdoor existence.

Differential diagnosis and investigations

Photosensitive eczema and photoallergic contact dermatitis may present similarly and, indeed, may co-exist. CAD is characterised by abnormally low erythemal thresholds to UVB, often to UVA and occasionally also to visible irradiation. Patch and photopatch tests will establish any associated contact sensitivities.

Acquired Idiopathic Photodermatoses

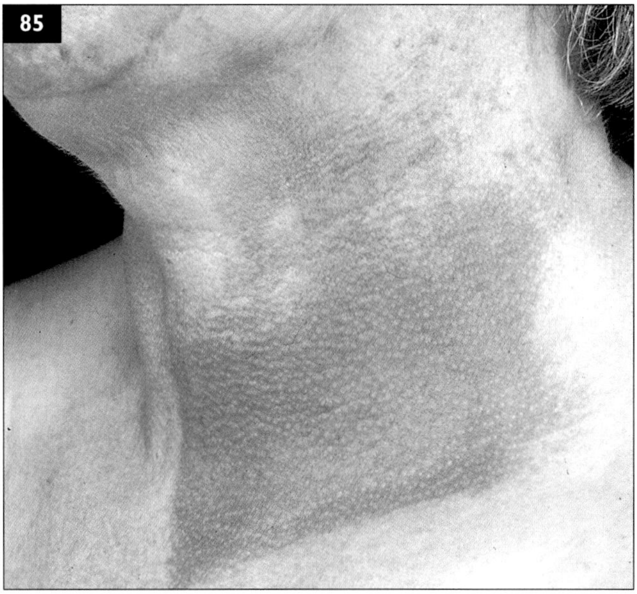

85 Solar urticaria.

Special points

Rigorous avoidance of UV and other known allergens and regular use of high protection factor sunscreens is important but is rarely sufficient. Intermittent courses of azathioprine or cyclosporin may be required.

SOLAR URTICARIA

Definition and clinical features

Solar urticaria (SU) is an uncommon photodermatosis in which UV irradiation leads to urticaria of exposed skin. SU appears to be an immediate (Type I) hypersensitivity response involving a circulating photoallergen, which is generated on absorption of light by a precursor. Within 5–10 minutes of exposure to sunlight, patients develop an itching or burning sensation that is rapidly followed by erythema and patchy or confluent wealing (**85**).

With sun avoidance SU resolves completely within 12 hours (unlike PLE). SU may affect only normally covered skin, sparing the face and hands, or all exposed sites. SU may be accompanied by systemic symptoms or even syncope. When severe this is an extremely incapacitating condition.

Epidemiology

SU is more common in females and usually begins between the ages of 20 and 40 years, persisting indefinitely or gradually improving.

Differential diagnosis

The history of an immediate reaction resolving rapidly should distinguish SU from PLE. Artificial irradiation testing may be able to induce typical lesions and demonstrate the wavelengths responsible.

Special points

Sunscreens are seldom sufficient. Non-sedative antihistamines in high doses may give reasonable protection. Regular exposure to the inducing wavelengths occasionally helps, and PUVA, given with fractionated doses under specialist supervision, may provide useful remissions.

HYDROA VACCINIFORME

Definition and clinical features

Hydroa vacciniforme (HV) is an exceedingly rare photodermatosis usually confined to childhood. HV is characterised by recurrent crops of vesicles on sun-exposed skin with subsequent vacciniform scarring. The aetiology is unknown.

Within hours of sun exposure, clusters of 2–3 mm erythematous macules appear on light-exposed sites, especially the face and the backs of the hands, often associated with a severe burning sensation. These rapidly progress to papules and then vesicles which umbilicate over a day or so; they then dry, form

Acquired Idiopathic Photodermatoses

86

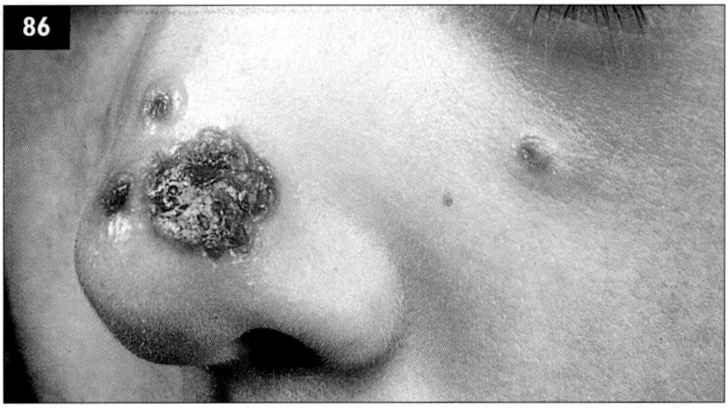

86 Hydroa vacciniforme.

87

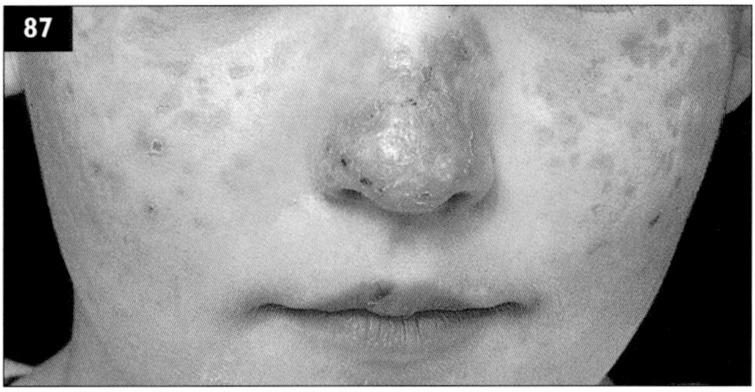

87 Varioliform scars.

88

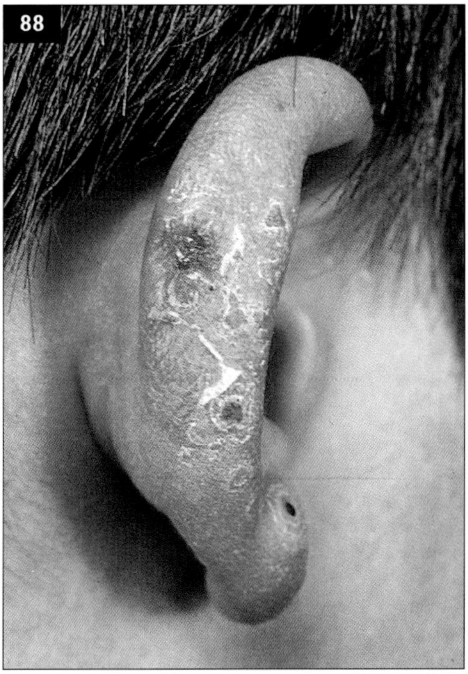

88 Juvenile spring eruption.

a crust (**86**) and heal into pitted, varioliform scars (**87**). Occasionally there are associated systemic features such as headache, fever or malaise. Remission often occurs during adolescence. Broad spectrum sunscreens with UVA protection should be prescribed.

Diagnosis

Diagnosis is clinical. Repetitive broad spectrum UVA and UVB will often induce typical lesions.

JUVENILE SPRING ERUPTION

This typically presents as itchy blisters arising on the light-exposed helices of young boys ears following sun exposure (**88**). This is probably a variant of PLE presenting in boys because of their short hair styles. Development of tolerance to UVR, as also seen with PLE, explains why it is typically restricted to the spring months.

Genetic and Metabolic Photodermatoses

CUTANEOUS PORPHYRIAS

The cutaneous porphyrias are disorders of haem synthesis in which excessive formation of porphyrins, secondary to partial enzyme deficiencies, produce photosensitisation. There are five main types:

- Porphyria cutanea tarda (PCT).
- Variegate porphyria.
- Hereditary coproporphyria.
- Erythropoietic protoporphyria (EPP).
- Congenital erythropoietic protoporphyria (CEP).

The erythemal action spectrum of cutaneous porphyria resembles the absorption spectrum of porphyrins, peaking at around 400 nm. Light absorption produces excited-state porphyrins within the skin that can transfer energy, particularly to oxygen to form singlet oxygen and free radicals that are highly toxic to adjacent molecules.

DNA REPAIR DEFICIENT PHOTODERMATOSES

Absorption of UV radiation by DNA in skin cells induces structural alterations in DNA, notably intra-strand pyrimidine dimer and 6–4 photo-adduct formation. Photosensitive dermatoses associated with established defects of DNA repair currently include xeroderma pigmentosum, Cockayne's syndrome, trichothiodystrophy and Bloom's syndrome. These rare autosomal recessive genodermatoses have a variable association with cancer.

PORPHYRIA CUTANEA TARDA

Definition and clinical features

Porphyria cutanea tarda (PCT) is the commonest porphyria, presenting with blisters and skin fragility of light-exposed sites. It is due to uroporphyrinogen decarboxylase deficiency and has a complex inheritance with iron-dependent inactivation of the enzyme contributing to one of four different types of familial predisposition.

The only consistent feature of PCT are lesions on exposed skin. These include hypertrichosis (**89**), pigmentation, erosions and subepidermal bullae (**90**). Patients may describe fragility of the exposed skin especially on their hands. Blisters tend to heal with scarring and milia. Acute photosensitivity is uncommon and acute porphyric attacks do not occur. The onset of PCT seems to require interaction between several acquired and inherited factors. Clinical

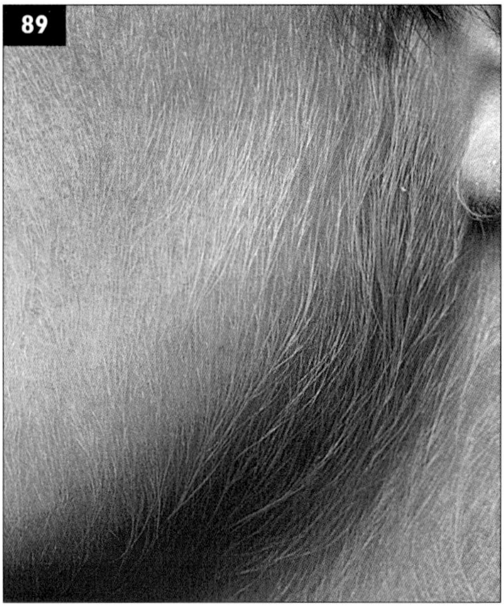

89 Hypertrichosis in porphyria cutanea tarda.

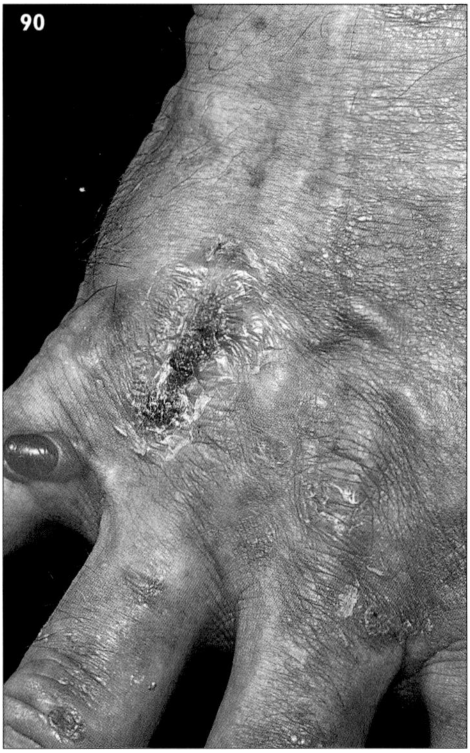

90 Subepidermal bullae.

Genetic and Metabolic Photodermatoses

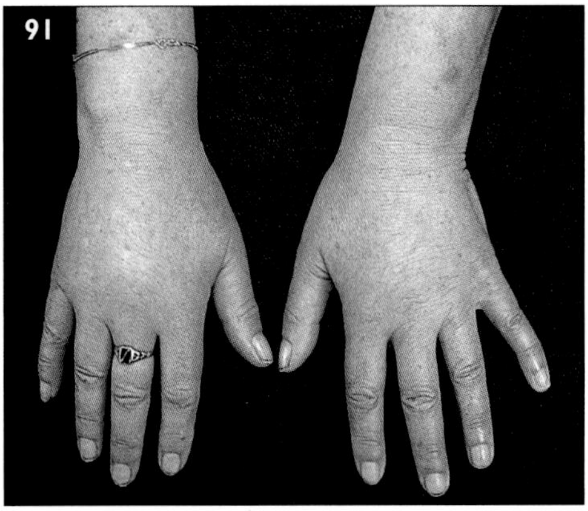

91 Erythropoietic protoporphyria (EPP).

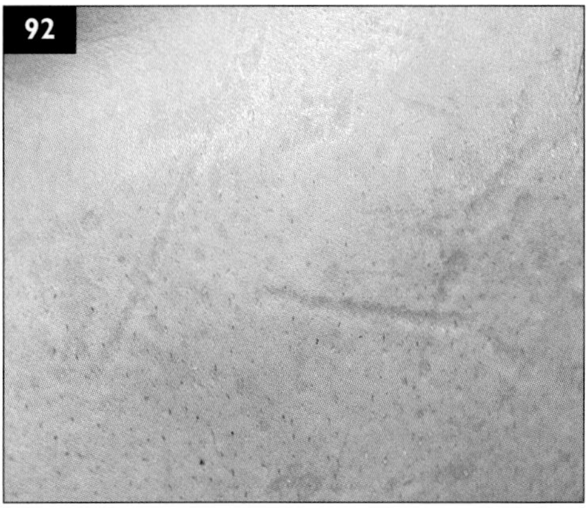

92 Scarring in EPP.

manifestations of PCT usually only occur in association with other disorders such as alcoholic liver disease or oestrogen ingestion.

Hepatic siderosis, associated with a high alcohol intake, may progressively inactivate hepatic uroporphyrinogen decarboxylase activity to a level where cutaneous disease develops.

Differential diagnosis

Diagnosis of PCT is confirmed by finding elevated levels of predominantly Type I uro- and coproporphyrin isomers in the urine and stools. Hepatoerythropoietic porphyria in children and late onset Gunther's disease will rarely confuse. Variegate porphyria may present with similar clinical features.

Special points

Apart from avoidance of alcohol and oestrogens, PCT will generally respond to either depletion of body iron stores by venesection or low-dose hydroxychloroquine.

ERYTHROPOIETIC PROTOPORPHYRIA

Definition and clinical features

Erythropoietic protoporphyria (EPP) is a relatively uncommon photosensitising porphyria of complex inheritance. It results from the accumulation of protoporphyrin secondary to decreased ferrochetalase activity.

Patents present with acute photosensitivity starting in early childhood, both of these features being rare in PCT. A typical history is of a young child screaming with pain whenever exposed to bright sunlight. An intense pricking, itching, burning sensation usually occurs within 5–30 minutes of sun exposure, although occasionally this is delayed for several hours. The patient experiences several hours of burning pain often with no visible signs although severe attacks produce erythema, oedema and occasionally later crusting, petechiae or even small vesicles (**91**).

Acute photo-onycholysis may occur and after repeated attacks the skin characteristically becomes thickened, waxy and pitted with small circular or linear scars, especially over the bridge of the nose, around the mouth and over the knuckles (**92**).

Liver damage from the accumulation of protoporphyrin crystals in hepatocytes commonly gives abnormal liver biochemistry. Progressive hepatic failure and porphyrin gallstones are rare.

Differential diagnosis

Diagnosis of EPP is established by demonstrating increased free protoporphyrin in erythrocytes. It may be necessary to distinguish this from increased zinc protoporphyrin found in iron deficiency, lead poisoning and some anaemias, which may coexist fortuitously with photosensitivity.

Special points

Sunlight avoidance is the only effective treatment. High factor UVA-protecting sunscreens and oral β-carotene help marginally.

Genetic and Metabolic Photodermatoses

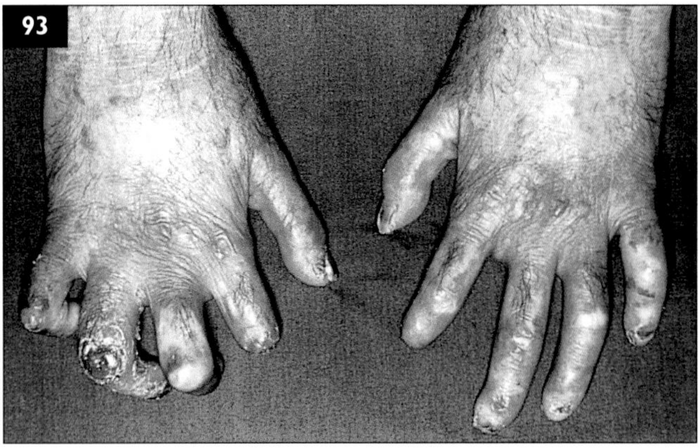

93 Congenital erythropoietic protoporphyria.

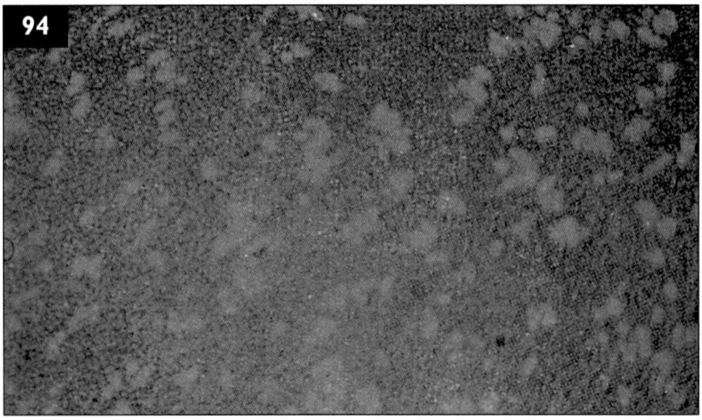

94 Fluorescing erythrocytes.

CONGENITAL ERYTHROPOIETIC PROTOPORPHYRIA

Definition and clinical features

Congenital erythropoietic protoporphyria (CED), also known as Gunther's disease, is a rare autosomal recessive disorder with severe photosensitivity, scarring and deformity resulting from uroporphyrinogen III synthase deficiency and consequent accumulation of Type I uro- and coproporphyrin isomers in the blood and tissues.

Classic CEP presents in early childhood with acute painful erythema, swelling and blistering after sunlight exposure. Severe photosensitivity leads to extensive scarring and photomutilation (**93**). The urine is pink from the excessive amounts of porphyrin, and the teeth stain brown and show red fluorescence (erythrodontia). Erythrocytes also fluoresce (**94**) and haemolytic anaemia with splenomegaly, probably caused by photodamage of porphyrin-laden erythrocytes, is common. Chronic changes include face and hand deformities, eye damage and hypertrichosis. A fatal outcome from hepatic cirrhosis or haemolytic anaemia is not unusual.

Epidemiology

There are early and late onset forms. Early onset CEP is clinically severe with mutilating disease, while the probably commoner late onset CEP is much less severe and may be mistaken for PCT.

Differential diagnosis

Diagnosis is established by finding increased levels of uro- and coproporphyrin in urine, faeces and erythrocytes (RBCs). There are increased levels of both free and zinc-protoporphyrin in RBCs. Late onset CEP may be distinguished from PCT by the absence of RBC porphyrins and by the excretion of Type I rather than Type III uro- and coproporphyrin isomers.

Genetic and Metabolic Photodermatoses

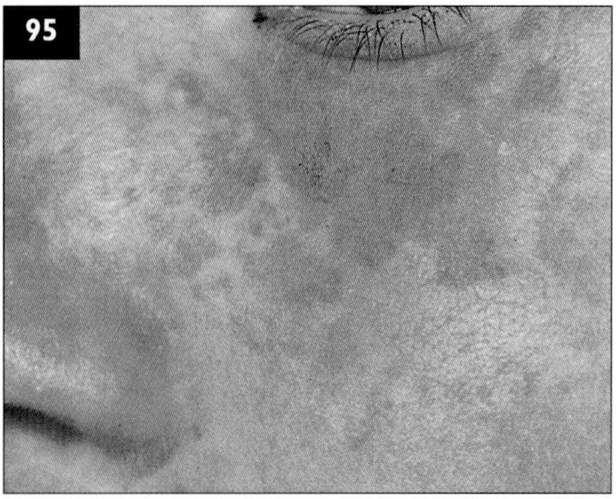

95 Xeroderma pigmentosum.

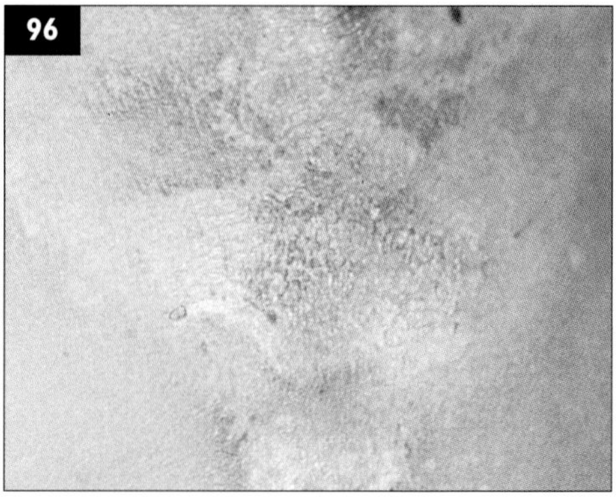

96 Casal's necklace in pellagra.

XERODERMA PIGMENTOSUM

Definition and clinical features

Xeroderma pigmentosum (XP) is a heterogeneous disorder associated with defective excision repair or daughter strand repair of UV-induced DNA damage. XP is characterised by extreme photosensitivity, accelerated photo-ageing and early death from cutaneous malignancy.

The cutaneous features usually begin at 1–2 years of age with exaggerated sunburning after minimal exposure, often with blister formation. Exposed skin is prematurely photo-aged with dryness, freckling and telangiectasia (**95**).

XP patients are prone to a variety of benign and malignant skin tumours with at least a thousandfold increased risk of melanoma and non-melanoma skin cancer. Most sufferers have developed a skin cancer by the age of ten. Chronic conjunctivitis, keratitis and iritis are common, and progressive neurological deterioration may occur.

Epidemiology

XP occurs in about one in 250 000 live births found in all races worldwide. Cell fusion studies have suggested at least seven different complementation groups, indicating that a number of different enzymes can be affected. Approximately 25% of XP patients are XP variants with an ill-defined deficiency in daughter strand repair and much milder clinical manifestations.

Differential diagnosis

In infants XP may need to be distinguished from other conditions, such as Cockayne's or Bloom's syndromes, that present with photosensitivity. Later, the pigmentary and photoageing changes can resemble the congenital poikilodermas.

Investigations

Diagnosis is by clinical assessment, by irradiation skin tests, which show enhanced delayed erythemal responses to UVB, and by demonstration of reduced DNA repair in cultured fibroblasts.

Special points

Patients must to minimise UV exposure with appropriate protective clothing and sunglasses, and the use of highly protective sunscreens.

OTHER METABOLIC PHOTODERMATOSES

Some metabolic and nutritional disorders are associated with photodermatitis. The most important of these is pellagra.

Pellagra

Definition and clinical features

Pellagra is caused by a cellular deficiency of niacin resulting from a dietary deficiency or, in the Western world, from an unbalanced diet due to alcoholism, gastrointestinal disease or psychiatric disturbance. Rare causes include functioning carcinoid tumours and Hartnup disease.

Pellagra produces the classic triad of dermatitis, diarrhoea and dementia. The dermatitis is typically photosensitive with redness, scaling and, subsequently, hypermelanosis of light exposed areas. A symmetrical butterfly rash on the face and a well-marginated eruption on the anterior chest (Casal's necklace) are characteristic (**96**). A dermatitis may be induced, similarly, by heat, friction or pressure. Abdominal pain with diarrhoea and depression or apathy are usually associated.

Genetic and Metabolic Photodermatoses

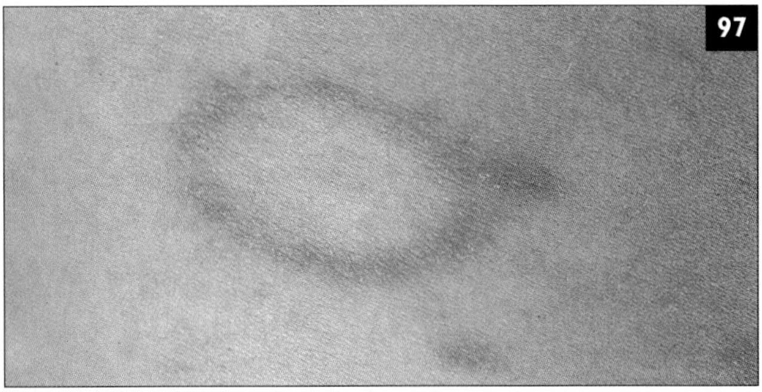

97 Herald patch in pityriasis rosea.

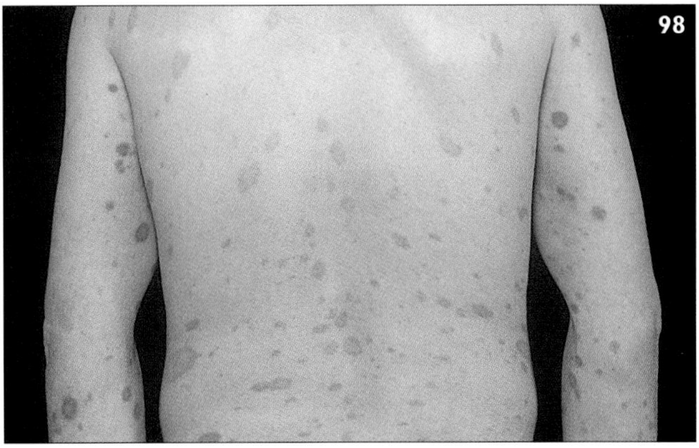

98 'Christmas tree' pattern in pityriasis rosea.

Differential diagnosis
The main differential diagnoses are a phototoxic drug eruption, porphyria or chronic actinic dermatitis. Zinc deficiency or other vitamin B deficiencies may co-exist.

Special points
Hartnup disease is a rare inborn error of metabolism characterised by a pellagrous eruption, an intermittent cerebellar ataxia and a characteristic renal amino aciduria with excessive indicanuria.

Pityriasis Rosea

Definition and clinical features
Acute, self-limiting, inflammatory dermatosis, probably of infectious origin, with a characteristic eruption affecting mainly young adults.

The first manifestation is usually the herald patch (**97**) which is larger than the subsequent oval pink scaly patches that appear in crops over a week or two, mainly, but not exclusively, on the trunk in a Christmas tree pattern (**98**). There may be slight to moderate itching. Spontaneous resolution usually occurs within 6 weeks and recurrences are rare.

Epidemiology
Most cases occur in the 10–35 year age group, equally in males and females.

Differential diagnosis
Seborrhoeic dermatitis, guttate psoriasis, lichen planus, pityriasis lichenoides, tinea corporis, drug reactions and secondary syphilis.

Investigations
Mycologic examination of skin scrapings and serological tests of syphilis should be considered.

Special points
Secondary syphilis is the classic trap – examine the genitals and mouth!

Psoriasis

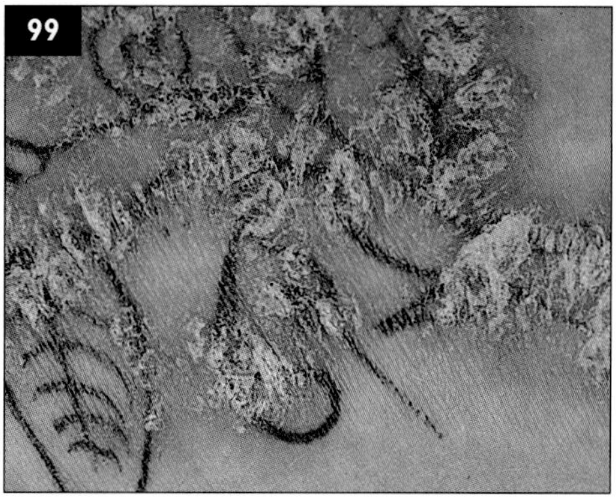

99 Köbner phenomenon.

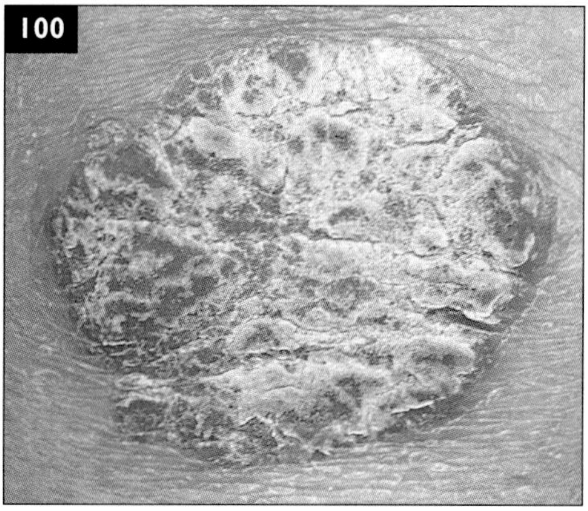

100 Psoriatic plaque.

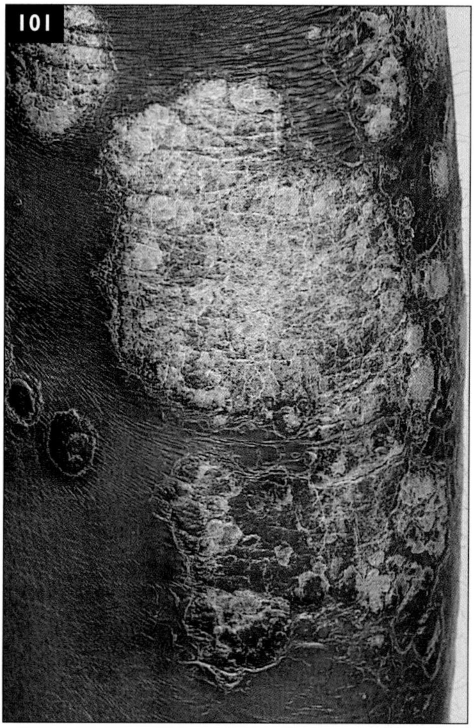

101 Psoriatic knee.

Definition and clinical features

A common inflammatory dermatosis, most frequently characterised by well-defined, red, scaly plaques on the extensor aspects of limbs and scalp. Severity and duration are variable and a wide variety of clinical patterns recognised.

Different forms of the disease may occur in the same patient at different times. Precipitating or exacerbating factors include trauma (Köbner phenomenon) (**99**), streptococcal infection, various drugs (particularly lithium, adrenergic blocking agents, antimalarials), stress and excessive alcohol intake.

Chronic plaque psoriasis (also called psoriasis vulgaris or nummular psoriasis), the commonest form, is characterised by well-demarcated, thickened, deep-red plaques, surmounted by silvery scale (**100**). They may be distributed anywhere, although characteristically occur on the extensor aspects of limbs, particularly the knees (**101**) and elbows, sacrum, scalp (along the hairline) (**102**) and ears. The plaques vary in size from small (1–2cm) to very large (e.g. covering the entire extensor aspect of a limb). The disease may be localised to one or two areas only, or cover most of the body (**103**).

Rupioid psoriasis describes a grossly hyperkeratotic form of chronic plaque psoriasis (**104**).

Guttate psoriasis classically occurs following a streptococcal throat infection in children and young adults: showers of red,

Psoriasis

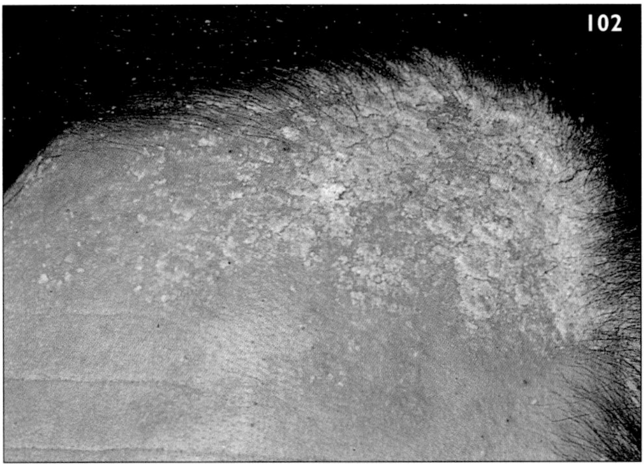

102 Psoriatic scalp.

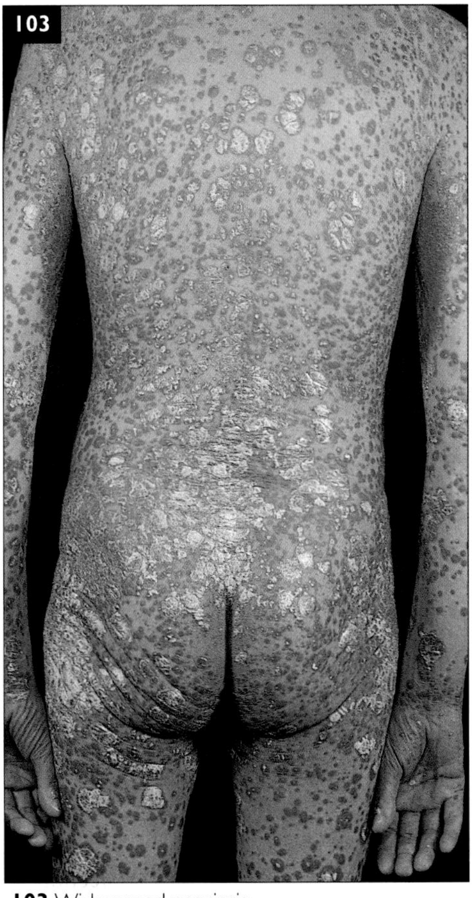

103 Widespread psoriasis.

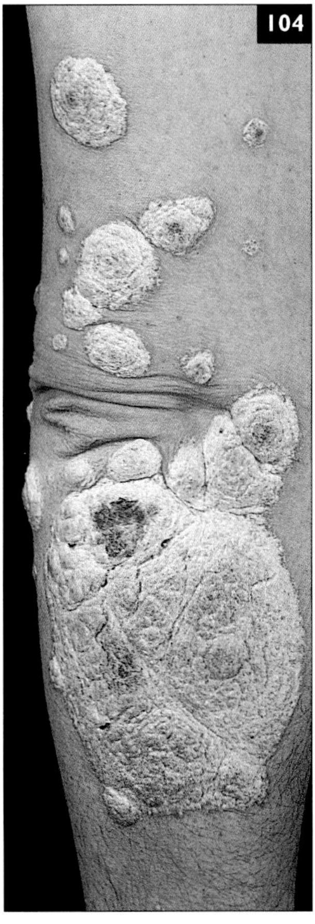

104 Rupioid psoriasis.

Psoriasis

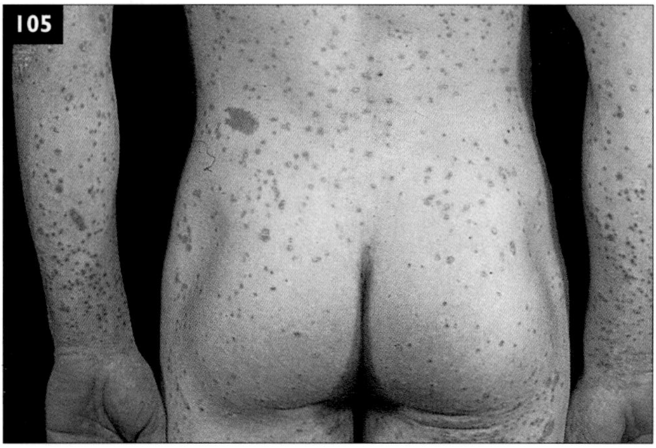

105 Guttate psoriasis.

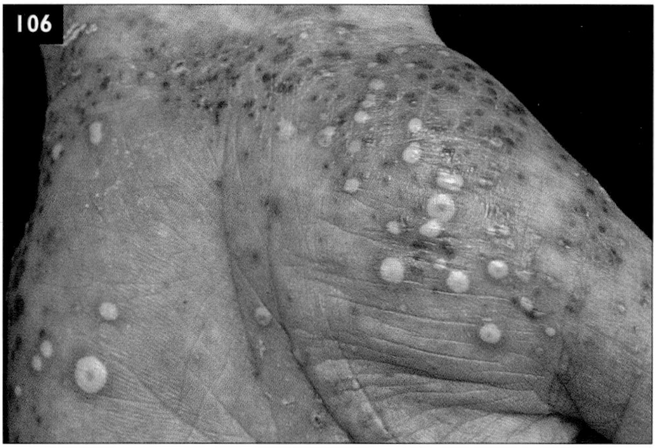

106 Pustular psoriasis.

oval or round, scaly plaques up to 1cm in diameter rapidly appear on the trunk and proximal limbs (**105**).

Pustular psoriasis may be localised or generalised. Chronic, localised pustular psoriasis (also called palmoplantar pustulosis) occurs predominantly in adults and manifests as recurrent crops of sterile yellow pustules, 0.1–0.5 cm in diameter, on the palms and soles (**106**). The pustules involute to leave red-brown stained macules which may scale before disappearing. Generalised pustular psoriasis is a serious, unstable form of psoriasis with a significant mortality. Erythematous plaques studded with pustules rapidly appear at any site and may become confluent (**107**). Fever and malaise are common.

Erythrodermic psoriasis describes generalised itching, erythema and scaling, and is similarly associated with systemic symptoms, unstable, poorly controlled disease, and a significant mortality (**108**). It may result from generalised pustular psoriasis or be triggered by infection, overtreatment with tar, dithranol or (possibly) the sudden withdrawal of corticosteroids. Patients are at risk of fluid and protein loss, poor temperature control and infection. The clinical features of psoriasis may be modified by site. Involvement of flexures leads to loss of scale, with erythema and maceration only (**109**).

Scalp psoriasis, particularly in children and young adults, may be associated with thick, white lumps of scale adhering to the scalp and

Psoriasis

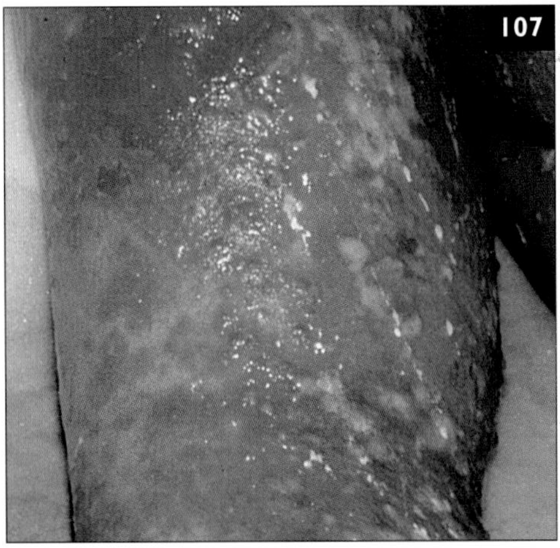

107 Generalised pustular psoriasis.

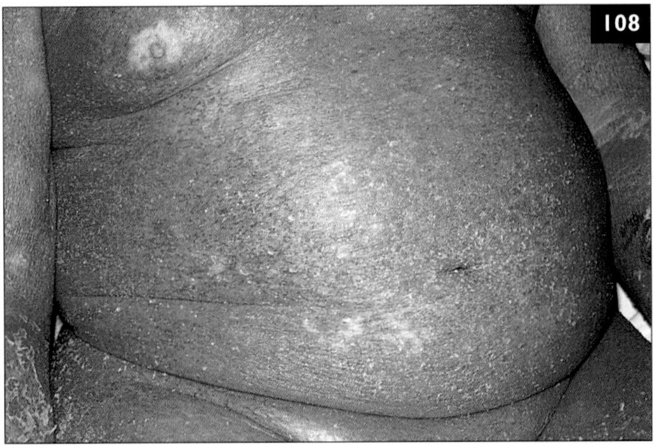

108 Erythrodermic psoriasis.

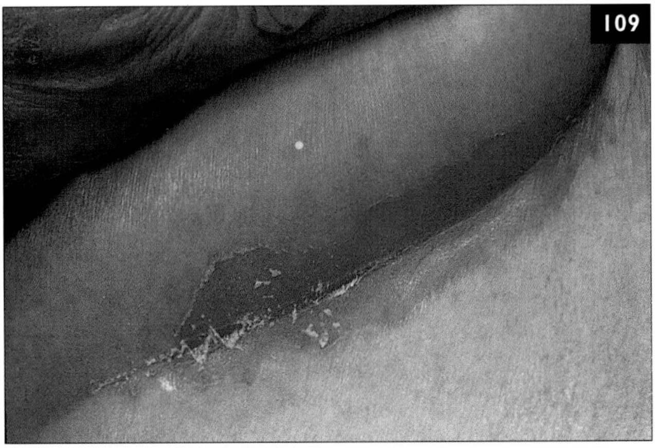

109 Flexural psoriasis.

Psoriasis

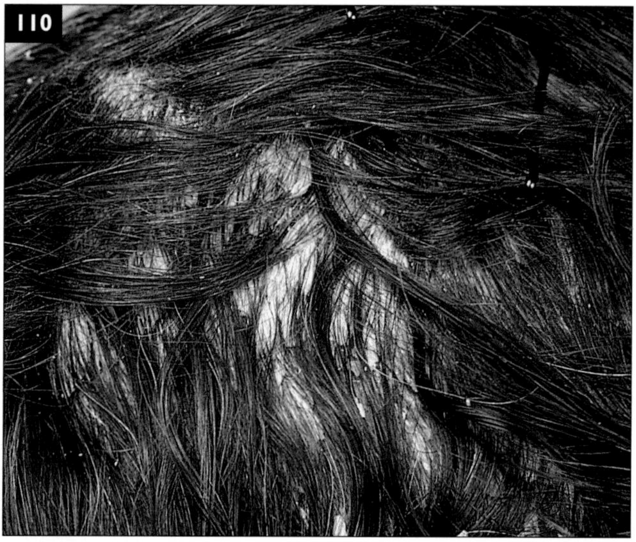

110 Pityriasis amiantacea.

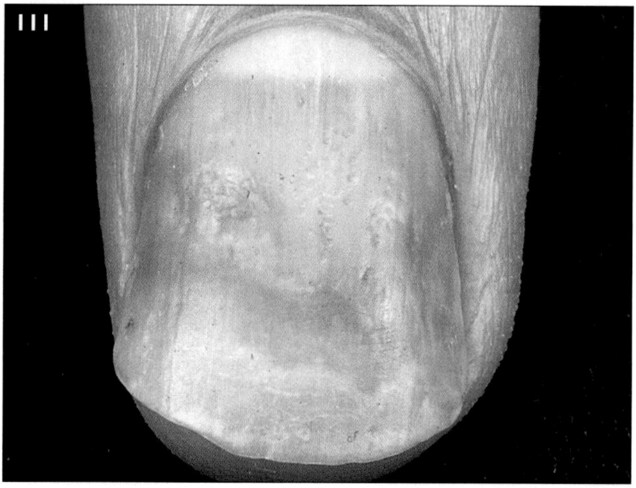

111 Psoriatic pitting, onycholysis and salmon patch

hair shaft (pityriasis amiantacea) (**110**). Nail changes are common, especially in association with arthropathy, and manifest as pitting, onycholysis, yellow-brown areas of discoloration (salmon patches or oil-drop sign) (**111**) and subungual hyperkeratosis (**112**).

Five clinical patterns of arthritis occur in association with psoriasis (**113**) although the incidence is uncertain:

- Small joint arthritis involving the distal interphalangeal joints of the hands and feet.
- Large joint, monoarthritis.
- Axial arthritis leading to ankylosis of the spine and sacro-iliac joints.
- A rheumatoid-like arthritis.
- Arthritis mutilans with gross joint destruction and consequent loss of function.

Epidemiology

Psoriasis affects approximately 2% of the UK population and has a peak age of onset between 10 and 20 years. It may be inherited in up to 40% of individuals, particularly in those developing the disease before the age of 40 years; an

Psoriasis

112

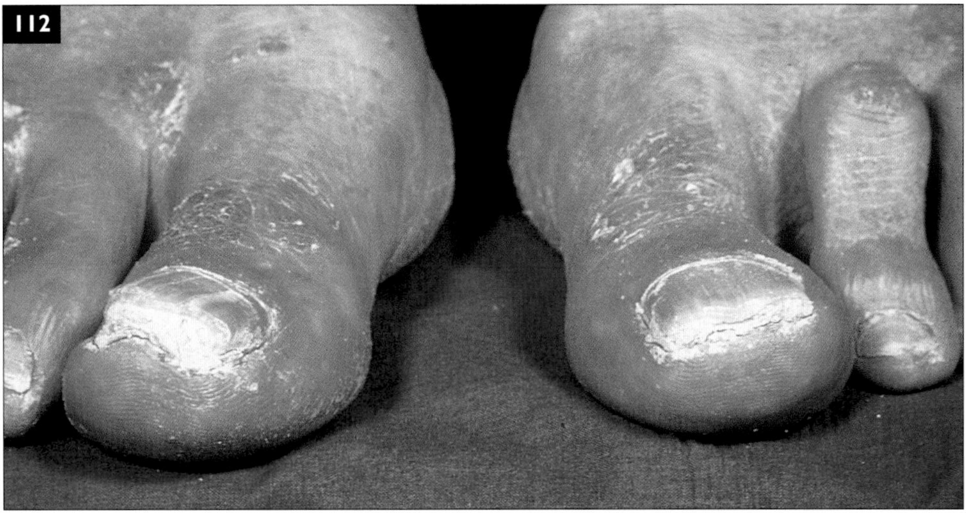

112 Subungual hyperkeratosis.

113 Psoriatic arthritis.

113

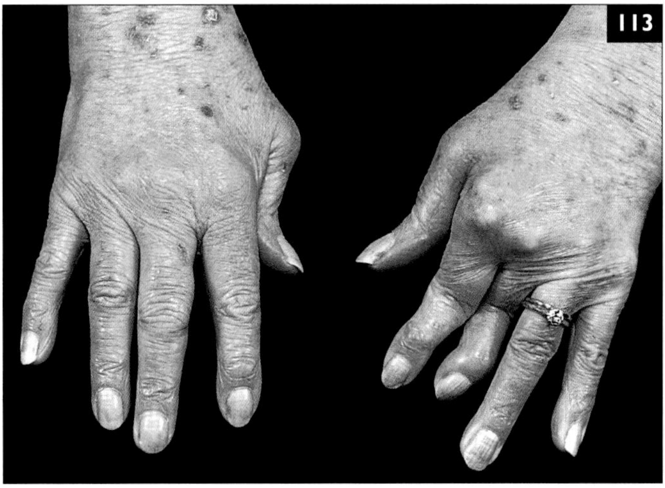

autosomal dominant pattern of inheritance with variable penetrance has been proposed. Strong associations with HLA-Cw6 have also been documented.

Differential diagnosis

Chronic plaque psoriasis confined to the palms or soles may be confused with chronic eczema or tinea manuum. Guttate psoriasis can simulate pityriasis rosea, pityriasis lichenoides and secondary syphilis. Flexural psoriasis is often misdiagnosed as chronic intertrigo.

Psoriasis may köbnerise co-existent areas of seborrhoiec dermatitis and, if the psoriasis is not present elsewhere, distinction between the two disorders is impossible. Erythrodermic psoriasis may be indistinguishable from other causes of erythroderma, particularly pityriasis rubra pilaris.

Investigations

Usually none – where the diagnosis is unclear, biopsy may be helpful.

Pityriasis Rubra Pilaris

114

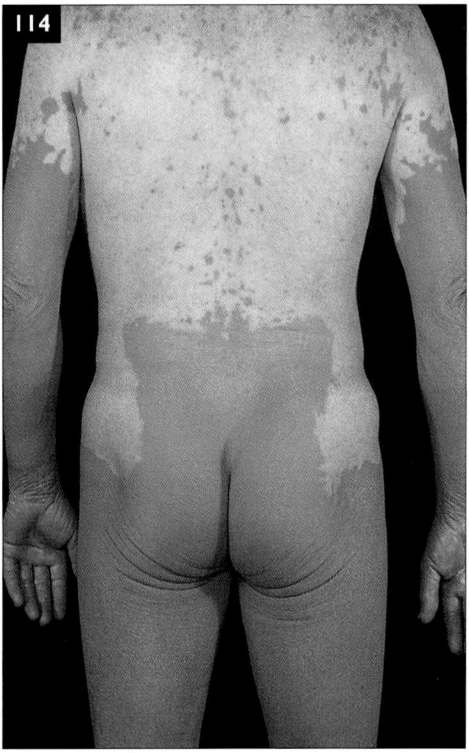

114 Pityriasis rubra pilaris.

Definition and clinical features

Pityriasis rubra pilaris (PRP) is a rare acquired inflammatory disorder of keratinisation of unknown cause. Griffiths' classification identifies five categories:

- Type 1 or classical adult PRP.
- Type 2 or atypical adult form.
- Type 3 or classical juvenile form.
- Type 4 which is circumscribed juvenile PRP.
- Type 5 which is atypical juvenile PRP.

PRP is characterised by patches of follicular erythema, hyperkeratosis and plugging on a background of orange erythema (**114**). It generally spreads from the head downwards over a period of weeks or months and produces a branny or pityriasiform scale. The extensor proximal digits are often affected producing a nutmeg-grater effect. Palmoplantar keratoderma and a nail dystrophy consisting of thickened nail plates may develop and, later in the course, an erythroderma with islands of spared normal skin may result. Mild pruritus and diffuse branny scaling are common. Many cases, especially Type 3, improve spontaneously but the disease can persist for years.

Epidemiology

It is commonest in middle age but can occur at any age. It affects the sexes equally.

Differential diagnosis

Early cases, in particular Type 4, may resemble psoriasis or erythrokeratoderma. Follicular ichthyosis, lichen spinulosus and keratosis pilaris may resemble it and atypical lesions can mimic seborrhoeic dermatitis.

Investigations

Histology of a typical lesion shows ortho- and para-hyperkeratosis and plugged hair follicles. Acanthosis and blunted rete ridges are seen and a mild lymphocytic dermal infiltrate is present.

Special points

There are isolated reports of abnormal circulating T-cell subsets in PRP. A number of cases in HIV-positive patients have been reported.

Pityriasis Lichenoides

Definition and clinical features

A disease of unknown aetiology characterised by multiple papules and plaques which develop in crops on the trunk and limbs. In the acute form (pityriasis lichenoides acuta et varioliformis), lesions evolve from erythematous papules into haemorrhagic vesicles and necrotic ulcers, and heal with chickenpox-like scars (**115**). Systemic upset with fever and malaise may occur rarely (febrile ulceronecrotic variant). The chronic form (pityriasis lichenoides chronica) is characterised by small reddish-brown papules with an adherent scale, and scarring is unusual (**116**). Both acute and chronic forms may follow a relapsing course over several months or years. Success has been reported with long-term erythromycin or tetracycline treatment or phototherapy.

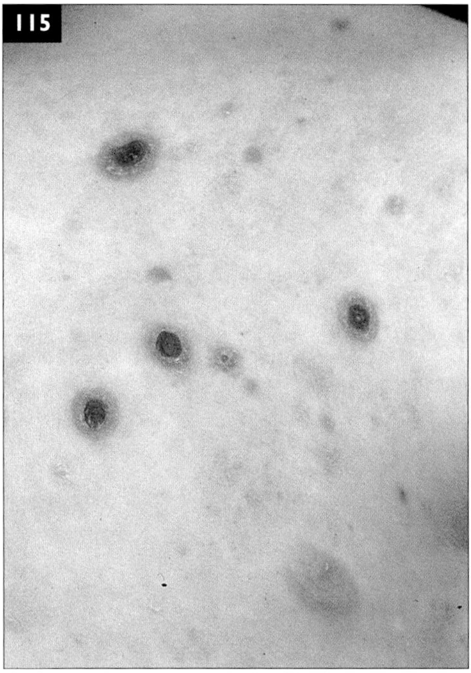

115 Acute pityriasis lichenoides.

Epidemiology

Pityriasis lichenoides predominantly affects children (especially the acute form) and young adults, with a male preponderance.

Differential diagnosis

The acute form is usually distinctive, but may resemble other vesicobullous disorders, including viral eruptions and insect bites. The chronic form should be differentiated from other papulosquamous disorders, including psoriasis, lichen planus and secondary syphilis.

Investigations

Histology usually helps support the diagnosis, with features varying according to the stage of the lesion. Early lesions show a dense lymphocytic infiltrate with dilated superficial blood vessels and purpura. In chronic lesions, the infiltrate is less dense, with epidermal changes such as spongiosis, acanthosis and parakeratosis.

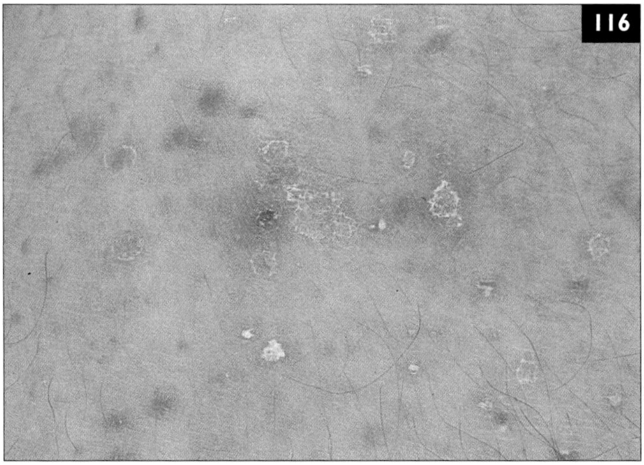

116 Chronic pityriasis lichenoides.

Chronic Superficial Scaly Dermatitis

117

117 Chronic superficial scaly dermatitis.

Definition and clinical features

A chronic eruption of small, superficial, pink–yellowish plaques with fine surface scaling on the trunk and limbs, often showing a characteristic digitate pattern (**117**). Lesions may show signs of atrophy. The cause is unknown, and the condition is usually asymptomatic with a tendency to improve on sun exposure. Emollients and mild topical corticosteroids can be used if there is any associated pruritus. This condition was once classified amongst so-called pre-mycotic eruptions, and termed 'small plaque parapsoriasis', but it is now considered to be a benign entity that does not evolve into cutaneous lymphoma.

Epidemiology

Typically, this affects middle-aged adults.

Differential diagnosis

Other eczematous disorders, and psoriasis. In early (patch stage) mycosis fungoides, lesions are usually larger and show evolving, histological features of cutaneous lymphoma.

Investigations

Histology shows mild eczematous features with spongiosis, variable parakeratosis and a sparse, dermal lymphocytic infiltrate. There is no epidermotropism, or lymphocyte atypia, and there is no change in the histological features with time (*cf.* mycosis fungoides).

Lichen Planus

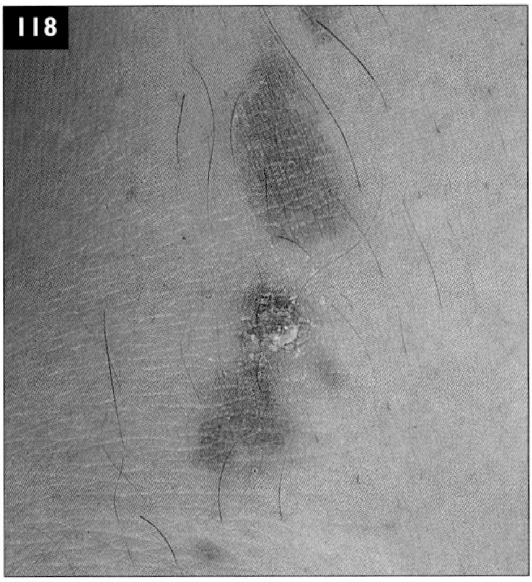

118 Lichen planus hyperpigmentation.

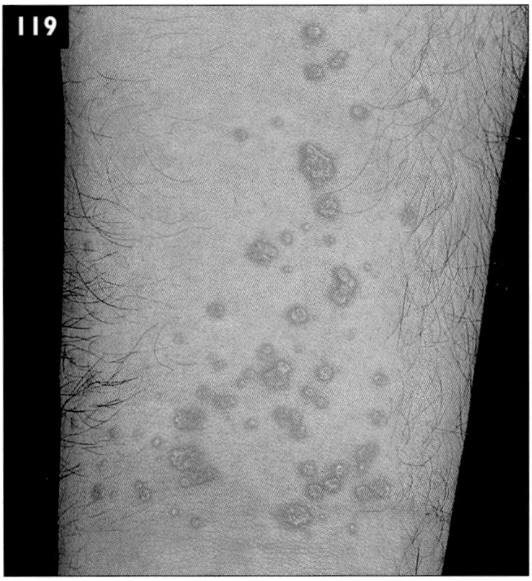

119 Flat-topped papules.

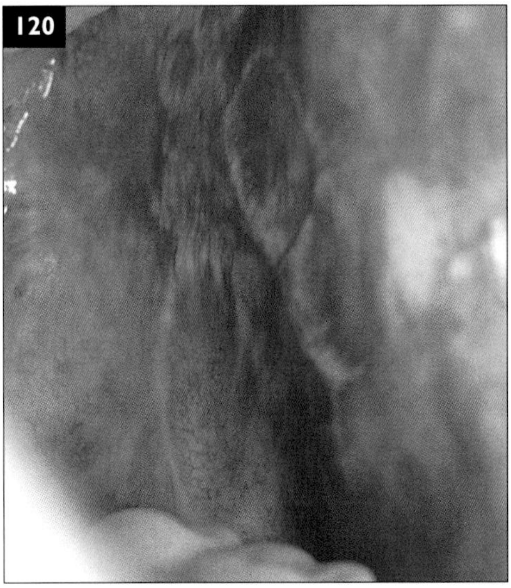

120 Oral lichen planus.

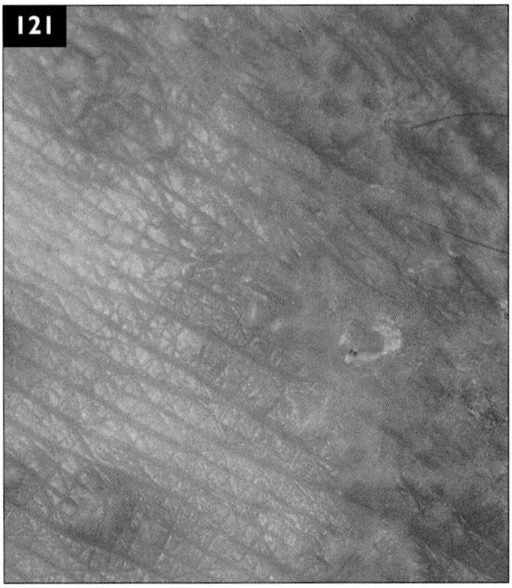

121 Wickham's striae.

Definition and clinical features

Lichen planus is a pruritic eruption of characteristic papules that usually resolves spontaneously, leaving temporary hyperpigmentation frequently (**118**) and scarring infrequently.

It presents as typical pruritic, discrete, violaceous, flat-topped papules (**119**) or plaques symmetrically involving the flexor surfaces of the wrists, forearms, ankles and lower back. The mucous membranes are often affected and may produce erosions (**120**). White streaks (Wickham's striae) (**121**) overlie the lesions and hyperkeratosis

Lichen Planus

may occur in plaques on the legs (**122**), palms (**123**) and soles. Scalp involvement produces scarring alopecia (**124**) and nail involvement causes increased longitudinal striations, variable atrophy and permanent scarring (pterygium) (**125**). Lesions occur at sites of trauma (Köbner phenomenon) (**126**) and more rarely lichen planus may cause bullae or annular lesions (**127**). Spontaneous recovery is usual within 6 months; recurrence is rare. An uncommon variant may, however, cause recalcitrant erosions of the orogenital mucosa.

Epidemiology

All races and ages are susceptible, although the greatest incidence is from 20 to 50 years of age. The cause is unknown though an autoimmune basis is suggested. Some drugs can induce lichen planus-like eruptions (e.g. antimalarials, heavy metals, antituberculous therapy). An association with hepatitis C infection has also been reported.

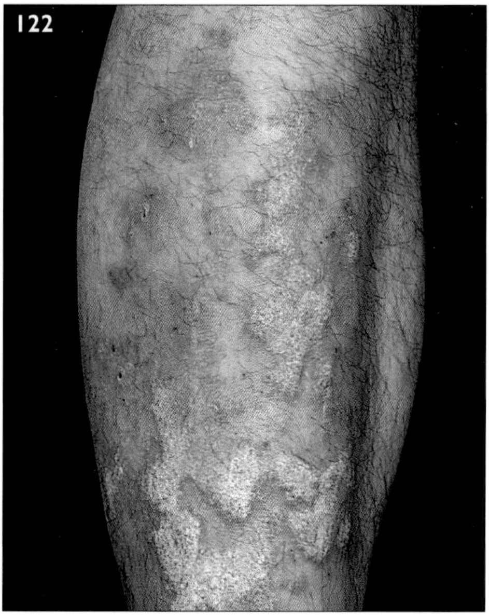

122 Hyperkeratotic lichen planus.

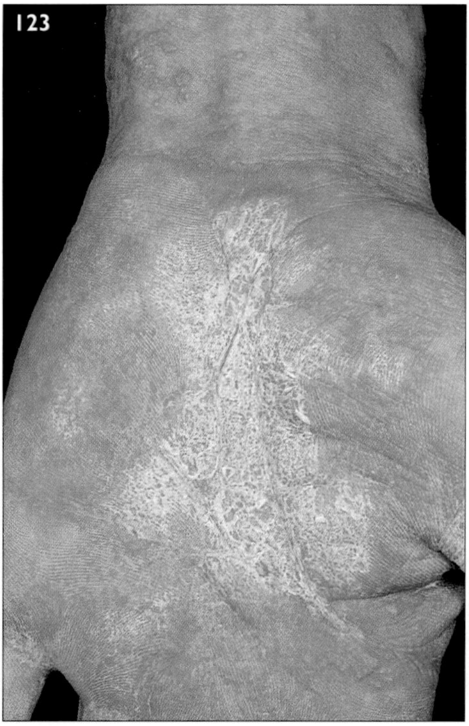

123 Palmar lichen planus.

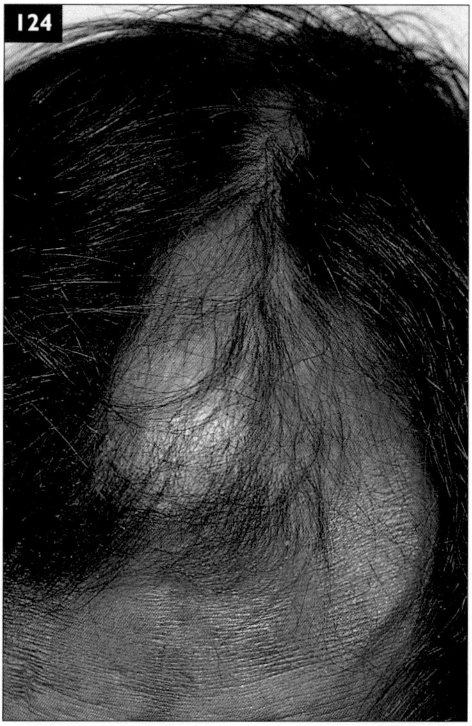

124 Scarring alopecia.

Lichen Planus

Differential diagnosis
Lichen simplex and lichenified eczema on the lower legs. A drug history is important in lichenified eruptions. *Candida albicans* produces white streaks on the oral mucosa.

Investigations
Biopsy is supportive, with variable hyperkeratosis, granular cell layer thickening, sawtooth pattern of rete ridges, increased prickle cell layer, basal cell degeneration, colloid body formation and a subepidermal bank of mononuclear infiltration.

Special points
Potent topical, intralesional or occasionally systemic corticosteroids are helpful.

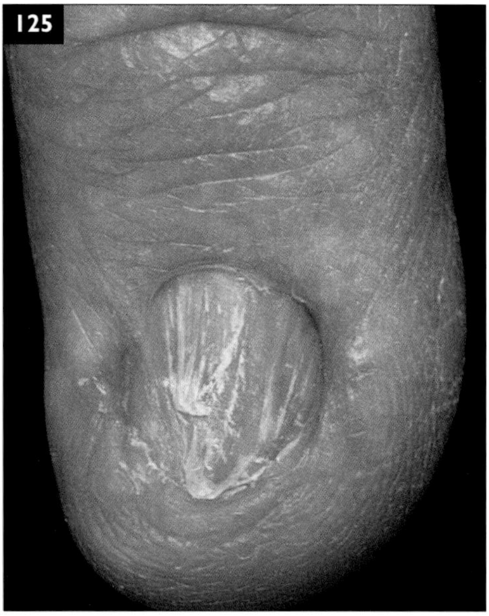

125 Pterygium.

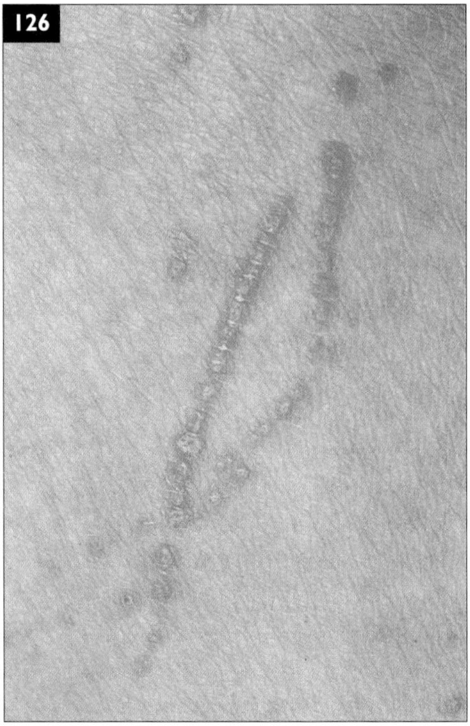

126 Köbner phenomenon.

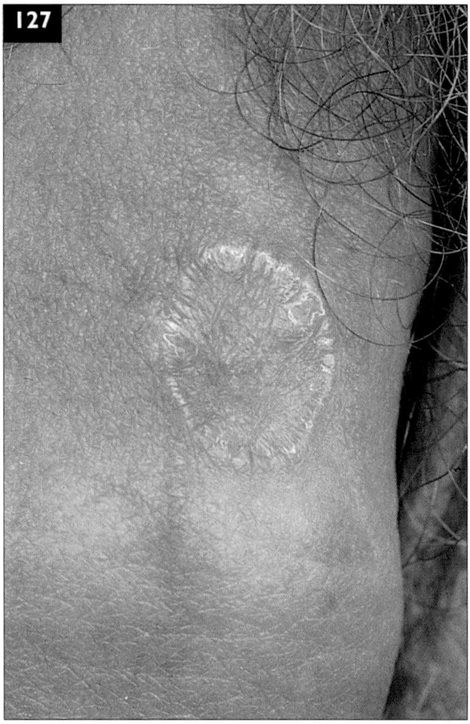

127 Annular lichen planus.

Bacterial Infections

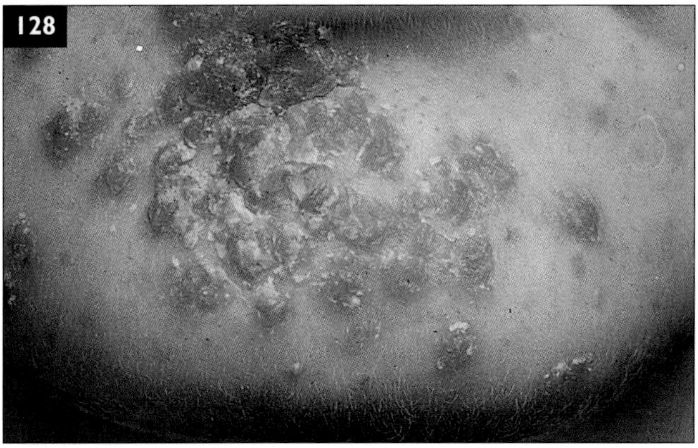

128 Impetigo.

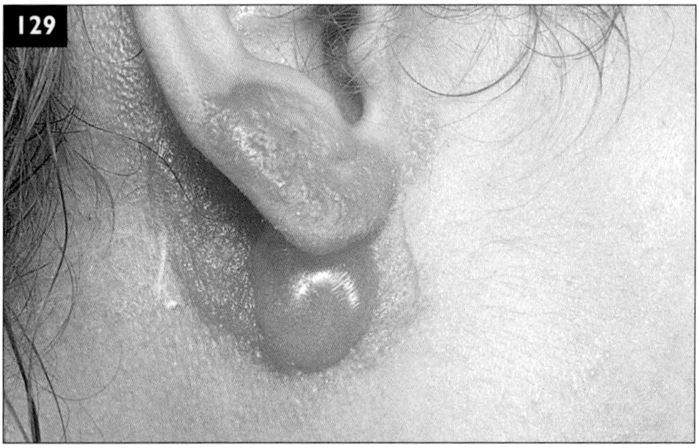

129 Bullous impetigo.

IMPETIGO

Definition and clinical features

An acute superficial infection of the skin caused by *Staphylococcus aureus* or, less commonly, group A β-haemolytic streptococci.

It presents as golden-yellow crusts, formed from exuding serum, usually affecting the face (**128**). The lesions spread locally and may coalesce; multiple lesions are common. Blisters can be a feature (**129**) and, as they rupture, typical crusts form at the edge of the lesion. Systemic upset is not usual but glomerulonephritis has been reported following streptococcal impetigo.

Epidemiology

Children are most commonly affected but no age group is exempt. Breaks in the skin, including those caused by eczema, predispose to impetigo. It is contagious.

Differential diagnosis

Fungal infection, herpes simplex.

Investigations

Microbiology if clinically atypical.

Special points

Treatment with topical mupirocin or fusidic acid is effective for localised impetigo. For more extensive lesions systemic antibiotics are necessary.

ECTHYMA

Definition and clinical features

Ecthyma is a deeper and more prolonged infection than impetigo but is also caused by *Staphylococcus aureus* and *Streptococcus* spp.

Bacterial Infections

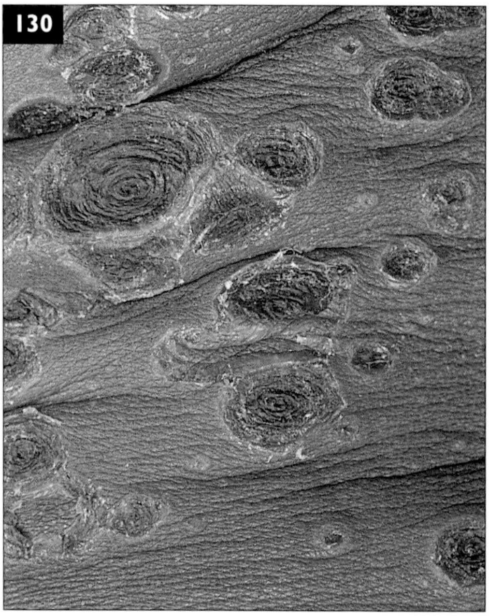

130 Ecthyma.

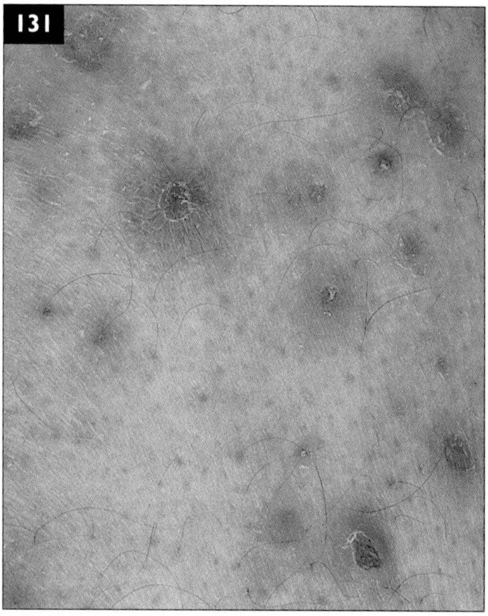

131 Folliculitis.

This condition presents as hard black crusts and eschars overlie localised areas of necrotic skin, with surrounding inflammation (**130**). The lesions are usually on the limbs and bullae are sometimes seen. Healing takes 2–3 weeks and leaves scars. Ecthyma may follow trauma to the skin.

Epidemiology
Uncommon in temperate climates. Children, often from disadvantaged backgrounds, are usually affected.

Differential diagnosis
Vasculitis, pityriasis lichenoides.

Investigations
Microbiology.

Special points
Treatment is with systemic antibiotics.

FOLLICULITIS
Definition and clinical features
Superficial inflammation within hair follicles caused by *Staphylococcus aureus*, coagulase negative *Staphylococcus*, *Pityrosporum* yeasts or a variety of chemical and traumatic factors.

Its clinical features are small pustules which, on close inspection, can be seen to be centred on hair follicles (**131**). There are variable degrees of inflammation in surrounding skin.

Epidemiology
A common problem, seen most often in young adults, but all ages are susceptible depending on aetiology.

Differential diagnosis
Follicular disorders, such as lichen planopilaris, and non-follicular pustules, as in psoriasis.

Investigations
Microbiology.

Special points
In susceptible individuals keloidal scarring can result.

FURUNCLES AND CARBUNCLES
Definition and clinical features
A furuncle (or boil) is an abscess caused by *Staphylococcus aureus* within a single hair follicle. Carbuncles are more extensive lesions with

Bacterial Infections

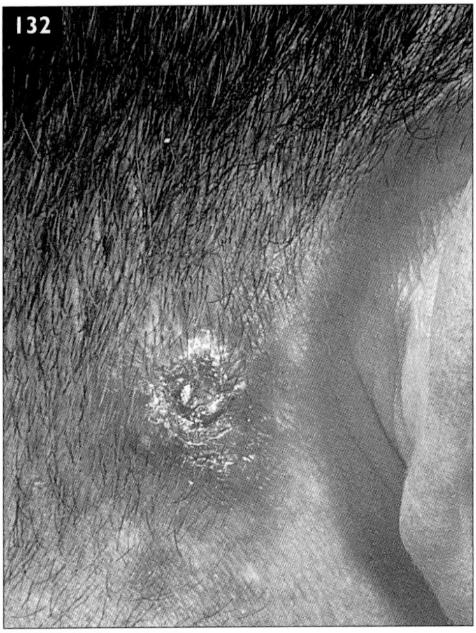

132 Furunculosis.

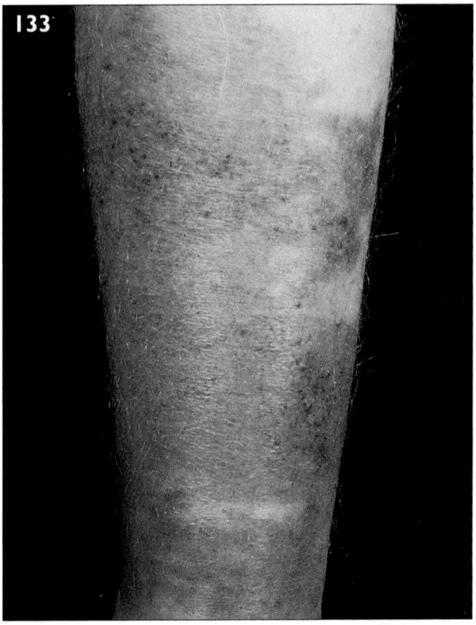

133 Cellulitis.

infection and necrosis spreading to several follicles and to surrounding soft tissues.

An inflammatory nodule develops into a follicular pustule which will point and discharge (**132**). Furuncles are often multiple; carbuncles are similar but more extensive with multiple openings – they may reach more than 1cm in diameter. Discharge leaves a deep ulcer. Fever and malaise can occur with both furuncles and carbuncles but are usually more severe with the latter.

Epidemiology

Furuncles typically affect healthy, young adults although recurrent boils can be a sign of poorly controlled diabetes. Carbuncles usually affect older patients with concurrent illness.

Differential diagnosis

Acne, hidradenitis suppurativa.

Investigations

Microbiology of the skin and carrier sites. Exclude underlying illness.

Special points

Early furuncles can be treated with topical antibiotics but more established lesions and carbuncles need systemic antibiotics. Recurrent furunculosis can be a taxing problem and involves identifying and eradicating carriage sites of *Staphylococcus*, and treatment with antiseptics and antibiotics.

ERYSIPELAS, CELLULITIS AND NECROTISING FASCIITIS

Definition and clinical features

Infection of the dermis and subcutaneous tissue usually caused by *Streptococcus pyogenes*, although a wide variety of organisms have been reported as causing cellulitis. There is no clear distinction between cellulitis and erysipelas: in the latter the infection is more superficial, but in necrotising fasciitis the infection is deeper still, reaching the fascia.

Infection is heralded by malaise and fever, and after a few hours to days the affected area becomes red, tender and swollen (**133**). Bullae, sometimes haemorrhagic, can appear in acute

Bacterial Infections

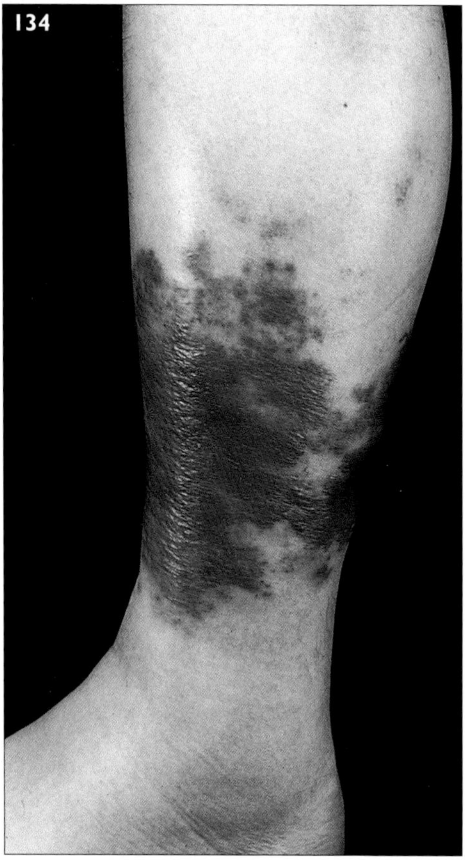

134 Erysipelas.

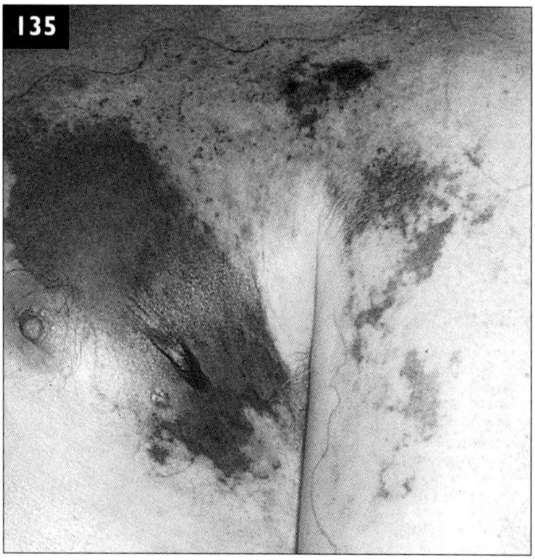

135 Necrotising fasciitis.

cases. Red streaks of lymphangitis and tender lymphadenopathy are common. In erysipelas the margins of erythema are usually more clearly demarcated than in cellulitis (**134**). In necrotising fasciitis the erythema is often dusky, and deep haemorrhagic bullae develop with necrosis of the skin and soft tissues (**135**).

Epidemiology

In all three conditions predisposing factors are important, with both systemic and local disease allowing infection to become established. Oedema, particularly lymphoedema, is an important predisposing factor and can lead to recurrent attacks.

Differential diagnosis

Deep venous thrombosis.

Investigations

Microbiology of the affected skin is often negative. Blood cultures. Serology: ASOT; anti DNAase B.

Special points

Treatment of all three conditions is with systemic antibiotics; these often need to be given parenterally. In necrotising fasciitis urgent surgery to debride necrotic tissue is essential to preserve life and limb. Management of recurrent cellulitis may require long-term antibiotics, and skin care to avoid entry portals.

SCARLET FEVER

Definition and clinical features

Infection with a toxin-producing *Streptococcus pyogenes*. The usual portal of entry of the streptococcus is the upper respiratory tract, hence the disease presents with sore throat and lymphadenopathy. The erythematous rash appears on the trunk and becomes generalised. The face is flushed but the perioral area shows relative pallor. The tongue becomes red with swollen papillae, the strawberry tongue.

Bacterial Infections

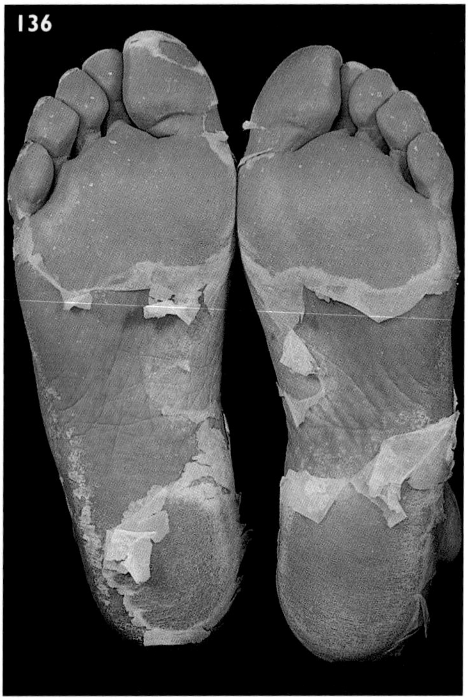

136 Skin peeling following toxic shock syndrome.

Epidemiology
Scarlet fever is usually seen in children. From being an endemic and epidemic problem it has become relatively uncommon.

Differential diagnosis
Staphylococcal toxic shock syndrome, Kawasaki disease, viral exanthems, drug eruptions.

Investigations
Throat swab.

Special points
Scarlet fever has become less severe than in previous decades. With systemic antibiotics the prognosis is good.

TOXIC SHOCK SYNDROME
Definition and clinical features
Infection with a toxin-producing *Staphylococcus aureus*. The vagina is the usual site of initial, often asymptomatic, infection. Presentation is with fever and widespread erythema. Conjunctivitis and swelling of the hands and feet are commonly seen. The rash fades within a few days and peeling of the hands and feet may occur after a week (**136**). Multisystem involvement and circulatory collapse are typical features.

Epidemiology
Women of childbearing age are usually affected at the time of menstruation. The use of tampons has been implicated. Staphylococcal infection at other sites, including the skin, has also been reported.

Differential diagnosis
Kawasaki disease, scarlet fever.

Investigations
Microbiological examination of swabs from appropriate sites.

STAPHYLOCOCCAL SCALDED SKIN SYNDROME
Definition and clinical features
Infection with epidermolytic toxin-producing strains of *Staphylococcus aureus* producing a widespread superficial blistering eruption.

Bacterial Infections

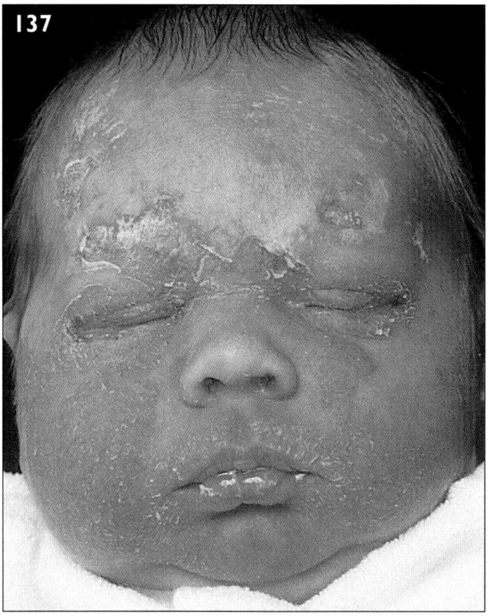

137 Staphylococcal scalded skin syndrome.

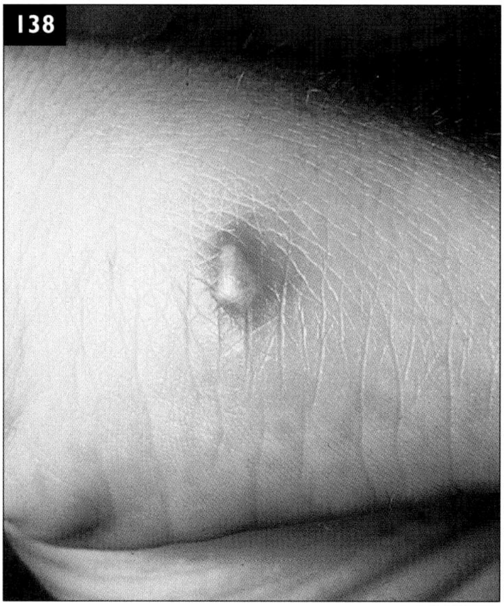

138 Haemorrhagic pustule in gonococcal septicaemia.

The causative staphylococcus can be on the skin (or an occult infection) which becomes red and tender and peels away to form raw areas (**137**). The trunk and flexures are often affected, as is the face. Healing takes place in about a week. Although the condition is not so severe as toxic epidermal necrolysis, in extensive cases there is an appreciable mortality.

Epidemiology
Children are usually affected. Adults may develop localised areas, usually in the context of renal failure.

Differential diagnosis
In toxic epidermal necrolysis the split in the epidermis is deeper resulting in a more serious condition with higher morbidity and mortality.

Investigations
Identification of the causative organism.

GONOCOCCAL SEPTICAEMIA
Definition and clinical features
Chronic occult infection with *Neisseria gonorrhoeae* can result in bacteraemia and give rise to a multisystem illness. Skin lesions, fever and arthralgia are presenting features. Haemorrhagic pustules and vesicles appear in crops, typically on the fingers (**138**).

Epidemiology
Predominantly affects women.

Differential diagnosis
Meningococcal septicaemia, vasculitis and subacute bacterial endocarditis.

Investigations
Microbiological examination of genital secretions and blood.

Special points
Sexual contacts need to be traced and screened for infection.

MENINGOCOCCAL INFECTION
Definition and clinical features
Meningococcal septicaemia and meningitis caused by *Neisseria meningitidis* can present with a purpuric exanthem. Widespread purpura occurs early in the course of fulminating meningococcal septicaemia or

Bacterial Infections

139
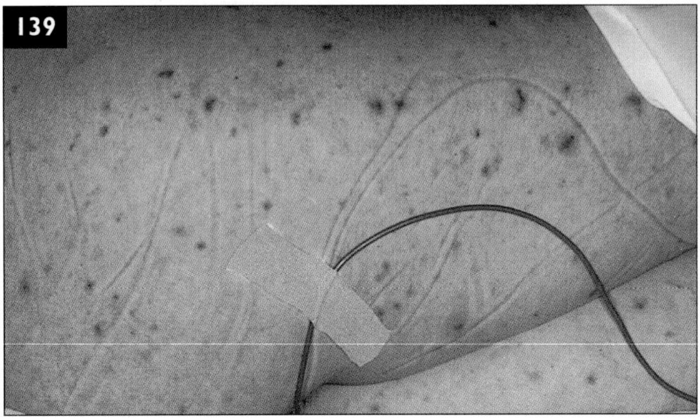

139 Purpuric lesions in meningococcal septicaemia.

140
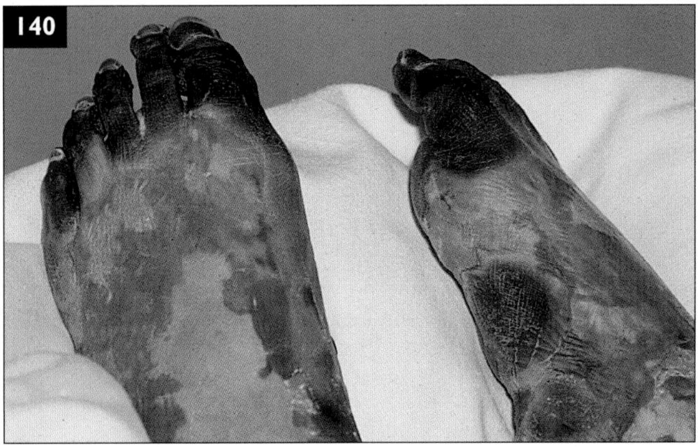

140 Gangrenous lesions in meningococcal septicaemia.

meningitis (**139**). In cases where the onset is less acute, the initial rash may be urticated or morbilliform. Large, patches of purpura with ragged-edged can occur at any site. In the rarer chronic infection, vasculitic nodules may occur.

Epidemiology
Children and young adults are most commonly affected. Cases are usually sporadic but small epidemics may occur.

Differential diagnosis
Severe vasculitis, viral meningitis with exanthem.

Investigations
Microbiological culture of blood, CSF and skin lesions can all reveal the organism.

Special points
Infection is rapidly progressive (**140**) and death can occur in the early stages. It is recommended that antibiotic treatment is given as soon as the diagnosis is suspected and the patient admitted to hospital.

ERYTHRASMA

Definition and clinical features
Chronic superficial infection with *Corynebacterium minutissimum* producing an eruption in the flexures. This presents as red or brown, well-marginated, slightly scaly or glazed patches (**141**). Sites most commonly affected are the axillae and groins. Lesions are asymptomatic or mildly pruritic.

Epidemiology
Adults are affected more often than children, and it is more common in tropical climates and in diabetics. Asymptomatic carriage of C. *minutissimum* is common.

Differential diagnosis
Pityriasis versicolor does not usually affect flexures. Candida is more inflammatory. In

Bacterial Infections

141
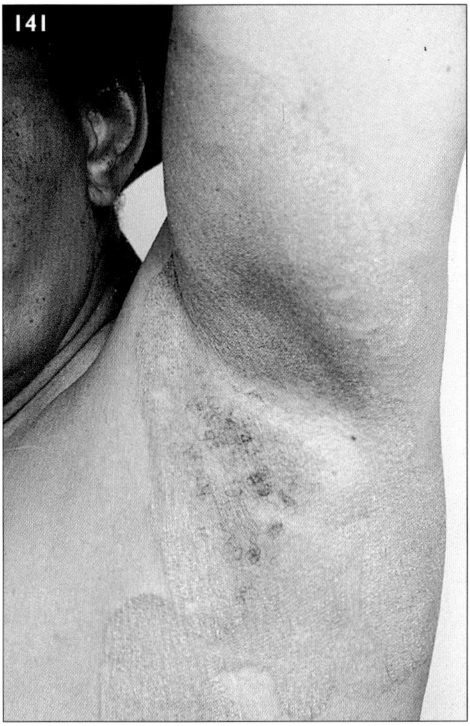

141 Erythrasma.

flexural psoriasis there are usually signs on the non-flexural skin.

Investigations
Coral red fluorescence under Wood's light may help confirm the diagnosis.

Special points
Topical antibiotics are usually effective unless infection is extensive.

PITTED KERATOLYSIS
Definition and clinical features
Chronic superficial infection with *Corynebacterium minutissimum* producing small, pitted erosions on the soles of the feet. Presents as shallow, punched-out erosions in the keratin on the soles (**142, 143**). Occlusive footwear and sweaty feet usually precipitate the problem, which is usually asymptomatic.

Epidemiology
Most frequent in young men, especially when occlusive footwear is worn.

142
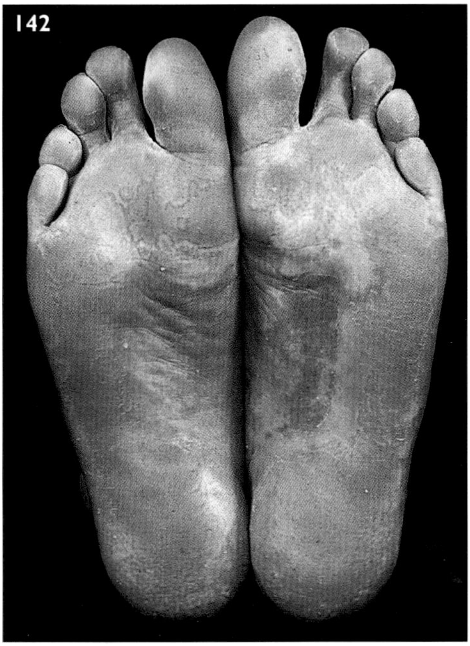

142 Pitted keratolysis.

143
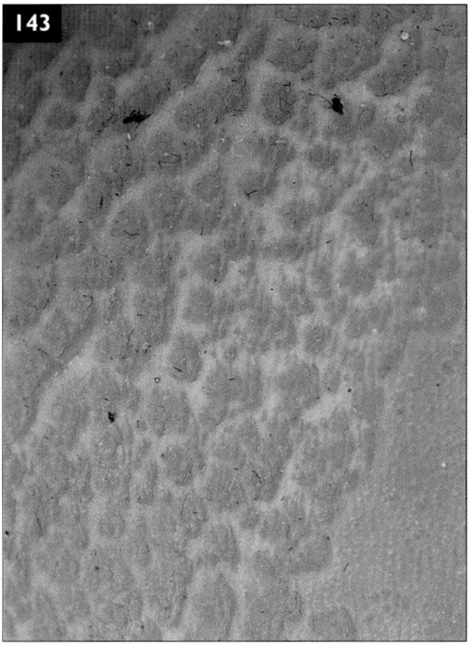

143 Pitted keratolysis.

Bacterial Infections

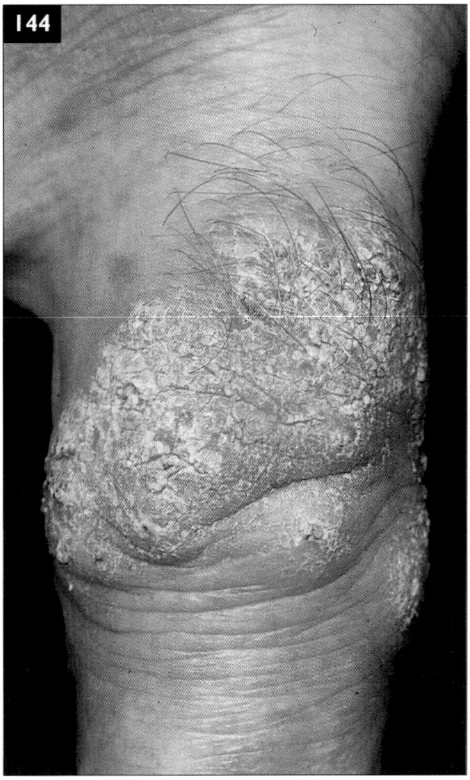

144 Warty TB.

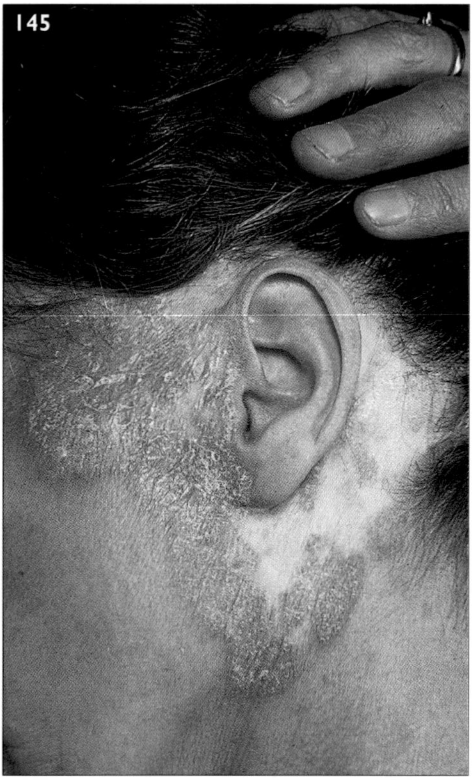

145 Lupus vulgaris.

Differential diagnosis
Tinea pedis.

Special points
Treatment with topical antibiotics such as fusidic acid must be combined with measures to reduce sweating of the feet.

CUTANEOUS TUBERCULOSIS (TB)
Definition and clinical features
Cutaneous infection with *Mycobacterium tuberculae*. Clinical appearance varies with mode of infection, which can be direct, metastatic or from draining lymph nodes.

Lupus vulgaris is the most frequent clinical variant. Tuberculous chancre, warty TB (**144**) (both from direct contact) and cutaneous spread from infected lymph nodes and bones are rarely seen. Lupus vulgaris typically affects the head and neck. It presents as progressive red–brown, soft papules and plaques, described as 'apple jelly' nodules (**145**). The disease spreads slowly over many years with resultant scarring.

Epidemiology
Cutaneous tuberculosis is now uncommon in the UK but is still frequent in Asia.

Differential diagnosis
Lupus erythematosus, leprosy, sarcoid.

Investigations
Culture of *Mycobacterium* is not usually possible. Histology shows granuloma but caseation is unusual in lupus vulgaris.

Special points
Treatment is with anti-tuberculous therapy. Squamous cell carcinoma can occur in long-standing lupus vulgaris.

Bacterial Infections

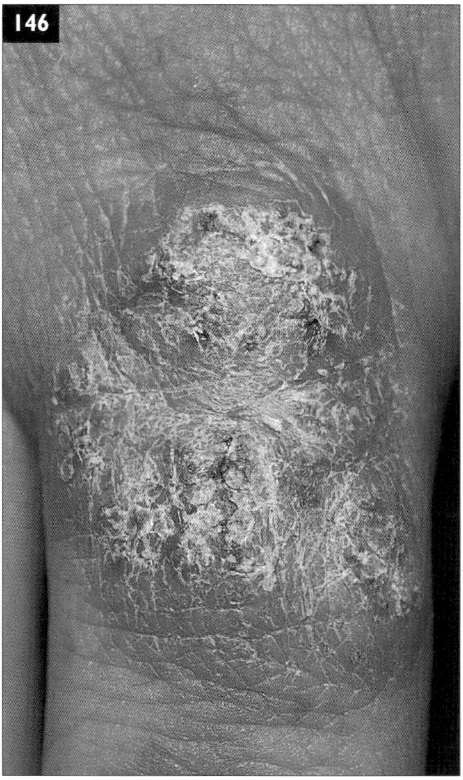

146 Fish-tank granuloma.

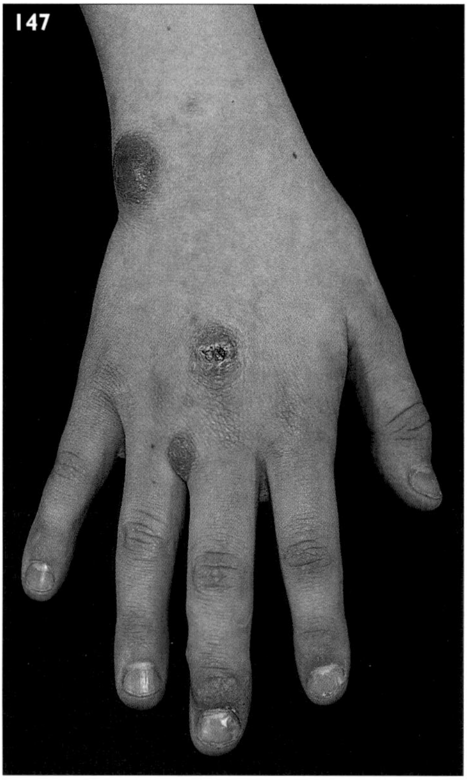

147 Sporotrichoid spread (see p. 72).

MYCOBACTERIUM MARINUM (FISH-TANK GRANULOMA)

Definition and clinical features

A chronic cutaneous infection with *Mycobacterium marinum*, an organism that occurs in warm water, especially tropical aquaria. Lesions arise in broken skin on exposed areas such as the hands. Pustules or nodules become crusted and warty (**146**). Spread along lymphatics causes lines of nodules and lymphadenopathy (**147**). The lesions may heal over a period of months.

Epidemiology

An uncommon condition usually seen in fish fanciers. The organism is endemic in most tropical fish.

Differential diagnosis

Sporotrichosis, leishmaniasis.

Investigations

Culture of affected skin is often positive. Histology is helpful but does not always distinguish from sporotrichosis.

Special points

Response to antibiotics is slow but lesions usually respond to a prolonged course of minocycline or co-trimoxazole.

Bacterial Infections

148

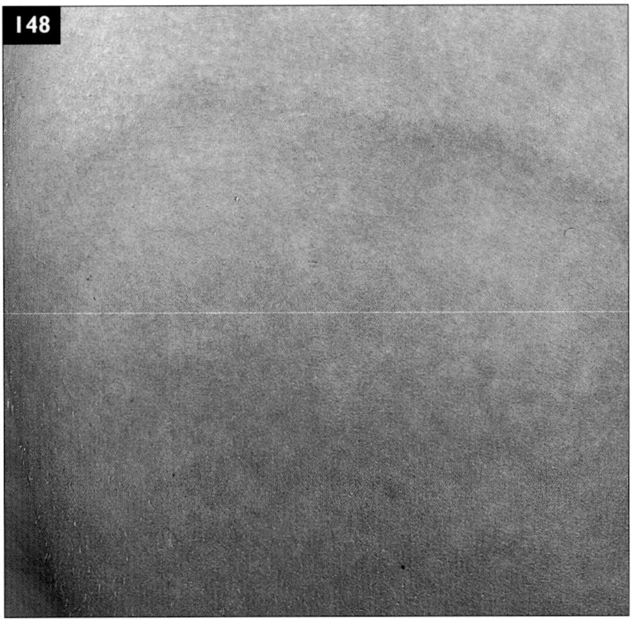

148 Erythema chronicum migrans.

LYME DISEASE

Definition and clinical features

A chronic multisystem infection often presenting with dermatological changes and progressing to involve the joints and nervous system. Lyme disease is caused by *Borrelia burgdorferi*, a tick-borne spirochete.

The early signs of infection are seen in the skin around the site of the bite, as a spreading annular erythema known as erythema chronicum migrans (**148**). Without treatment some patients develop a chronic infection which affects the joints and nervous system.

Another cutaneous manifestation, acrodermatitis chronica atrophicans, may occur in the later stages. This is seen as nodules and plaques, usually on the feet or hands, that spread leaving central atrophy. Other skin conditions, such as morphoea, are thought sometimes to be secondary to borrelial infection.

Epidemiology

The *Ixodes* tick is endemic in certain parts of the United States, Scandinavia and in some areas of the UK, such as the New Forest and the East Anglian Brecklands. Acrodermatitis is almost exclusive to European cases.

Differential diagnosis

Tinea corporis is more scaly than erythema chronicum migrans. Other annular erythemas must be distinguished by the history of a tick bite or from having travelled in a tick-endemic area.

Investigations

Serology: complement fixation tests and fluorescent antibody titres. False positives can occur.

Special points

Adequate treatment with antibiotics may prevent later multisystem illness.

Fungal Diseases

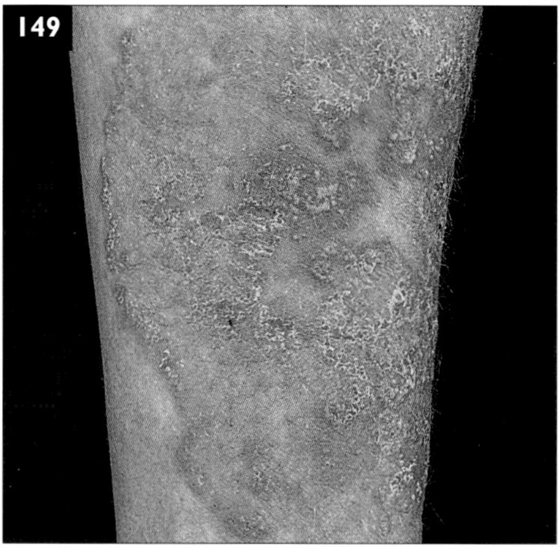

149 Tinea corporis.

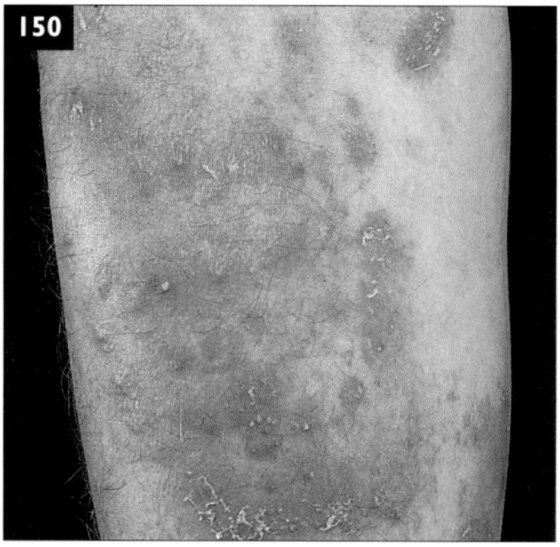

150 Tinea incognito.

DERMATOPHYTE INFECTION AND TINEA

Definition and clinical features

Dermatophytes are fungi that infect the stratum corneum of the skin producing ringworm. There are three genera – *Microsporum*, *Trichophyton* and *Epidermophyton*.

Skin signs vary with the site of infection and species of infecting fungus, but fungi transmitted from animals usually produce more inflammation than those that are exclusively human pathogens.

Tinea corporis, tinea of non-hair-bearing skin, is an infection that can be caused by any of the dermatophytes. *Trichophyton rubrum* and *Microsporum* canis are frequent offenders. Any part of the body can be involved from which spreading to other sites, such as the feet or scalp, is common. Lesions are circular, becoming annular, clearly defined and with a raised, scaly edge (**149**).

Treatment with topical or systemic corticosteroids can alter the appearance; such ill-defined lesions are known as tinea incognito (**150**).

Tinea cruris, affecting the groins and natal cleft (**151**), is often more itchy than tinea corporis but is otherwise similar.

Tinea pedis (athlete's foot) is extremely common. The moist skin of the web spaces provides ideal conditions for *Trichophyton interdigitale*, *T. rubrum* and *Epidermophyton floccosum*, often coexisting with bacteria (**152**). Soggy scaling and fissuring spreads from the

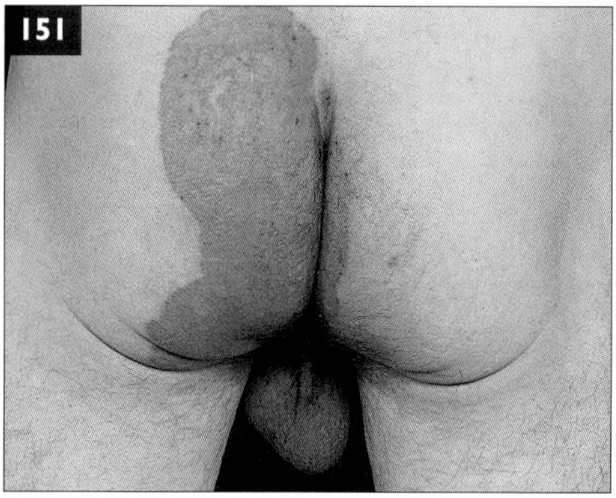

151 Tinea cruris.

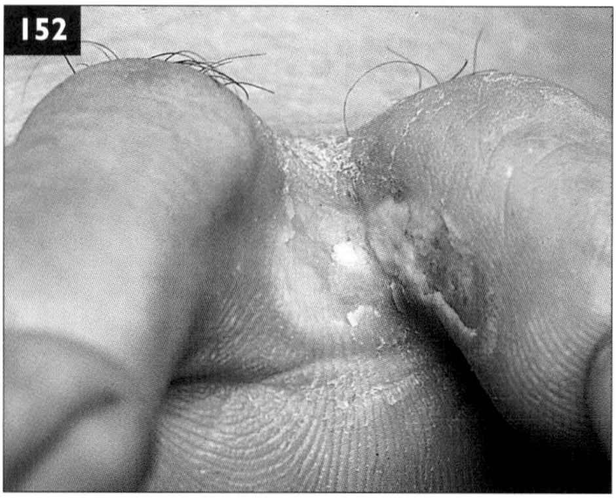

152 Tinea pedis ('athlete's foot').

Fungal Diseases

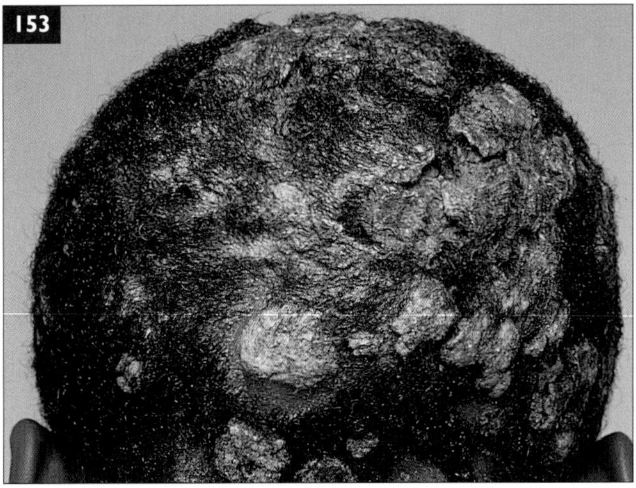

153 Tinea capitis.

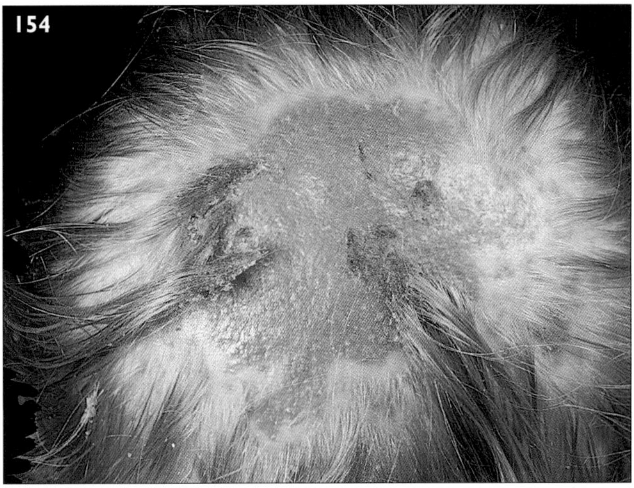

154 A kerion.

toe webs to the soles and dorsae of the feet.

Tinea capitis is the result of *Microsporum canis*, *M. audounii* and some species of *Trichophyton* invading hair shafts. The inflammatory reaction depends on the type of infecting fungus. M. canis produces patches of alopecia with broken hairs, scaling and inflammation (**153**). Animal dermatophytes such as *T. verrucosum* cause the most inflammation, producing a painful, swollen, boggy, purulent plaque known as a kerion (**154**). Malaise, lymphadenopathy and scarring alopecia are common.

Infection of the beard, tinea barbae, causes similar problems to tinea capitis, but, as the infecting agent is often an animal dermatophyte, inflammatory reactions can be marked (**155**).

Tinea manuum, affecting the hands, is usually caused by *T. rubrum* and causes particular diagnostic difficulties. Inflammation is often minimal. The palm becomes dry with

Fungal Diseases

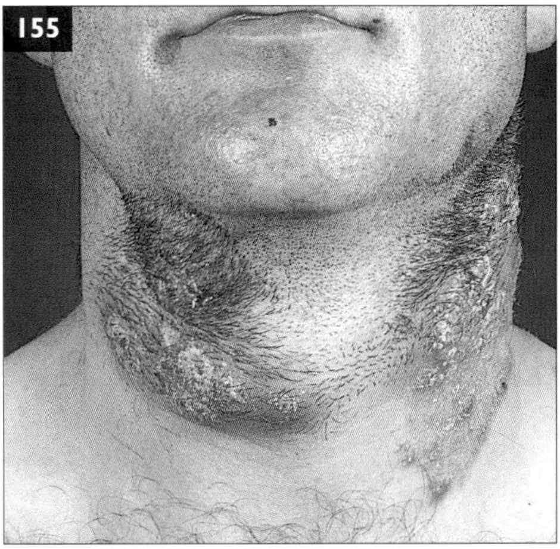

155 Tinea barbae.

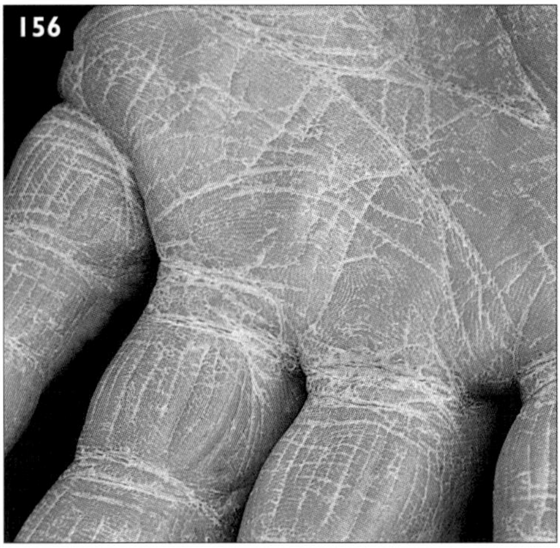

156 Tinea manuum.

mild scaling which is most obvious in the palmar creases (**156**). Infection is often unilateral.

Nail infection, tinea unguium, is very common and often an incidental finding. It is frequently associated with tinea pedis. A white or yellow discoloration first affects the free edge of the nail and spreads down towards the cuticle (**157**). The nail becomes thickened and crumbly. Toenails are most commonly affected.

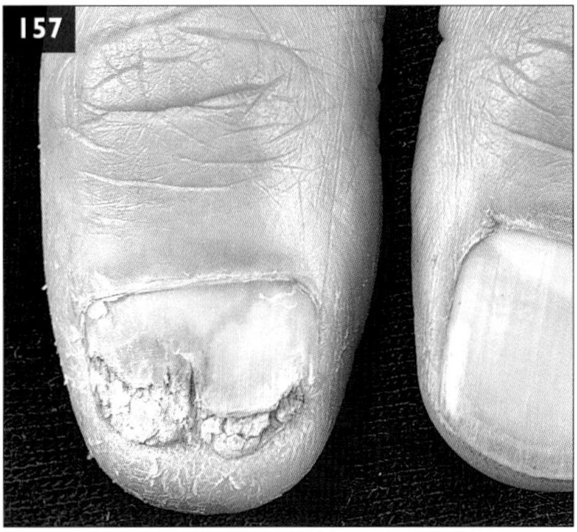

157 Tinea unguium.

Epidemiology

Superficial fungal infections are very common. Tinea capitis is chiefly a disease of childhood whereas infection at other sites is more often seen in adults. Shared showering or bathing facilities encourage the spread of tinea pedis. The endemic species of fungi varies from country to country.

Differential diagnosis

Tinea corporis should be distinguished from psoriasis and discoid (nummular) eczema. Candidal infection is less clearly demarcated than tinea cruris. Non-inflammatory scalp ringworm shows scaling and broken hairs, in contrast to alopecia areata. Tinea pedis may resemble bacterial infection when affecting the toe webs, and eczema or psoriasis when affecting the soles. Unilateral involvement helps differentiate tinea manuum from psoriasis, eczema and keratoderma.

Investigations

Direct microscopy and culture of skin scrapings and nail or hair clippings. Hair infected by *M. audounii* and *M. canis* shows bright green fluorescence under Wood's light (UV 365 nm). This is of particular use in tracing affected individuals in epidemics.

Special points

Localised infection of glabrous skin can be treated with topical antifungals. Infection of hair, nails and palms requires systemic antifungals.

Fungal Diseases

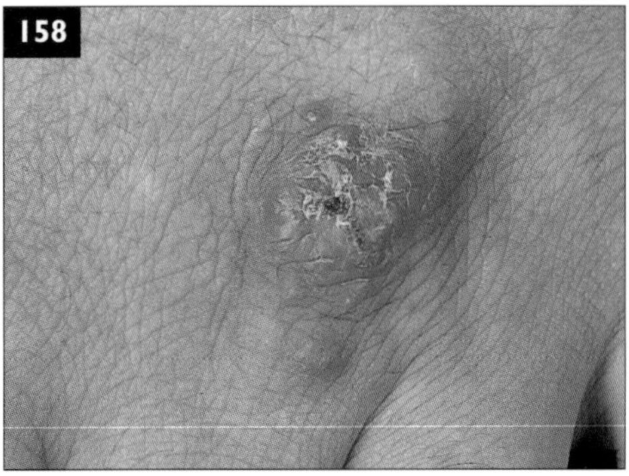

158 Sporotrichosis nodule.

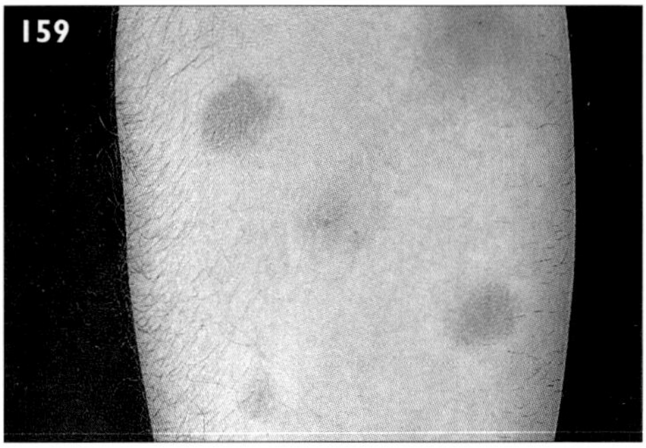

159 Nodules along local lymphatics in sporotrichosis.

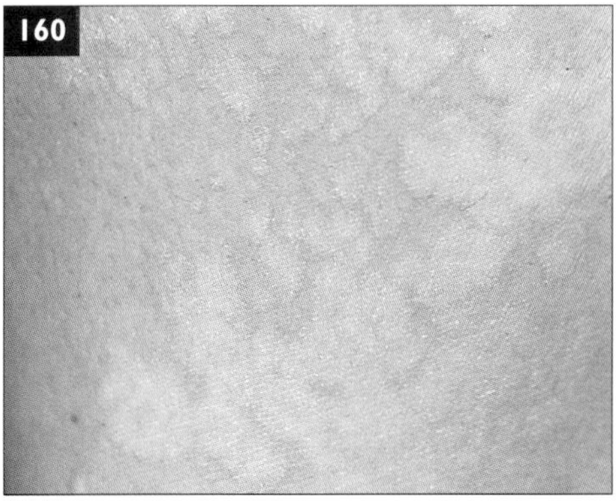

160 Pityriasis (tinea) versicolor.

SPOROTRICHOSIS

Definition and clinical features

An uncommon deep fungal infection caused by *Sporothrix schenckii*. This infection is usually acquired following injury, often from decaying wood. A nodule or warty plaque forms at the site of injury (**158**) and then, characteristically, nodules appear along local lymphatics (**159**).

Epidemiology

The fungus is widely distributed in decaying vegetation.

Differential diagnosis

Individual lesions can be mimicked by leishmaniasis and foreign body granulomas. The spread of lesions along lymphatics has been seen with fish tank granuloma and is known as sporotrichoid spread.

Investigations

Mycological culture. Histological examination is often non-specific.

Special points

Treatment is with systemic antifungals.
Other deep mycoses are rare in the UK.

PITYRIASIS (TINEA) VERSICOLOR

Definition and clinical features

Superficial chronic cutaneous infection with a yeast, *Pityrosporum orbiculare*. This presents as slightly scaly, or pale brown patches or macules that fail to tan on sun exposure. Usually asymptomatic. Affects trunk and sometimes the proximal parts of the limbs (**160**).

Epidemiology

P. orbiculare is a coloniser of normal skin. It thrives on warm, moist, oily skin and so is best suited to young adults and warm climates.

Differential diagnosis

Erythrasma, seborrhoeic eczema, vitiligo.

Investigations

Microscopy of skin scrapings.

Special points

Responds to topical antifungal preparations but tends to be recurrent.

CANDIDAL INFECTION

Definition and clinical features

Candida is a yeast that is an asymptomatic coloniser of mucosal surfaces. It causes infection of moist skin in susceptible individuals.

Fungal Diseases

161

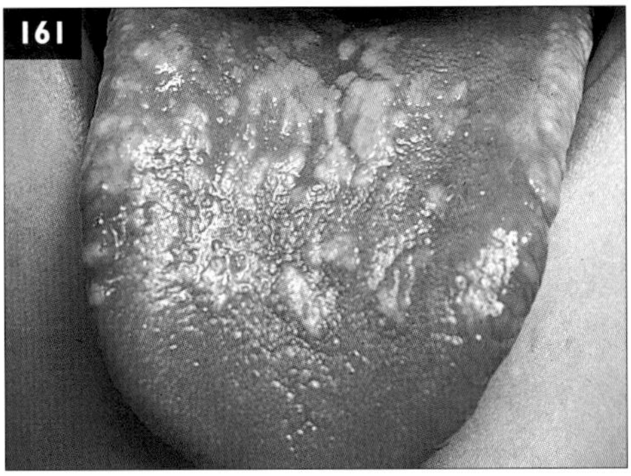

161 Oral candidiasis.

162

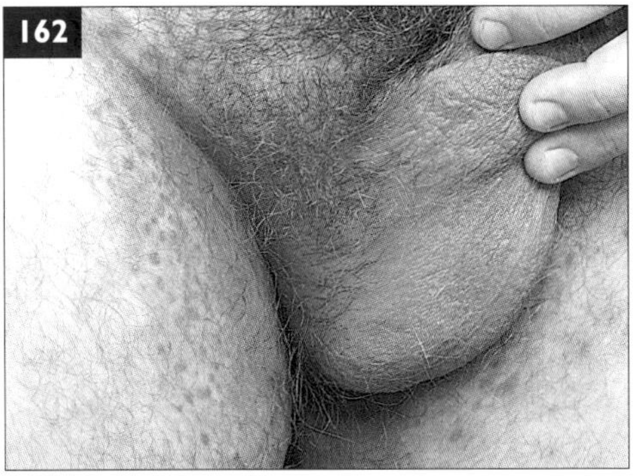

162 Flexural candidiasis with satellite lesions.

Candida can infect the flexures, mouth, genital mucosa and nail folds. Systemic spread may occur in the immunosuppressed. The mucosal surfaces show white plaques that detach and leave erythematous areas (**161**). Submammary and groin flexures become sore and itchy with glazed erythema, often with satellite lesions (**162**).

Chronic paronychia caused by candidal infection results in a painful swelling of the nail folds and usually of the fingers (**163**). Candidal paronychia often affects nail folds that are already damaged by trauma, irritants and eczema.

Chronic mucocutaneous candidiasis is a hereditary immunodeficiency resulting in the destruction of the nails (**164**) and in a chronic mucosal infection with spread to the oesophagus.

Candidal septicaemia is seen in debilitated patients, usually in intensive care.

Epidemiology
Candida is frequently found as a non-pathogenic coloniser. Infection is seen more commonly in immunosuppression of all types, after antibiotic or steroid therapy, and in diabetics.

Differential diagnosis
Flexural candidiasis must be distinguished from erythrasma, tinea cruris and flexural psoriasis. Oral lesions may be confused with lichen planus, dysplasia and hairy leukoplakia.

Investigations
Culture of swabs. Blood cultures in candidal septicaemia.

163

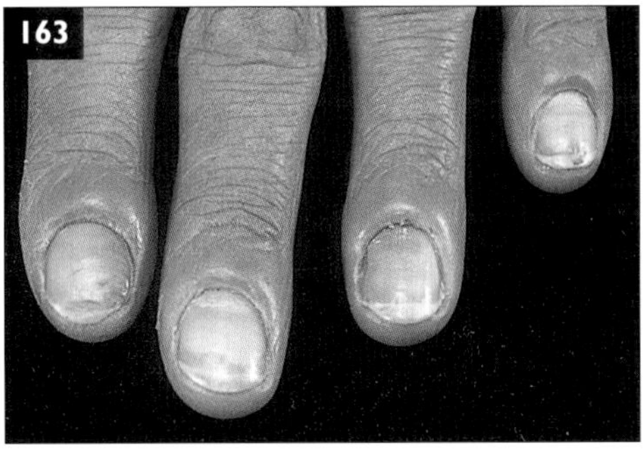

163 Candidal paronychia.

164

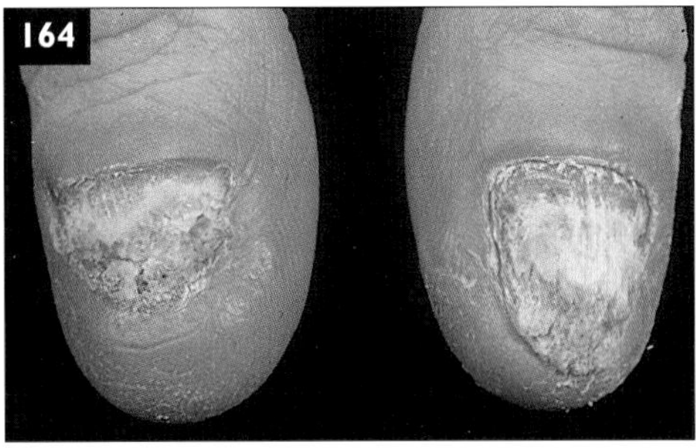

164 Chronic mucocutaneous candidiasis destroying the nails.

Special points
Treatment with either topical or systemic anti-candidal agents depends on the site of infection. Further management depends on the exclusion of underlying factors.

Viral Infections

MEASLES

Definition and clinical features

This is an infection with an RNA myxovirus, giving rise to upper respiratory symptoms, rash and fever.

The clinical features are fever, catarrh and conjunctivitis, followed after 3 or 4days by the appearance of Koplik's spots (pale spots on a red base) on the buccal mucosa. The rash usually develops a day or two later. It first shows behind the ears but rapidly becomes generalised as a maculopapular rash (**165**). After 7–10 days the rash fades with fine peeling. In immunosuppressed or malnourished patients the rash can either be more severe with purpura or may be minimal with rapid spread of the virus to the lungs and brain.

Epidemiology

Measles is usually contracted in childhood. It has become less common with effective immunisation.

Differential diagnosis

Kawasaki disease, scarlet fever, drug eruptions.

Investigations

Clinical appearance is usually sufficient. Serology may confirm diagnosis retrospectively.

Special points

Incubation period is about 10 days.

RUBELLA

Definition and clinical features

This is an infection with an RNA togavirus, giving rise to a macular exanthem, with mild constitutional symptoms.

Rubella presents as a fever, sore throat, conjunctivitis and sometimes arthritis which precede the rash by a few days, particularly in older children and adults. Younger children often present with the exanthem which is a red macular eruption starting on the face and spreading downwards. As it progresses a confluent, blotchy erythema develops (**166**). Lymphadenopathy, characteristically affecting the occipital nodes, may be a presenting feature and often occurs before the rash. The eruption disappears in about 4 or 5 days, clearing from the face downwards.

Epidemiology

Epidemics were a regular occurrence before the introduction of immunisation.

Differential diagnosis

Other viral exanthems.

Investigations

Paired serology or raised IgM against rubella.

Special points

Incubation period is 2–3 weeks. Congenital rubella produces multisystem abnormalities.

ERYTHEMA INFECTIOSUM (FIFTH DISEASE OR 'SLAPPED CHEEK' DISEASE)

Definition and clinical features

Parvovirus infection causing rash and sometimes arthralgia. The first sign of infection is a rash on the cheeks. Initially there are red papules that later coalesce to give a raised, red slapped cheeks appearance. Reticulate rash may also affect the buttocks and upper arms, and spread proximally and distally (**167**). The palms and soles may be involved with the rash lasting 7 days. Mucous membranes may show red spots. Low-grade fever is common. Older children and adults may develop arthralgia, often with minimal or absent rash. Sickle cell crisis may occur in susceptible children.

Epidemiology

Epidemics occur, usually in the spring. Infectivity is low. Females are more commonly affected.

Differential diagnosis

Other exanthems. Rash may suggest Kawasaki disease but systemic upset is less marked.

Investigations

IgM to parvovirus B19.

Special points

Incubation period is 1–2 weeks.

HAND, FOOT AND MOUTH DISEASE

Definition and clinical features

A viral infection with Coxsackie A strains giving rise to stomatitis and blisters on the

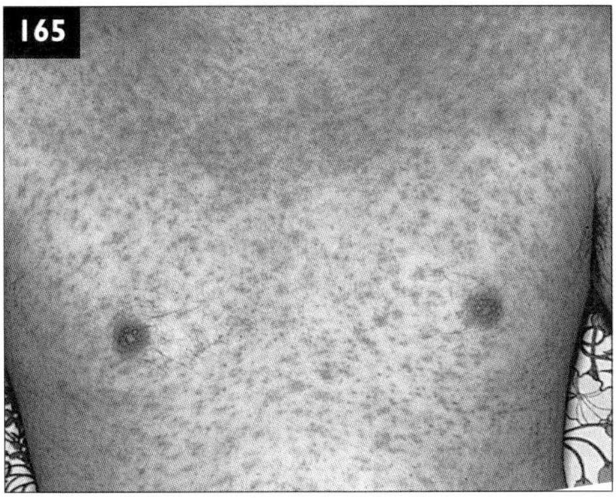

165 Generalised maculopapular measles rash.

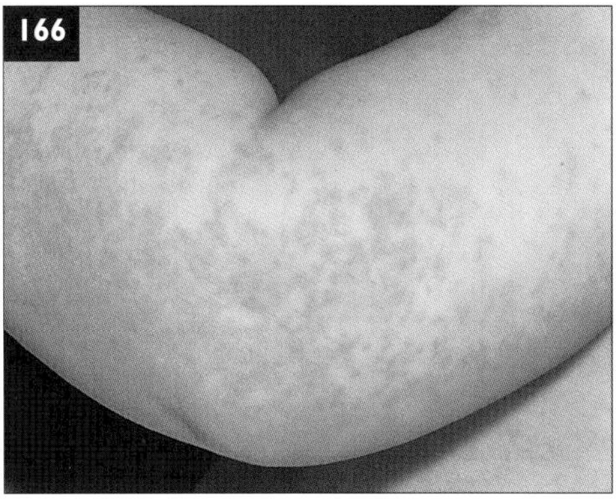

166 Rubella.

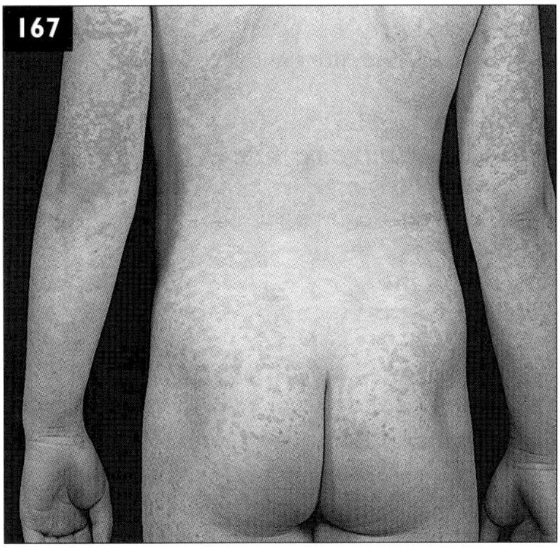

167 Erythema infectiosum (fifth disease or 'slapped cheek' disease).

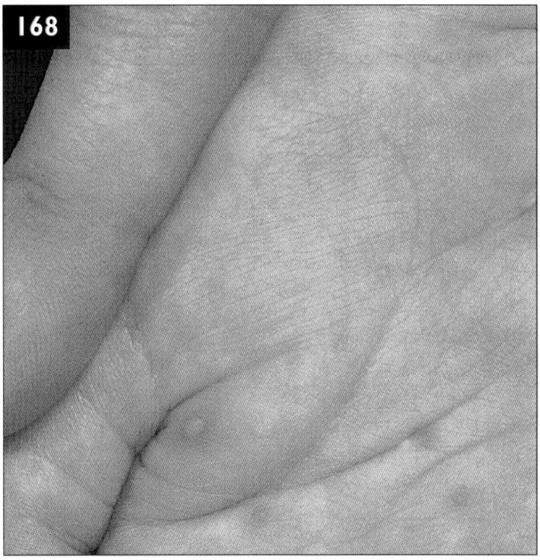

168 Hand, foot and mouth disease.

hands and feet. Mouth lesions are rapidly ulcerating vesicles which break to form painful ulcers. The hands and feet show oval grey blisters with surrounding erythema (**168**). The sides and backs of the digits, and the palms and soles can be affected. Fever is mild. The condition lasts up to a week. Oral lesions are most marked in adults.

Epidemiology
Occurs in epidemics, usually affecting children.

Differential diagnosis
The fully developed condition is characteristic.

Special points
The incubation period is 1 week.

GLANDULAR FEVER, INFECTIOUS MONONUCLEOSIS

Definition and clinical features
This is an infection with the Epstein–Barr virus causing fever, sore throat and lymphadenopathy.

Viral Infections

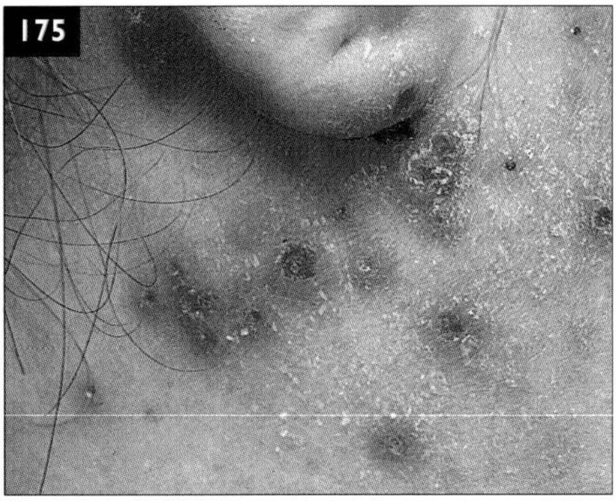

175 Eczema herpeticum.

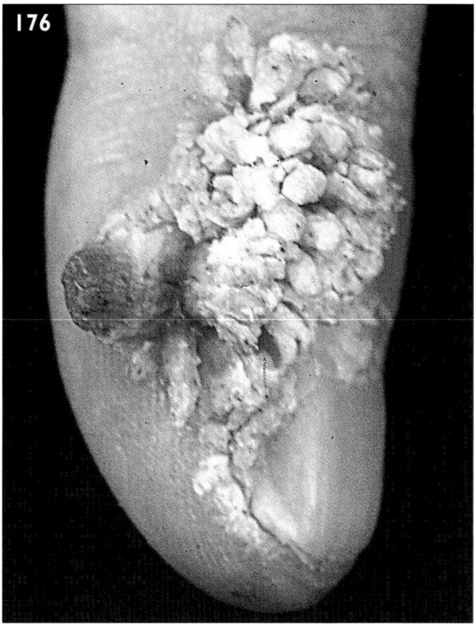

176 Common warts.

heralded by a tingling of the affected skin. The vesicles crust over and, in the absence of any secondary infection, clear in a week. When the skin is damaged, as in eczema and some other skin conditions, the herpes can spread widely and become life threatening (eczema herpeticum (**175**), Kaposi's varicelliform eruption). Immunosuppression can result in atypical widespread lesions with the risk of systemic spread. Chronic ulcerative lesions are sometimes seen in AIDS patients.

Genital herpes is usually caused by the Type 2 virus (see pp. 209–210).

Epidemiology
Primary infection with herpes Type 1 occurs in about 50% of individuals by the time they reach adult life. Incidence increases with overcrowded conditions.

Differential diagnosis
Severe aphthous ulcers and some strains of Coxsackie virus can resemble primary herpes stomatitis. Herpetic whitlow must be distinguished from bacterial infection. Herpetic cold sores can resemble impetigo; severe infections should be distinguished from herpes zoster and chickenpox.

Investigations
Electron microscopy and/or culture or immunological examination of vesicle fluid.

Special points
Severe infection, particularly in the context of eczema or immunosuppression, requires treatment with systemic antiviral agents such as acyclovir. Spread of infection into the eye can result in potentially blinding keratoconjunctivitis.

VIRAL WARTS, VERRUCA
Definition and clinical features
Infection of the skin and mucous membranes with human papilloma virus, resulting in skin-coloured papules. Appearance and site is determined by the subtype of virus. The main types of wart are as follows:

- Common warts are usually found on the hands but may develop on any area. Their spread is by direct contact, especially to abraded or damaged skin. Lesions are spread from the hands to the elbows, knees and face. Lesions are hard, rough, skin-coloured lumps that range from a few millimetres to large confluent masses (**176**).
- Filiform or digitate warts are commonly found on the face and are finer and more thread-like than common warts (**177**). If they spread into the shaving area then eradication can be difficult.
- Plantar warts (i.e. verrucas) are found on the soles of the feet and sometimes cause pain (**178**).

Viral Infections

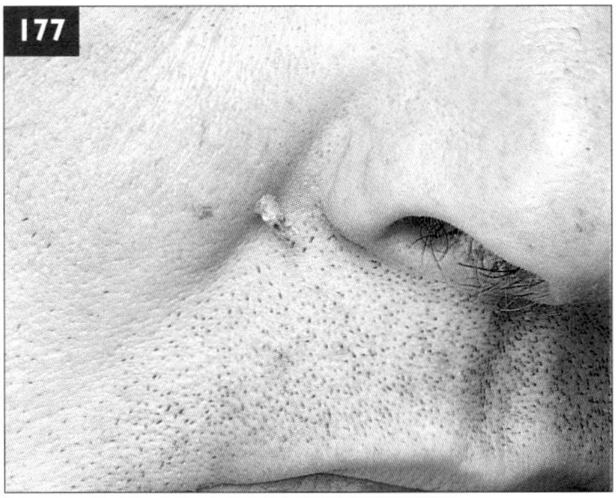
177 Filiform or digitate wart.

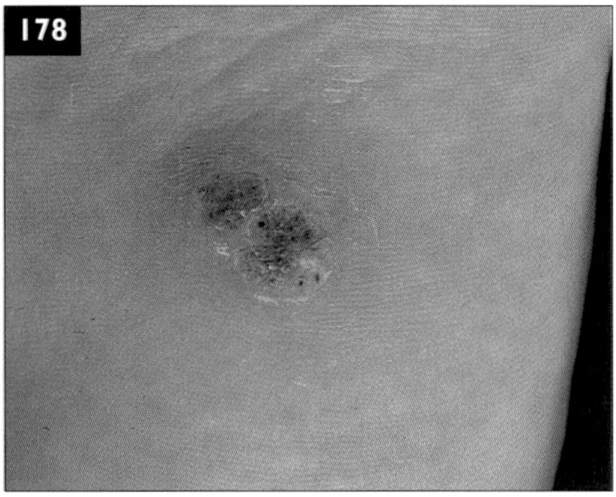
178 Plantar warts (verrucas).

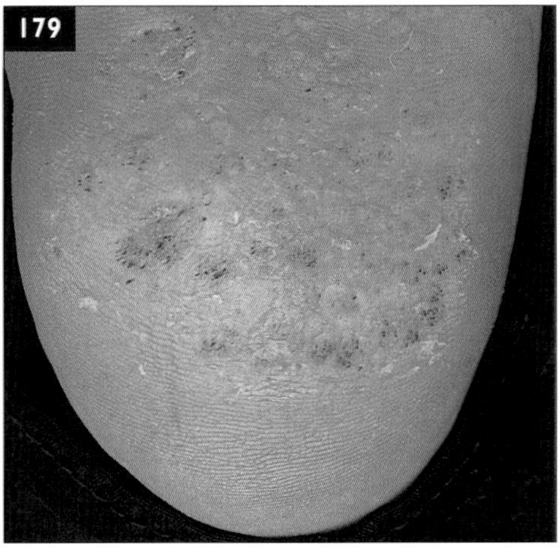
179 Mosaic warts.

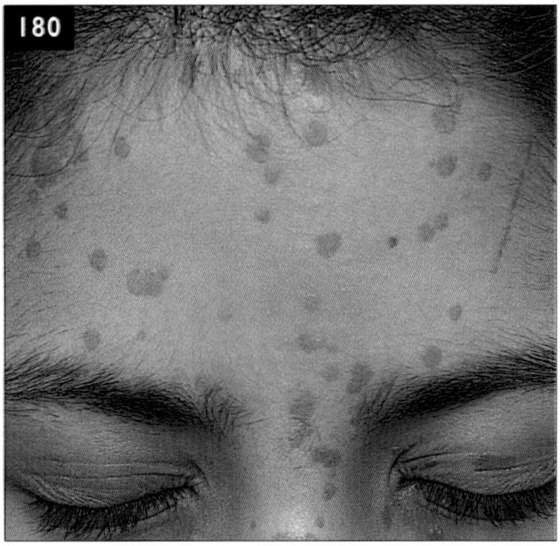
180 Plane warts.

- Mosaic warts, found on the soles of the feet, are numerous individual warts grouped together to form a plaque (**179**).
- Plane warts are smaller and flatter than the other types and may spread widely, usually on the face and dorsal surfaces of the hands (**180**).
- Genital warts.

Epidemiology
Viral warts are extremely common, most often in children but no age group is exempt. Immunosuppression results in more widespread and numerous lesions. Hand warts are more common on the hands of raw meat and fish handlers.

Differential diagnosis
Non-viral papilloma, solar and seborrhoeic keratoses can resemble warts.

Special points
Most warts, particularly in children, clear spontaneously in 2–3 years. Treatment for recalcitrant lesions includes keratolytic paints and destructive measures such as cryotherapy.

MOLLUSCUM CONTAGIOSUM
Definition and clinical features
Benign papules caused by a poxvirus that present as shiny, umbilicated, slightly translucent, pink or skin-coloured papules. They grow slowly, usually

Viral Infections

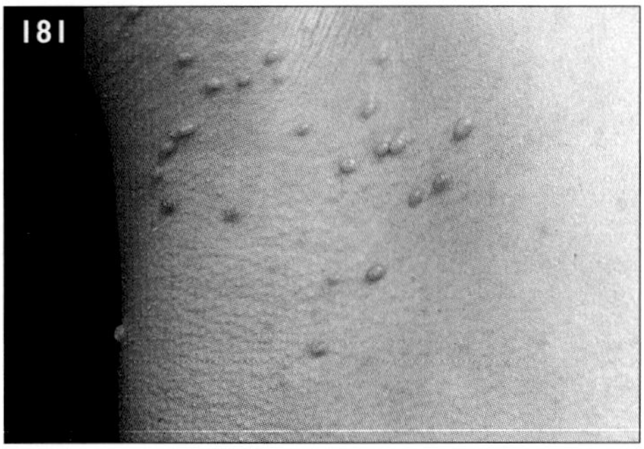

181 Molluscum contagiosum.

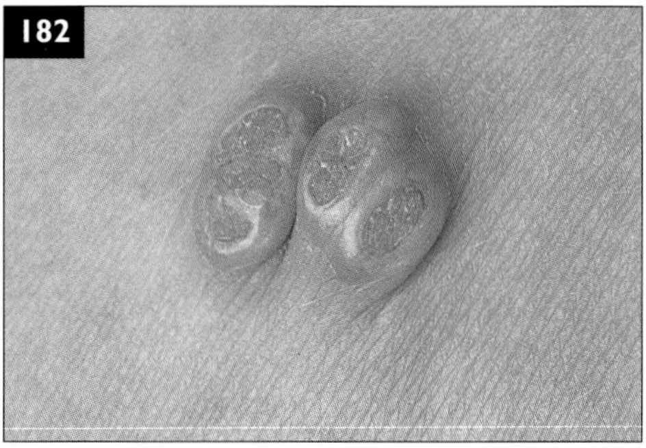

182 Molluscum contagiosum.

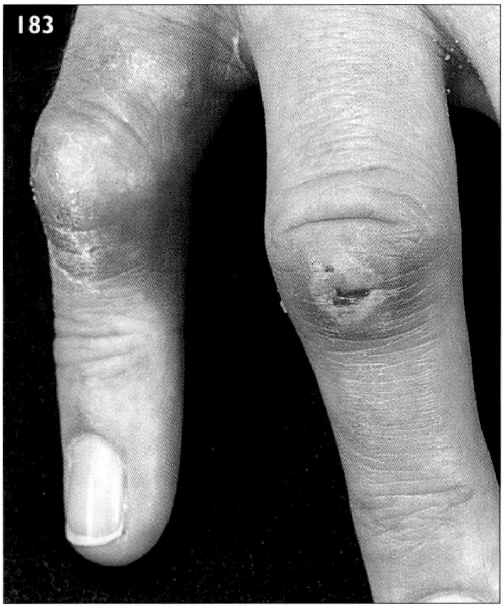

183 Orf.

being less than 1 cm in diameter (**181**, **182**). Lesions can occur at any site, usually on the head, neck and flexures; they are more widespread and larger in immunosuppressed patients. Rarely, grouped lesions can form large plaques.

Epidemiology
Mainly occur in childhood. May be sexually transmitted in adults.

Differential diagnosis
Solitary giant lesions can be confused with a wide variety of lesions including keratoacanthoma, basal cell carcinoma and viral warts.

Special points
Treatment is usually not necessary. Troublesome lesions can be treated by curettage, cryotherapy or by gently expressing or disrupting the contents. The incubation period is several months.

ORF
Definition and clinical features
A poxvirus infection of lambs that may infect humans by direct contact causing vesicopustular nodules. Early lesions are purplish papules. Over a few days these become umbilicated, haemorrhagic vesicopustules with central crusting, surrounded by a grey halo on an erythematous base (**183**). The lesions are usually solitary, on the hands and may reach 2–3 cm in diameter. They heal spontaneously in 3–5 weeks.

Epidemiology
Orf is common in sheep, goats and deer. Infection is typically acquired following contact with lambs.

Differential diagnosis
Herpetic whitlow, bacterial infection.

Investigations
Not usually necessary. Electron microscopy of vesicle fluid.

Special points
Treatment of secondary infection is all that is required.

Infestations

INSECT AND MITE BITES (PAPULAR URTICARIA)

Fleas, gnats and mosquitoes are the most common biting insects, with geographical and seasonal variation. Reaction depends on individual response, from none, through innocuous itchy papules, to blisters. Season and circumstance are usually sufficient to identify bites from gnats and mosquitoes. Flea and mite bites, when numerous and recurrent, can cause diagnostic difficulty and the term papular urticaria is used.

Definition and clinical features

Multiple weals, papules, excoriations and sometimes bullae as a reaction to insect or mite bites.

Lesions are most numerous on the legs and lower trunk (**184**) but any area can be affected. Pruritic papules and weals may be grouped, sometimes linearly. A punctum may be seen at the centre of a lesion but this is usually obliterated by scratching. Bullae may occur, particularly on the legs (**185**).

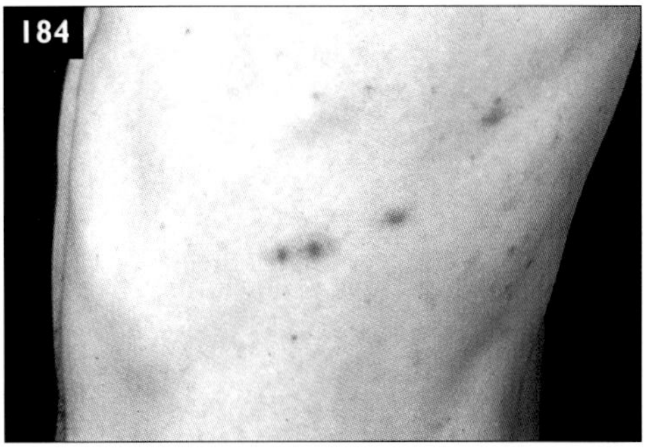

184 Papular urticaria.

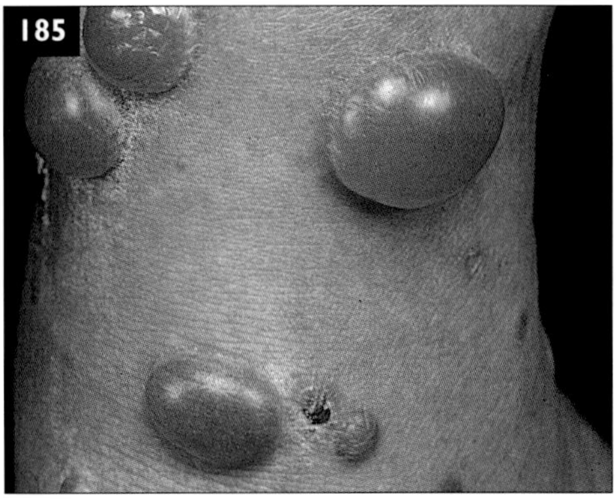

185 Bullous papular urticaria.

Epidemiology

The condition is more common in children, though adults may also be affected. Continued exposure may lead to hyposensitisation. Cat and dog fleas are the most common pests. Bird fleas and mites can also cause problems.

Differential diagnosis

Follicular eczema, dermatitis herpetiformis.

Investigations

Inspection of brushings from the cat or dog, and its bedding. Examination of the animal itself rarely shows infestation.

Special points

Tracking down the causative agent is often difficult.

INSECT STINGS

Definition and clinical features

A local and sometimes systemic reaction to stings from insects, including wasps, bees and ants. The injection of venom causes immediate pain, with gradually increasing swelling and erythema. Systemic reactions, such as wheeze, hypotension and anaphylaxis, as well as florid local reactions (**186**) are usually caused by hypersensitivity to insect antigens.

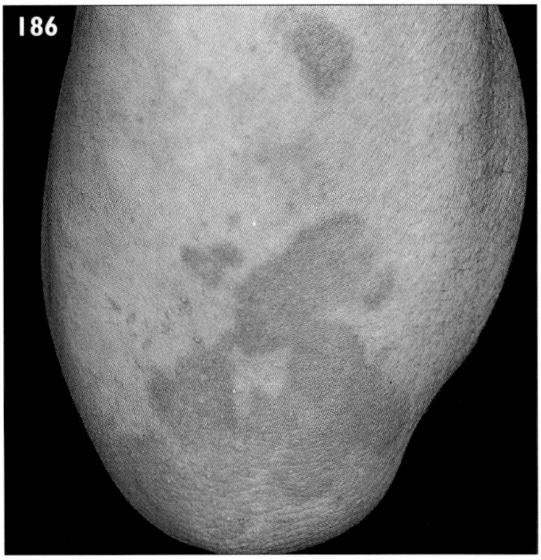

186 Insect sting reaction.

Infestations

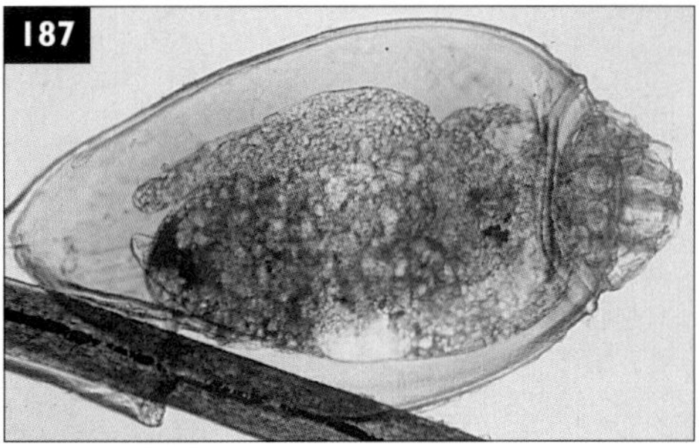

187 Head lice nit (egg).

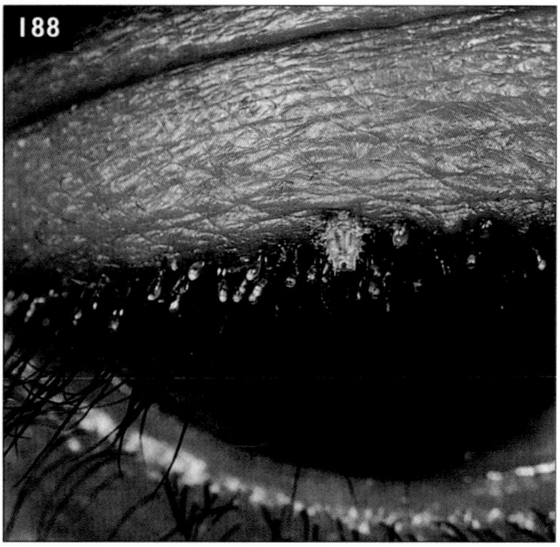

188 Crab louse in the eyelashes.

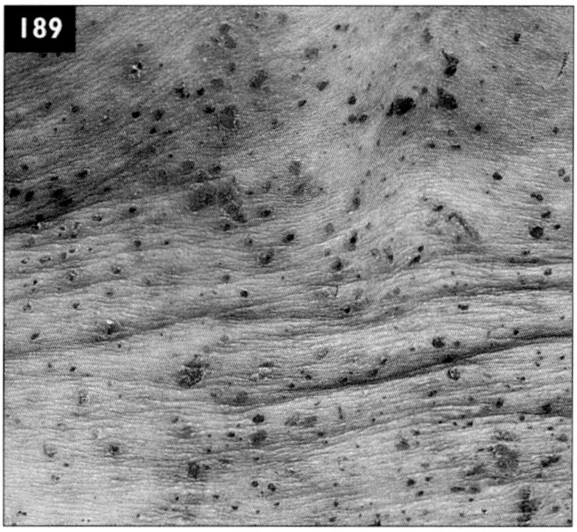

189 Body lice lesions.

Investigations
Radioallergosorbent tests (RASTs) can identify raised IgE levels to wasp or bee venom.

Special points
Systemic hypersensitivity reactions need rapid treatment with adrenaline and supportive care; systemic antihistamines are sufficient for local reactions. Hyposensitisation may be undertaken in those with a history of life-threatening reactions but only if resuscitation equipment is available.

HEAD LICE (PEDICULOSIS CAPITIS)
Definition and clinical features
This is an infestation of the scalp with the head louse *Phthirus humanus capitis*. Pruritus may lead to excoriations and secondary infection. The lice themselves are usually scanty but their nits (the white oval eggs) can be found adhering to hair shafts (**187**).

Epidemiology
Endemic in school children.

Special points
To avoid lice becoming resistant to insecticides most regions have a recommended treatment that is changed periodically.

PUBIC LICE (PEDICULOSIS PUBIS)
Definition and clinical features
An infestation of the pubic area by *Phthirus pubis*, the crab louse, which presents with an itching in the pubic area. Lice and nits can be seen.

Epidemiology
Crab lice are transferred during sexual contact.

Special points
Crab lice can also affect the eyelashes (**188**).

BODY LICE (PEDICULOSIS CORPORIS)
Definition and clinical features
Infestation of the body and clothing by *Phthirus hominis*. Itching, usually of the trunk, can result in excoriations, lichenification, secondary infection and pigmentation (**189**). Red macules and papules can sometimes be seen. Inspection of clothing reveals lice, often in small numbers, in the seams (**190**).

Infestations

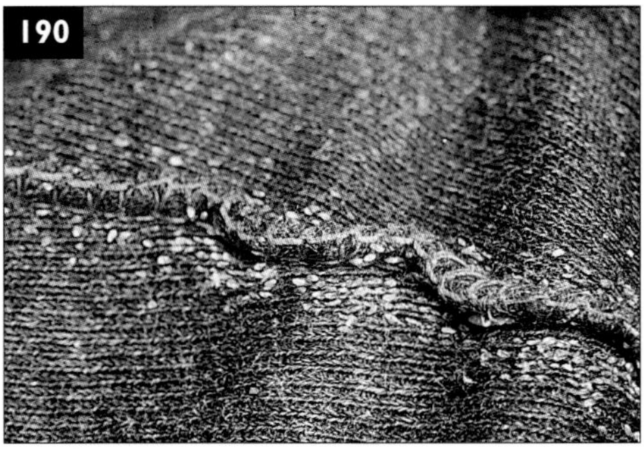

190 Body lice in a seam.

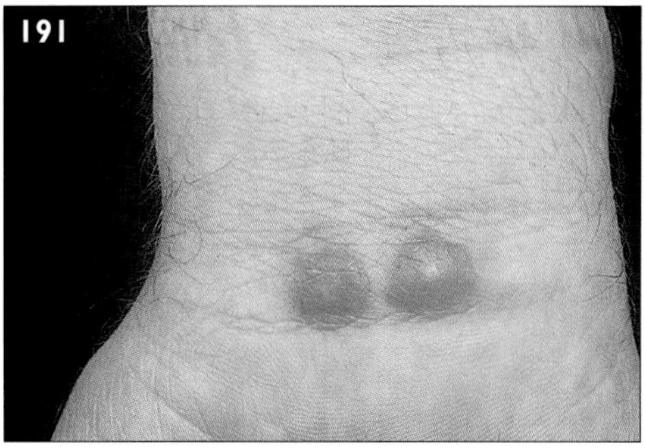

191 Bed bug bites.

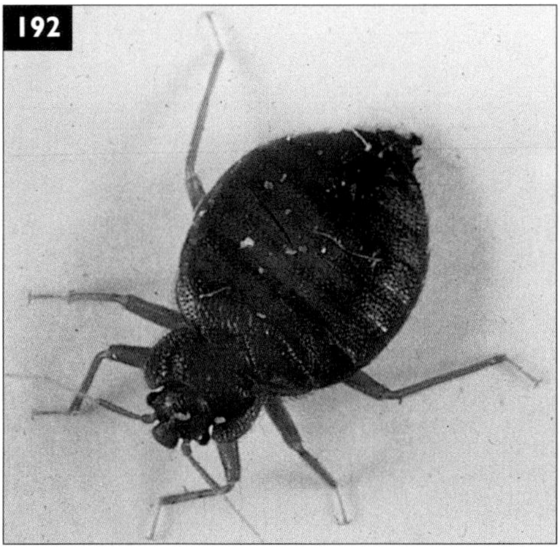

192 Bed bug.

Epidemiology
Body lice is a condition of homelessness and poverty as the lice only survive if clothing is left unchanged for weeks at a time.

Differential diagnosis
Pruritus of systemic disease may be confused, particularly in a hospitalised patient in clean pyjamas.

Special points
Topical insecticides will only be effective if the clothes are destroyed completely or thoroughly treated.

BED BUGS
Definition and clinical features
Bites from blood sucking insect *Cimex lectularius*. Bed bugs feed at night, the bites normally occurring on the face and hands. Itchy papules, with a central punctum, are often grouped or linear (**191**).

Epidemiology
Bed bugs live in cracks in walls and furnishings and under loose wallpaper. They can travel from house to house in search of food.

Differential diagnosis
Bites from flying insects.

Investigations
Bed bugs are visible to the naked eye – they are brown, oval, wingless bugs with flattened bodies (**192**). Similar bugs, normally affecting birds, can bite humans.

SCABIES
Definition and clinical features
Infestation with *Sarcoptes scabiei*, a mite that burrows within the skin, giving rise to an intensely pruritic eruption.

Infestations

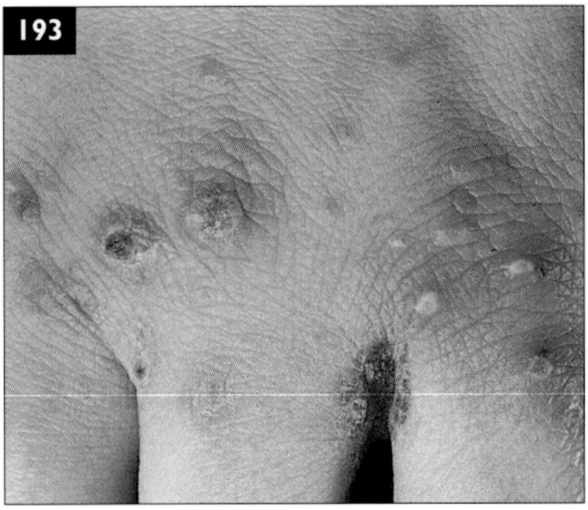

193 Scabies.

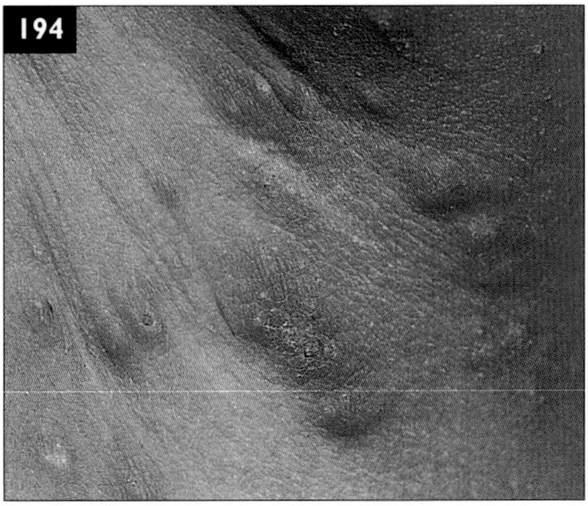

194 Scabietic nodules.

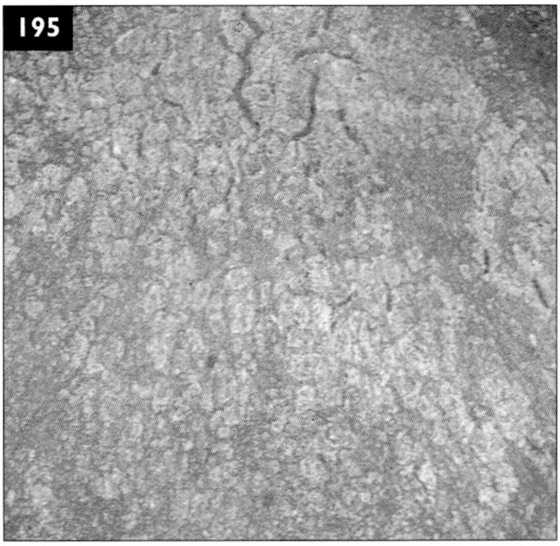

195 Crusted scabies.

The itching is so severe that sleep may be disturbed. Burrows containing the mite can often be found on the hands or genitals but are often sparse. The pruritus, urticated papules and occasional vesicles are thought to be a hypersensitivity reaction (**193**). Red pruritic nodules are sometimes found, often on the genitals. Scabietic nodules do not usually contain mites (**194**).

Norwegian or crusted scabies is an uncommon subtype in which a deficient immune response allows huge numbers of scabies to multiply. The crusts and psoriasiform scale, loaded with scabies mites, affect the hands, scalp, face and trunk (**195**). Itching may be minimal. Susceptible individuals are often only marginally immunosuppressed and may simply be elderly, pregnant or have learning difficulties. It is not uncommon in patients with AIDS.

Epidemiology

The incidence of scabies has been rising and it is now very common as it passes from person to person by direct contact. Its spread is facilitated by the latent period during which the scabies mite is carried asymptomatically.

Cases of Norwegian scabies are highly contagious and may give rise to outbreaks within hospitals and institutions.

Differential diagnosis

Diagnosis is not difficult in the presence of typical burrows. Papular urticaria, eczema, pemphigoid and many other itchy dermatoses have all been misdiagnosed. Animal scabies and mites can cause similar urticated erythematous papules without burrows.

Investigations

Microscopy of a mite or scrapings from a burrow confirms the diagnosis.

Special points

A range of topical scabicides are available. Recurrence is inevitable unless all contacts are treated simultaneously.

In cases of Norwegian scabies, the mites are shed onto clothing, bedding and furnishings, so these must be de-infested.

Acne Vulgaris

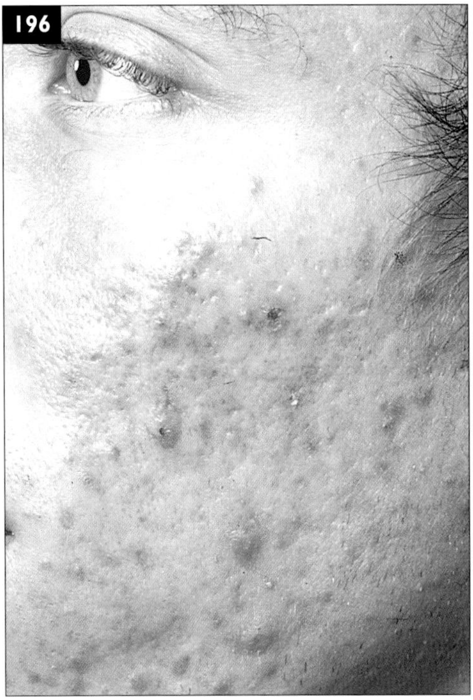

196 Acne vulgaris.

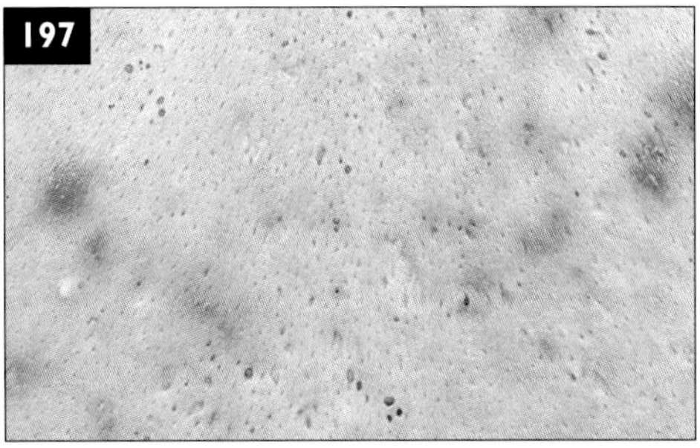

197 Comedones (blackheads) in acne vulgaris.

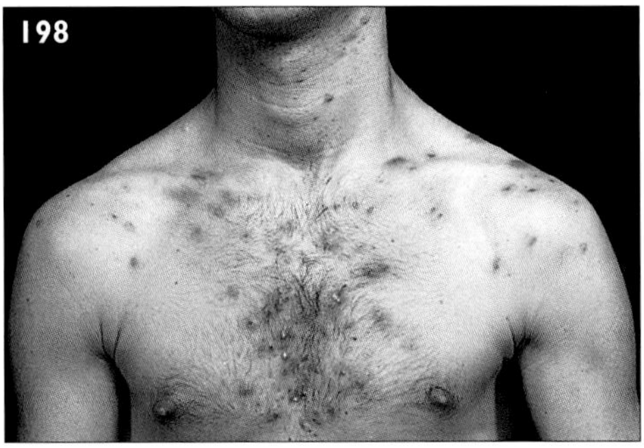

198 Scarring in acne vulgaris.

Definition and clinical features

A chronic inflammatory condition of pilosebaceous units characterised by excessive production of sebum and the presence of comedones, papules, pustules and scarring. Lesions almost always occur on the face though the upper back and chest are involved in around 70% of cases. A shiny appearance due to excessive grease production (seborrhoea) is practically universal (**196**). Young people show a predominance of non-inflammatory lesions such as comedones (blackheads) (**197**). Inflammatory superficial papules and pustules are common but deeper nodules and cysts may also occur and these may give rise to considerable scarring (**198**).

Epidemiology

Acne vulgaris is a common disease affecting around 40% of people aged 16–18 years, although minor degrees are an almost universal finding throughout puberty. All races may be affected and onset is usually earlier in females. Most cases clear by the early twenties but around 5% of cases (especially females) may persist into the third decade. Acne accounts for a considerable burden of psychological disability in an otherwise healthy but vulnerable population. Increased production of thickened sebum, hypercornification of the pilosebaceous ducts and colonisation with *Propionibacterium acnes* are all important aetiological factors.

Differential diagnosis

Rosacea occurs in older patients and comedones, nodules and scarring are absent. Perioral dermatitis is usually itchy and comedones are not present.

Investigations

None are usually required.

Special points

The psychological impact of acne on a young person's life should not be underestimated. Acne is a treatable disease.

Other Forms of Acne

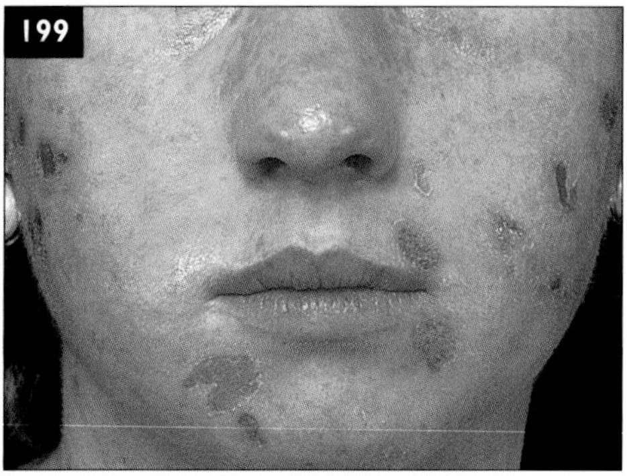

199 Acne excoriée.

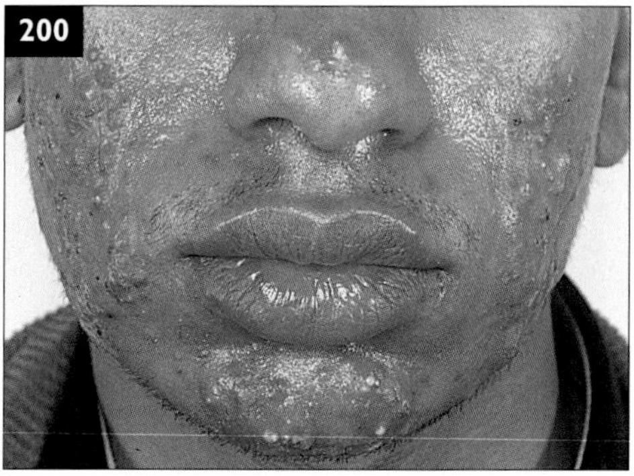

200 Nodulocystic acne.

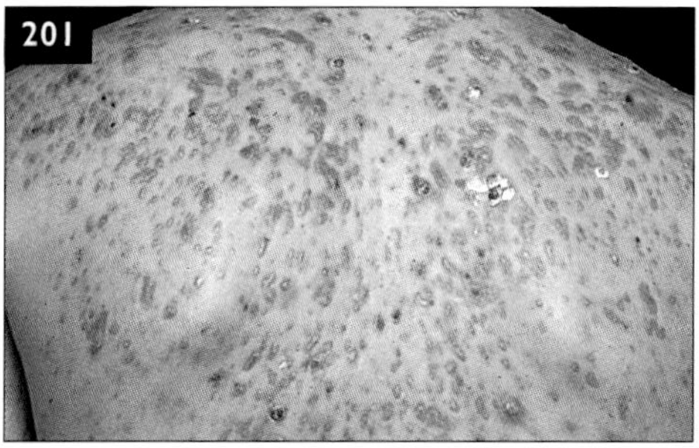

201 Nodulocystic acne.

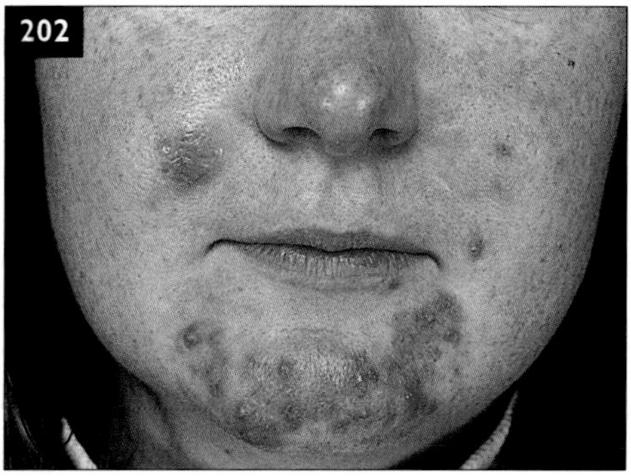

202 Endocrine acne.

ACNE EXCORIÉE

Some patients react to minor degrees of acne by constantly picking at the lesions giving rise to delayed healing and small linear scars. Lesions are usually present on the chin and cheeks, and the condition occurs predominantly in females (**199**).

NODULOCYSTIC ACNE

This variant of acne consists of large, tender nodules and cysts which eventually form deep scars (**200**). Extensive truncal involvement may occur and the condition rarely resolves (**201**). It is important to recognise this devastating form of acne early in life before extensive scarring has set in because treatment with oral isotretinoin produces excellent results.

POMADE ACNE

Various oils and cosmetics applied to the face and hair can exacerbate acne.

ENDOCRINE ACNE

Occasionally, acne is present as part of an endocrine disorder such as polycystic disease of the ovaries (**202**), Cushing's disease or adrenogenital syndrome.

DRUG-INDUCED ACNE

A number of drugs including isoniazid, oral steroids and gonadotrophins, lithium, phenytoin and iodides may give rise to a monomorphic acne which responds poorly to conventional treatment. Acne in body builders may occasionally indicate testosterone administration.

OCCUPATIONAL ACNE

This is illustrated on pp. 26–27.

Rosacea

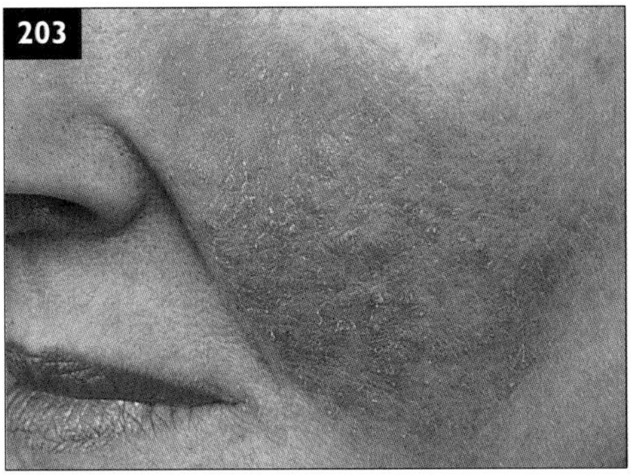

203 Rosacea.

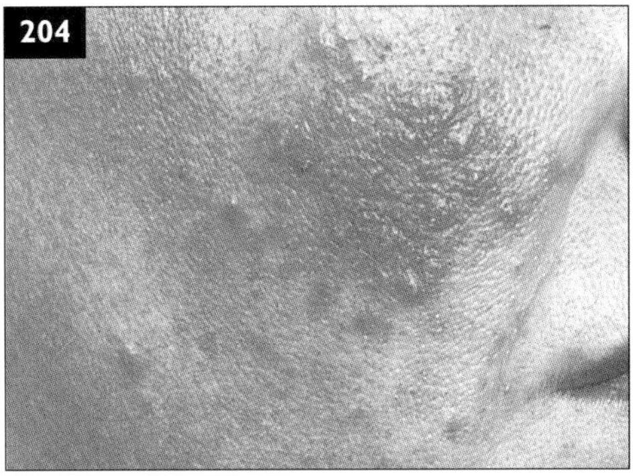

204 Papules and pustules of rosacea.

Definition and clinical features

This is a chronic inflammatory skin disorder, characterised by crops of papules and pustules on a background of erythema and fine telangiectasia, in which the convexities of the face are chiefly involved (**203**). During inflammatory episodes, papules and pustules are evident (**204**), and facial swelling may occur (**205**). Minor degrees of ocular involvement occur in around 50% of rosacea sufferers.

Conjunctivitis and blepharitis are the most frequent ocular complaints, and rosaceal keratitis can lead to corneal scarring.

Epidemiology

Acne rosacea typically begins in the third or fourth decade and may be commoner in females. It is seen less frequently in those with pigmented skins, and a fair skin complexion combined with chronic sun exposure may be important in the aetiology.

Rosacea is a persistent disease with episodic inflammatory flares.

Differential diagnosis.

Acne occurs in younger individuals and is distinguished by the presence of comedones and seborrhoea. Pustules and papules are not seen in facial seborrhoeic dermatitis.

Investigations

None are usually indicated.

Special points

Papules and pustules respond well to oral tetracyclines but the redness and telangiectasia may not improve. Occasionally, gross sebaceous gland hyperplasia develops and gives a bulbous craggy appearance to the nose (rhinophyma) (**206**). This can be treated surgically.

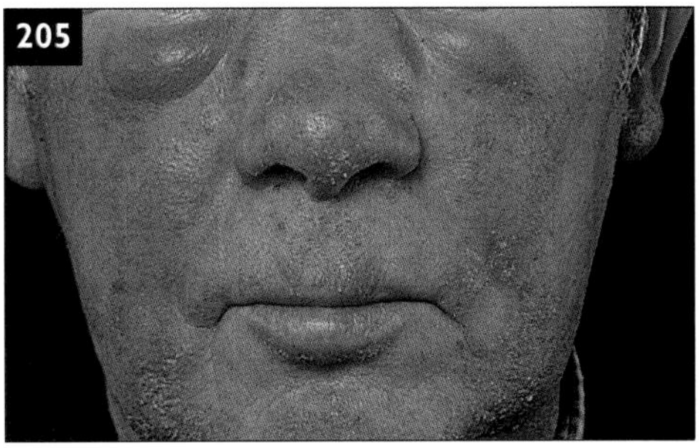

205 Facial swelling in rosacea.

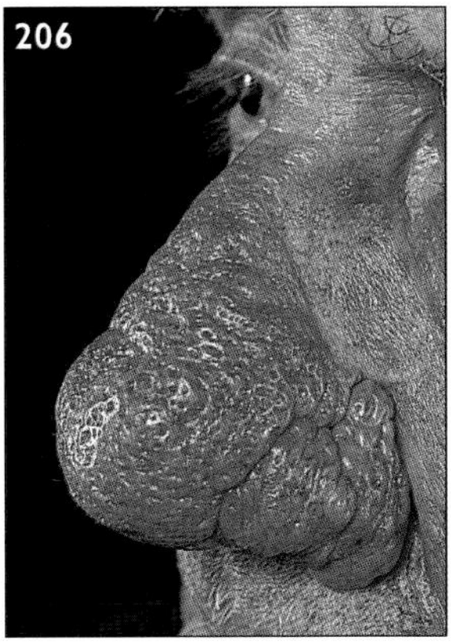

206 Rhinophyma.

Perioral Dermatitis

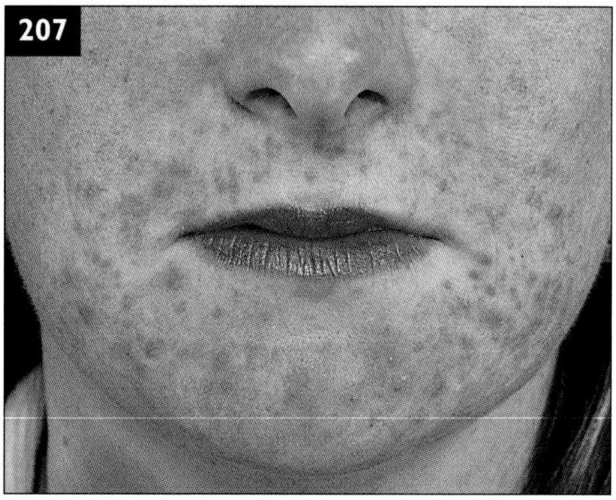

207 Perioral dermatitis.

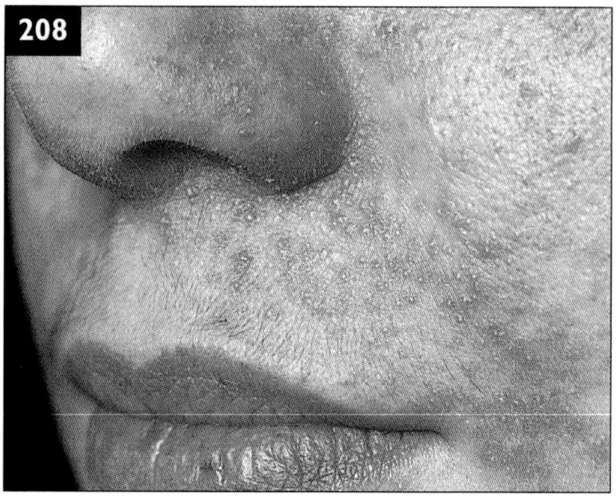

208 Perioral dermatitis showing sparing around the lips.

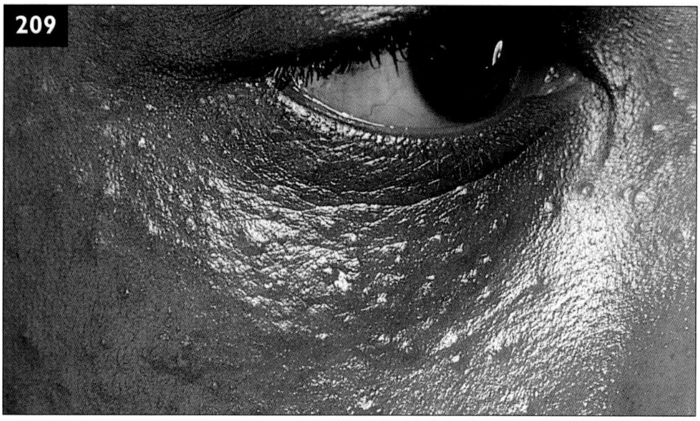

209 Periocular dermatitis.

Definition and clinical features

An eruption of multiple tiny papulovesicles around the mouth. The perioral distribution of this eruption is characteristic (**207**), and sparing of a small area around the vermilion of the lip is seen (**208**).

Epidemiology

This condition typically occurs in younger women where the previous use of topical steroids has been implicated as a causative factor in many cases.

Differential diagnosis

Rosacea tends to affect the upper face; the background erythema is striking. Contact dermatitis from lipstick or toothpaste is more localised and involves the lip vermilion. Irritant contact dermatitis secondary to lip licking is eczematous and not papular.

Investigations

None.

Treatment

Discontinuation of topical corticosteroids and a 6-week course of oral tetracyclines.

Special points

The condition responds rapidly to discontinuation of topical corticosteroids and oral tetracyclines. Periocular involvement may occasionally be seen (**209**).

Keratosis Pilaris

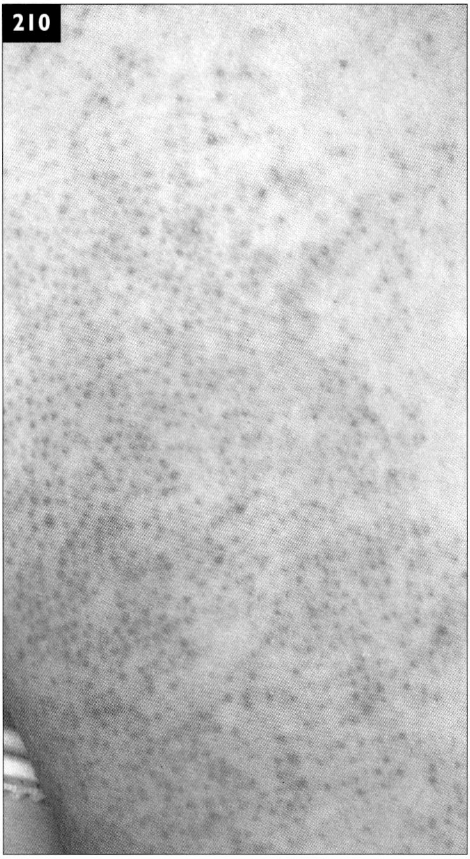

210 Keratosis pilaris.

Definition and clinical features

Keratosis pilaris is a common dry skin disorder due to abnormal keratinisation of hair follicle epithelium. Its features are prominent follicular hyperkeratosis with plugging that starts in early childhood and predominantly affects the extensor aspects of the upper arms (**210**) and legs, and the buttocks. Perifollicular erythema (keratosis pilaris rubra) may occur. Involvement of the eyebrows (ulerythema ophryogenes), cheeks (atrophoderma vermiculata) and even scalp can rarely lead to hair loss and pitted scars (keratosis pilaris decalvans or atrophicans).

Epidemiology

It is an autosomal dominant condition which may be associated with atopic eczema or ichthyosis vulgaris. It is common in patients with Down's syndrome. It improves in the summer months and lessens with age.

Differential diagnosis

A rough skin resembling mild keratosis pilaris frequently occurs in people with a tendency to dry skin. Phrynoderma is a more extreme form of follicular keratosis which affects bony prominences and results from nutritional deficiency. Pityriasis rubra pilaris and the various forms of minute or digitate keratoses are easily distinguished.

Investigations

Histology of a lesion shows follicular hyperkeratosis and plugging.

Darier's Disease

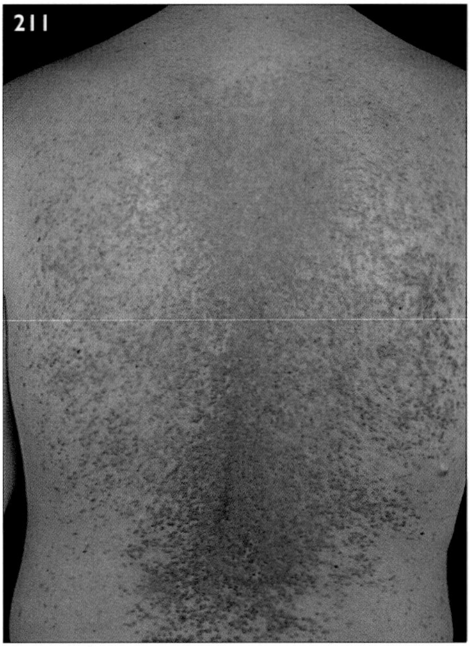

211 Darier's disease.

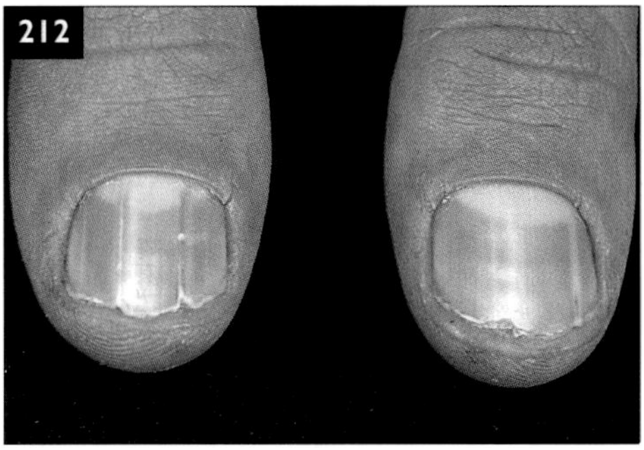

212 Nails in Darier's disease.

Definition and clinical features

First described in 1889, Darier's disease is a rare autosomal dominant disorder of keratinisation. It produces characteristic greasy papules and a variety of associated features in some patients. Although the precise molecular defect is unknown, studies to date suggest it is due to a mutation of an epidermal cellular protein responsible for desmosome–keratin adhesion.

Lesions generally develop in the seborrhoeic areas in childhood or early adult life but may not become apparent until later life. Brown, warty, greasy papules arise on the upper chest and back, lower neck, scalp and forehead and may coalesce into plaques (**211**). Occasionally hypertrophic plaques evolve in the major flexures and natal cleft and, rarely, bullous lesions can occur. Pruritus and body odour are common complaints and considerable cosmetic and social disability result.

The hands are involved with discrete skin-coloured papules similar to acrokeratosis verruciformis; palmoplantar pits are very common. The nails are longitudinally ridged with notching at the free edges (**212**). Many patients have white patches on the oral mucosa. Bacterial and viral infections especially with staphylococcus and herpes simplex are not uncommon. The condition is also aggravated by warmth and sunlight.

An increased incidence of depression, epilepsy and mild mental retardation have been noted in families with Darier's disease.

Epidemiology

Its incidence in the UK is estimated to be approximately 1 in 50 000. Males and females are equally affected.

Differential diagnosis

Clinically, early lesions may resemble acne vulgaris, seborrhoeic dermatitis or epidermal naevi. Histologically, other acantholytic disorders may cause confusion, in particular Hailey–Hailey benign familial pemphigus and Grover's acantholytic dermatosis.

Investigations

Typical histologic changes include acantholysis of suprabasal keratinocytes leading to clefting in the epidermis and dyskeratotic cells showing premature keratinisation (corps ronds and grains). Ultrastructurally, desmosomes are reduced in lesional skin, and perinuclear keratin clumps are seen.

Special points

The genetic defect has been mapped to chromosome 12, but the resultant abnormality is still unknown.

Erythrokeratodermas

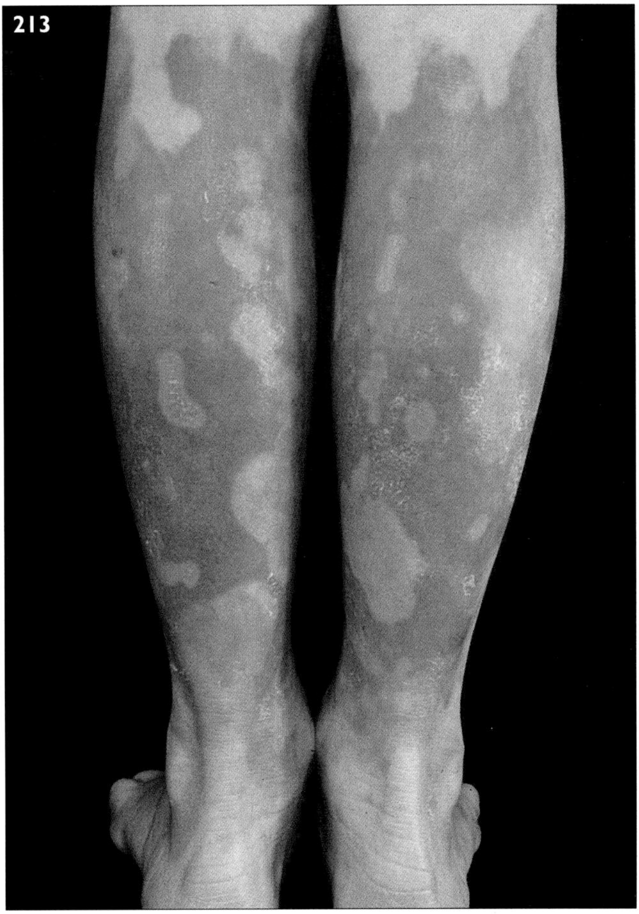

213 Erythrokeratoderma progressiva symmetrica.

Definition and clinical features

Erythrokeratodermas are a group of rare disorders whose typical lesions are persistent circumscribed, hyperkeratotic, erythematous plaques.

In erythrokeratoderma variabilis there is an association with transient and migratory patches of polycyclic erythema which fade within weeks, and with fixed scaly demarcated plaques which occur on the limbs and trunk. In erythrokeratoderma progressiva symmetrica there are symmetric orange-red plaques with fine scale (**213**) distributed on the extensor aspects of the limbs, over the trunk and buttocks and across the face. The palms may be involved and, rarely, lesions may remit spontaneously.

Epidemiology

They are either sporadic or autosomal dominant and usually start in childhood.

Differential diagnosis

Pityriasis rubra pilaris and psoriasis are the main contenders.

Investigations

The lesional skin shows acanthosis, ortho- and parakeratosis and an intact granular layer. Ultrastructurally distorted mitochondria have been observed.

Kyrle–Flegel Disease

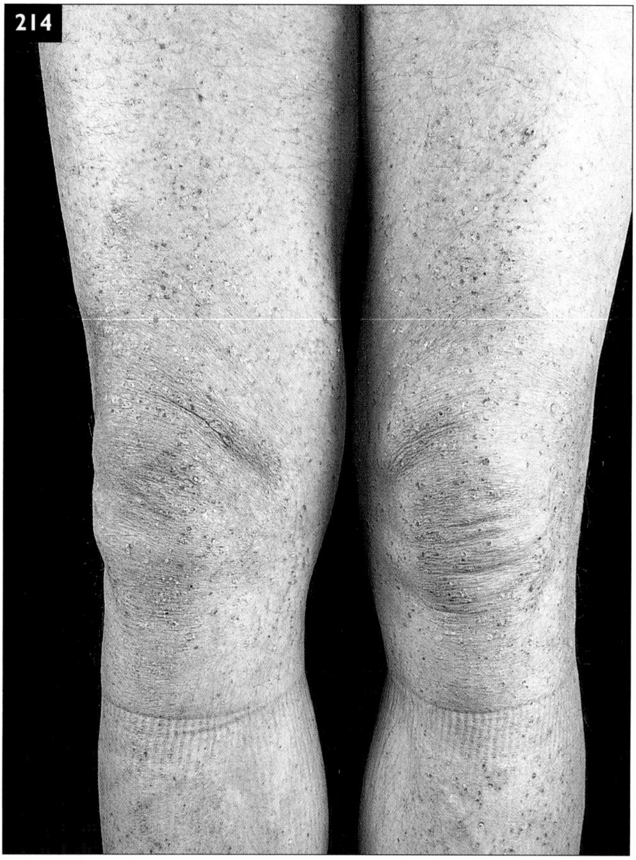

214 Kyrle–Flegel disease.

Definition and clinical features

Kyrle's disease (also known as hyperkeratosis follicularis et parafollicularis in cutem penetrans) and Flegel's disease (hyperkeratosis lenticularis perstans) are sufficiently similar to be treated as one entity, hence Kyrle–Flegel disease. It is a chronic disorder of keratinisation characterised by acral hyperkeratotic lesions.

Individual lesions begin as keratotic and scaly papules (**214**) which may enlarge to plugs greater than 1 cm across, with surrounding erythema. They occur on the lower legs, thighs and arms but may rarely involve the pinnae and trunk.

Epidemiology

Typical lesions develop late in life and it is sometimes familial. There is an occasional association with chronic renal or hepatic diseases and diabetes.

Differential diagnosis

Lesions may resemble stucco-keratoses, actinic or arsenical keratoses or disseminated actinic porokeratosis.

Investigations

Histology of a lesion may show ortho- or parakeratosis in an otherwise atrophic epidermis. There is a variable band-like lymphocytic infiltrate and disruption of some follicular walls.

Laboratory tests to exclude associated renal, liver or endocrine diseases should be carried out.

Palmoplantar Keratodermas

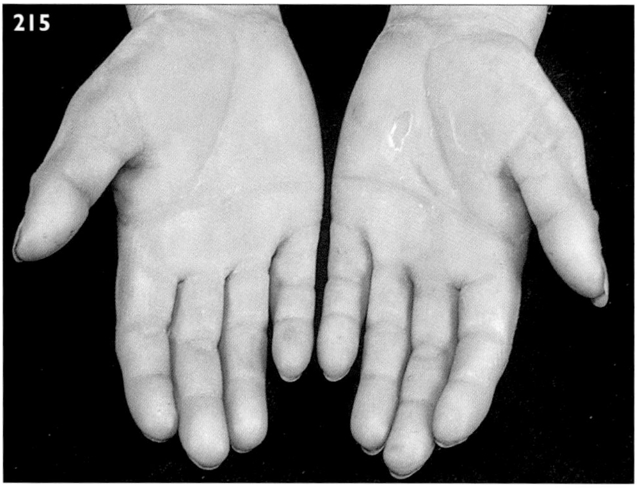

215 Thost–Unna PPK.

There are several acquired and hereditary forms of persistent diffuse or focal palmoplantar hyperkeratosis or tylosis. Most can be classified according to their specific features such as age at onset, family history, clinical pattern, presence of tissue destruction and association with other skin, ectodermal or systemic disease.

ACQUIRED PALMOPLANTAR KERATODERMA

This form commonly complicates pityriasis rubra pilaris and Reiter's disease and occurs in some patients with psoriasis, eczemas, lichen planus, porokeratosis, viral warts, tinea manuum, lupus erythematosus, iododerma, hypothyroidism, internal malignancy, treponemal and HIV disease.

A perimenopausal plantar keratoderma keratoderma climactericum may develop in overweight women in their forties.

HEREDITARY PALMOPLANTAR KERATODERMA

A palmoplantar keratoderma (PPK) is a common associated feature of genetic disorders or syndromes such as hidrotic ectodermal dysplasia, epidermolysis bullosa simplex, ichthyosiform erythrodermas, pachyonychia congenita, dyskeratosis congenita, Rothmund–Thomson syndrome and other poikilodermatous disorders.

The commonest inherited isolated PPKs are Thost–Unna and Vorner keratoderma. Papillon–Lefèvre syndrome describes PPK with periodontitis and leucocyte defects. The rarer mutilating PPKs include Vohwinkel, Mal de Meleda, Greither and Olmsted keratodermas. Tyrosinaemia Type 2 and keratoderma areata of Siemens are rare conditions which produce painful callosities.

Focal acral hyperkeratosis and punctate palmar keratoses are common autosomal dominant conditions characterised by discrete warty papules in Afro-Caribbeans. They are not regarded as palmoplantar keratodermas.

HOWEL–EVANS–CLARKE SYNDROME

The association of an autosomal dominant familial PPK and oesophageal carcinoma in early adulthood in the majority of the affected family members was reported in two English families in 1958.

THOST–UNNA PPK

An autosomal dominant disorder that develops in early childhood and produces a diffuse, yellow, waxy hyperkeratosis over the palms and soles (**215**). There is associated hyperhidrosis of the affected areas and a characteristic inflammatory line at the margins of the keratodermatous plaques. Tinea infection and pitted keratolysis may occur.

Palmopantar Keratodermas

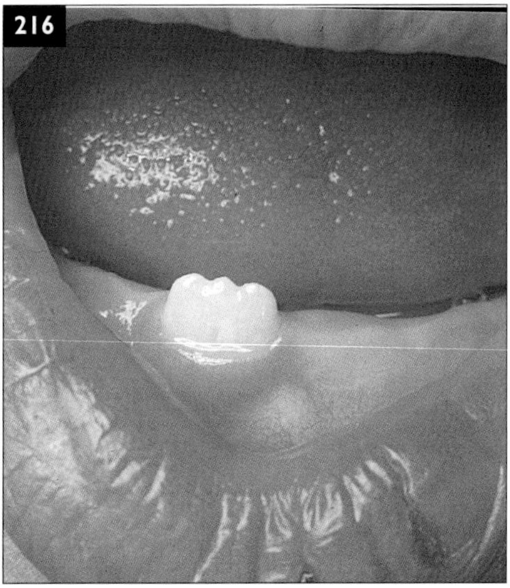

216 Papillon–Lefèvre syndrome.

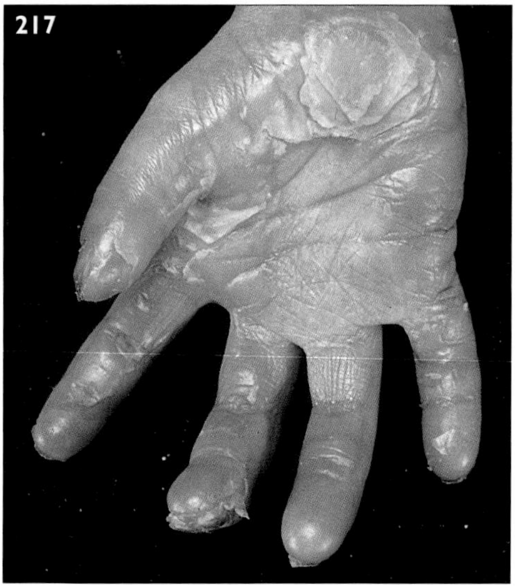

217 Vohwinkel PPK.

Histology shows orthokeratosis, acanthosis and an increased granular layer with a mild dermal lymphocytic infiltrate.

VORNER PPK

Also autosomal dominant, this condition resembles Thost–Unna PPK in onset and pattern. However, there is sometimes a history of blistering, and hyperhidrosis is absent.

Histology of the affected area shows typical epidermolytic hyperkeratosis and this can be regarded as a limited form of bullous ichthyosiform erythroderma.

PAPILLON–LEFÈVRE SYNDROME

An autosomal recessive condition that causes hyperhidrotic PPK from early childhood and is complicated by knuckle pads and skin infections. Progressive periodontal inflammation leads to early loss of teeth (**216**), possibly due to variable defects in leucocyte function.

VOHWINKEL PPK

An autosomal dominant mutilating keratoderma that starts in infancy and progresses. It produces a honeycomb-type ridging and is associated with starfish-like keratotic plaques on the digits and knees (**217**). A gradual spread onto the dorsal aspects of the hands and feet is termed transgrediens and is a feature of most mutilating keratodermas. From early adult life, fibrotic constrictions may cause digital contractures and partial loss of digits. Rarely, sensorineural deafness or alopecia are associated.

MAL DE MELEDA

An autosomal recessive syndrome of mutilating, transgredient, erythematous keratoderma sometimes associated with eczema, perioral erythema, nail dystrophy and syndactyly. It is commonest, due to inbreeding, on the island of Meleda in the Adriatic Sea.

GREITHER PPK

This autosomal dominant keratoderma is similar to Thost–Unna PPK but with mild transgrediens spread and a gradual improvement in later life.

OLMSTED'S SYNDROME

A very rare, severely mutilating congenital PPK with associated periorificial keratoderma affecting the face, groin and perianal regions. Other ectodermal defects such as alopecia occur and, in one report, a mother and son were affected.

Granuloma Annulare

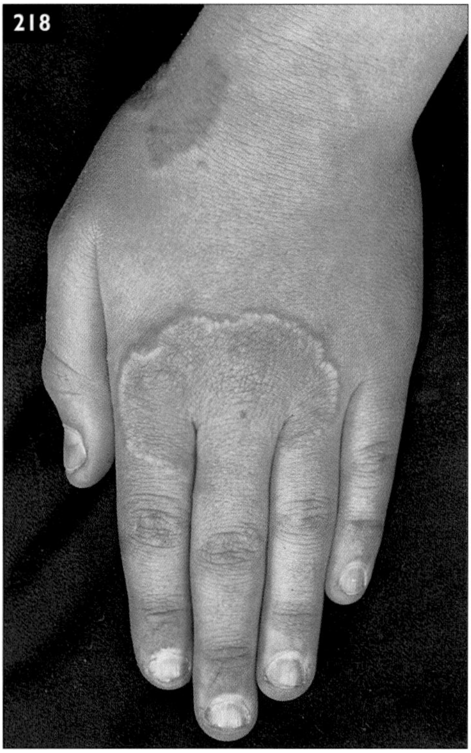

218 Granuloma annulare.

Definition and clinical features

Granuloma annulare is a disease characterised by the degeneration of dermal collagen and an associated lymphohistiocytic infiltrate.

The most frequent presentation of granuloma annulare consists of an asymmetrical annular lesion made up of individual dermal papules (**218**). These lesions are most commonly found on the dorsum of the hands and feet in children and young adults. The lesions are commonly asymptomatic apart from their appearance. They enlarge centrifugally and often persist for months or years before resolving without scarring.

Generalised or disseminated granuloma annulare consists of numerous small papules and macules which may be widespread on the trunk and limbs. They are often mildly hyperpigmented.

Epidemiology

Granuloma annulare is a relatively common idiopathic disorder. There is no association between the common form and diabetes. Diffuse granuloma annulare may have a weak association with diabetes mellitus.

Differential diagnosis

The clinical appearance is usually distinctive. On occasions other annular disorders, such as erythema annulare centrifugum, annular sarcoidosis and annular lichen planus, may be considered. The more diffuse form of granuloma annulare may be confused with sarcoidosis, mastocytosis and reticulate erythematous mucinosis. Histology should be diagnostic.

Investigations

Patients require no specific investigations when physical signs are characteristic. If the diagnosis is in doubt it can be confirmed on skin histology. Urine should be tested for glycosuria.

Rheumatoid Nodule

219

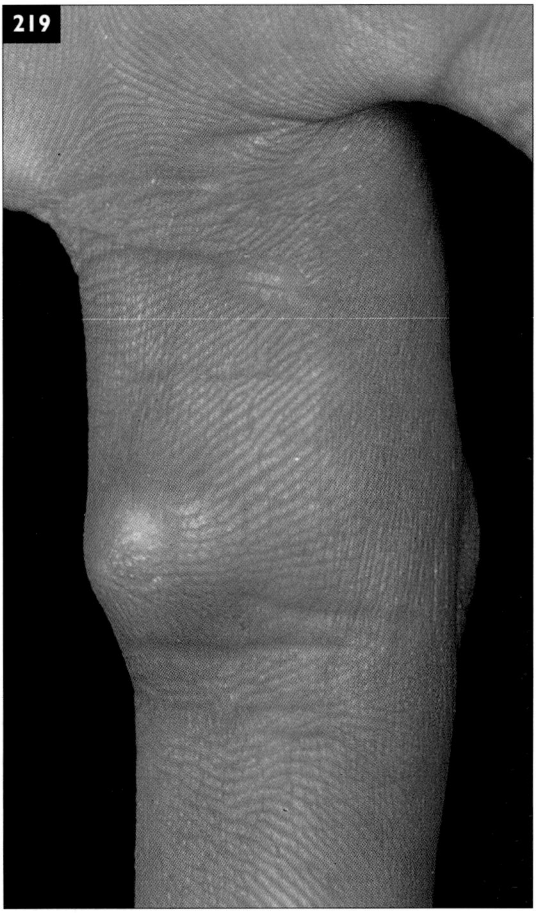

219 Rheumatoid nodule.

Definition and clinical features

Rheumatoid nodules consist of palisaded necrobiotic granulomas in the subcutis in patients with seropositive rheumatoid arthritis. They present as non-tender, subcutaneous nodules, occurring particularly over the ulnar border of the forearm, on the dorsum of the hands, the extensor aspect of the knees and elsewhere in patients with seropositive rheumatoid arthritis (**219**).

Epidemiology

Approximately 20% of patients with rheumatoid arthritis develop rheumatoid nodules at some stage during their disease.

Differential diagnosis

In the presence of established rheumatoid arthritis the diagnosis is usually easy. Subcutaneous granuloma annulare and the nodules of rheumatic fever have similar clinical and histologic appearances but are seen in a different clinical context.

Investigations

The diagnosis can be confirmed by serology for rheumatoid factor and histology.

Necrobiosis Lipoidica

220 Necrobiosis lipoidica.

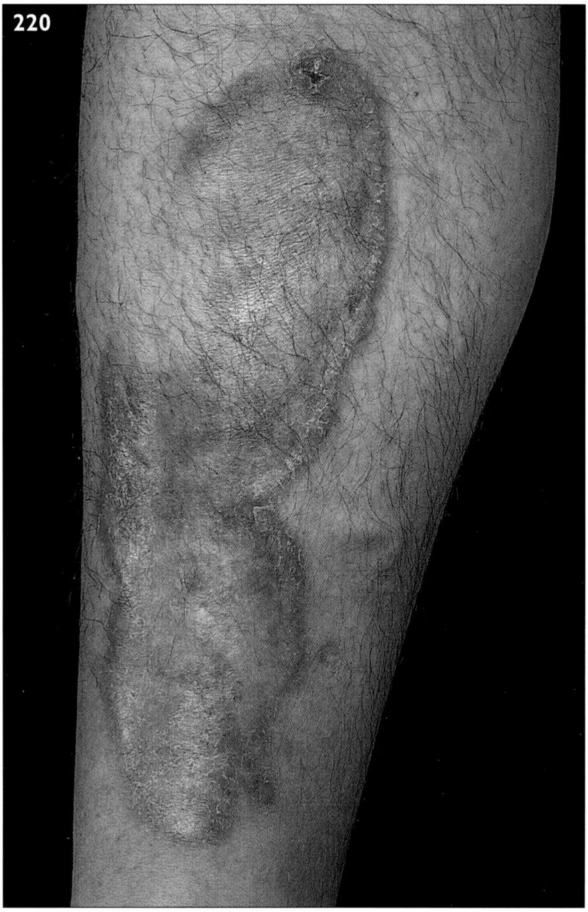

Definition and clinical features

Necrobiosis lipoidica consists of well-demarcated plaques of cutaneous atrophy with a yellowish discoloration associated with degeneration of collagen and a deep granulomatous infiltrate in the dermis and subcutis.

Necrobiosis lipoidica commonly occurs in young and middle-aged adults as atrophic plaques over the shins (**220**). The plaques enlarge by peripheral extension with central atrophy and may ulcerate. The borders of the lesions are brownish-red. The absence of cutaneous appendages within the plaques is prominent and, in some instances, sensation is reduced.

Epidemiology

Approximately two-thirds of patients with necrobiosis lipoidica have or will develop diabetes mellitus although there is no association with glycaemic control. The condition is uncommon, occurring in less than 1% of diabetics and is very uncommon in the non-diabetic population.

Differential diagnosis

Granuloma annulare, morphoea, sarcoid and planar xanthomata.

Investigations

A skin biopsy is only required in atypical cases where the signs are not characteristic. Patients should be investigated for diabetes.

Sarcoidosis

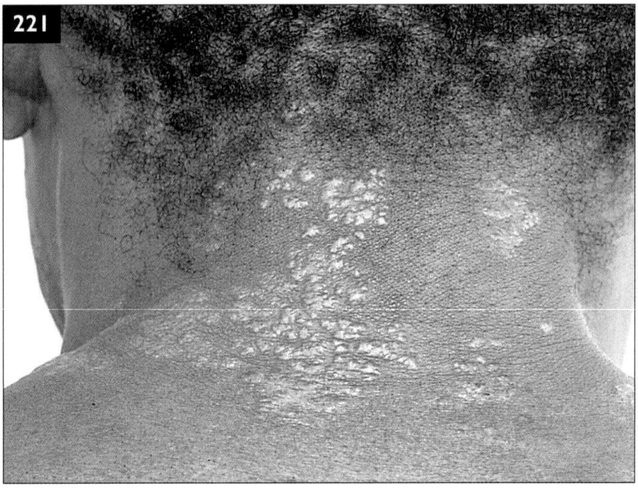

221 Sarcoidosis.

Definition and clinical features

Sarcoidosis is a disorder characterised by the development of non-caseating, lymphocyte-poor granulomatous inflammation of unknown aetiology in multiple organs. The manifestations are protean depending on the organs involved. The combination of erythema nodosum (aseptal panniculitis) and bilateral hilar lymphadenopathy in young people is a common presentation. Other patients with a more insidious onset commonly have respiratory symptoms and one or more of the following manifestations of cutaneous sarcoidosis.

Lupus pernio is the involvement of the nasal skin with an infiltrative erythema, commonly with involvement of the upper respiratory tract. Papular and nodular sarcoidosis consist of focal dermal infiltration with naked granulomas producing discrete nodules. Papular lesions are commonly symmetrical while nodular lesions are often asymmetrical; the papular lesions are commonly found around the nape of the neck (**221**) and may be symmetrically distributed on the trunk, buttocks and limbs. Nodules may be found at any site but have a particular predilection for periocular skin. Scar sarcoidosis consists of similar lesions involving old scars. Annular forms may be mistaken for granuloma annulare and plaque-like forms may be mistaken for necrobiosis lipoidica.

Epidemiology

Cutaneous involvement is found in approximately a quarter of patients with systemic sarcoidosis. Cutaneous sarcoidosis can be found in the absence of evidence of systemic disease.

Differential diagnosis

With the exception of erythema nodosum and lupus pernio, which have relatively characteristic clinical signs, sarcoidosis can be confused with granuloma annulare, necrobiosis lipoidica, infective granulomas including tuberculosis and, on occasion, lichen planus.

Investigations

Histological confirmation of the diagnosis of sarcoidosis is important and skin biopsy should be taken. Once the diagnosis is confirmed, the following investigations should be performed: chest radiograph; respiratory function tests; ECG; full blood count; serum calcium; urine electrolytes and creatinine; and liver function tests. Radiographs of the hands can be helpful if there are joint symptoms.

Special points

Careful examination and appropriate biopsies of the skin or conjunctiva can frequently spare a patient with systemic sarcoidosis a more invasive diagnostic procedure such as a transbronchial lung biopsy or liver biopsy.

Granulomatous Cheilitis

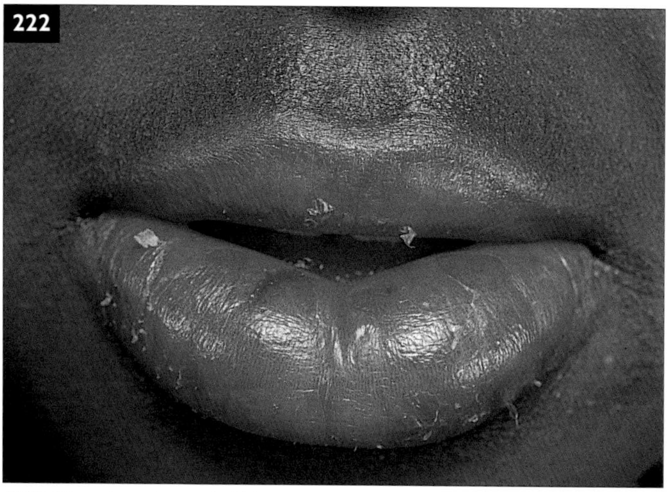

222 Granulomatous cheilitis.

Definition and clinical features

This is an uncommon condition characterised by chronic granulomatous inflammation of the lips which are markedly and persistently swollen and may have a purplish discoloration (**222**). Histology reveals chronic granulomatous inflammation and in idiopathic cases there may be no evidence of granulomatous disease elsewhere.

Epidemiology

Granulomatous cheilitis may be an isolated occurrence but sometimes it is the result of an adverse reaction to food additives including cinnamates. Other patients have underlying Crohn's disease or sarcoidosis.

Investigations

A lip biopsy is helpful to confirm the diagnosis. Patients should be patch tested to look for evidence of allergic contact dermatitis.

Special points

May be associated with fissured tongue and facial palsy (Melkersson–Rosenthal syndrome). Treatment with intralesional steroids is usually helpful but reduction cheiloplasty may be required in some cases.

Morphoea

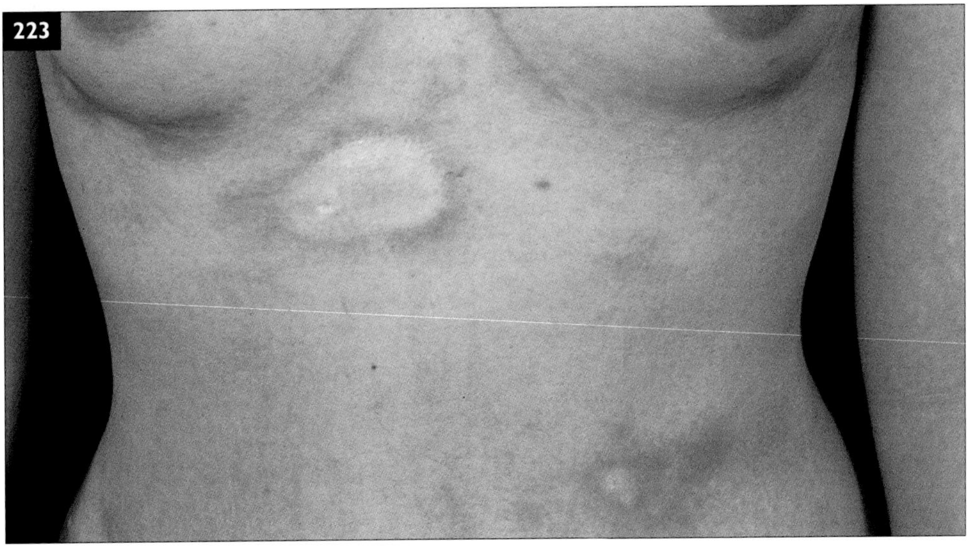

223 Morphoea.

Definition and clinical features

Morphoea is a disorder of unknown aetiology in which there is localised dermal fibrosis associated with atrophy of epidermal appendages.

Morphoea can be subdivided into four main clinical types:

- Circumscribed or localised morphoea which is by far the most common and presents with a slightly erythematous plaque which, over the course of several months, becomes thickened and waxy with associated loss of hair and eccrine glands (**223**).
- Linear morphoea which consists of a similar if more indolent process, usually affecting the limbs in childhood.
- Frontoparietal morphoea (or Parry–Romberg syndrome) which represents a similar linear process affecting half of the face, often in childhood or young adults ('coup de sabre').
- Generalised morphoea represents a similar process involving much of the skin but without other organ involvement.

Epidemiology

Localised morphoea is not uncommon. Other manifestations of morphoea are rare.

Differential diagnosis

This includes lichen sclerosus, necrobiosis lipoidica and acrodermatitis chronica atrophicans.

Investigations

The diagnosis can be confirmed with a skin biopsy. In some countries there appears to have been an association of morphoea with borrelia infection and *Borrelia burgdorferi* antibodies should be checked.

Special points

In patients with generalised morphoea the possibility of a toxic insult should be considered.

Systemic Sclerosis

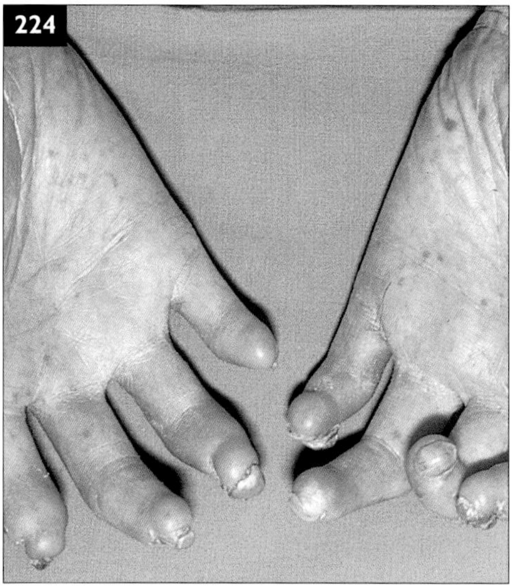

224 Systemic sclerosis.

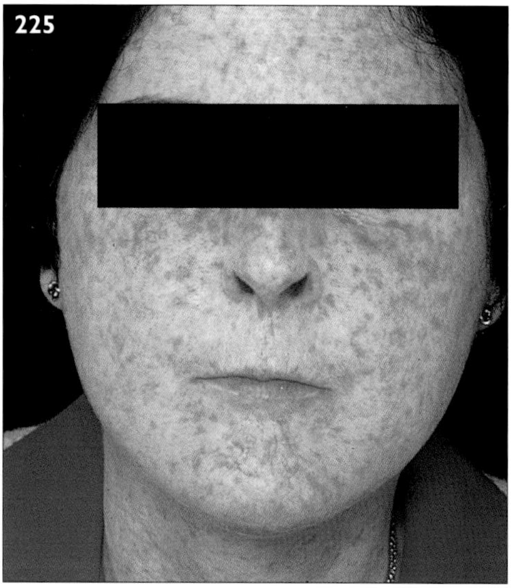

225 Systemic sclerosis.

Definition and clinical features

Systemic sclerosis is a disorder of unknown aetiology which causes progressive persistent fibrosis particularly in the skin, lower respiratory tract, gut and kidney. It frequently presents with cutaneous involvement. Early signs in the hands include swelling of the fingers; similar changes may occur on the feet. This is followed by progressive dermal fibrosis restricting the movement of the fingers and giving the skin a tight waxy appearance (**224**). There is resorption of the distal finger pulps associated with acro-osteolysis. Raynaud's phenomenon is common and digital gangrene may occur. Mat-like telangiectasia is often widespread and the face shows a beaked nose, a small mouth with restricted opening and radial furrowing (rhagades) (**225**). Involvement of other organs includes pulmonary fibrosis, oesophageal hypomotility causing dysphagia and aspiration, malabsorption and malignant hypertension.

Epidemiology

Systemic sclerosis is rare, affecting 1 in 20 000 women and 1 in 100 000 men.

Differential diagnosis

Occupationally and environmentally induced systemic sclerosis-like disorders, of which vinyl chloride disease is the prototype, may sometimes resemble idiopathic systemic sclerosis very closely. Always ask a patient with apparently idiopathic systemic sclerosis their job!

Investigations

The diagnosis of systemic sclerosis can be confirmed by evidence of involvement of several organs and a barium swallow, chest radiograph, respiratory function tests, creatinine clearance and serology for autoantibodies including ANA, ENAs such as anticentromere antibody and anti-SCL70, are helpful. Less specific autoantibodies include anticardiolipins and cold agglutinins. ESR is raised in some patients who exhibit an acute phase response. There is a particular association between the presence of anti-Jo-1 antibodies and pulmonary fibrosis, and anti-Ro antibodies and features suggestive of concurrent Sjögren's syndrome.

Special points

Patients with systemic sclerosis should not smoke and should be advised to modify their lifestyle/occupation in order to minimise their exposure to cold, which exacerbates their problems with Raynaud's syndrome. Blood pressure must also be carefully controlled.

Dermatomyositis

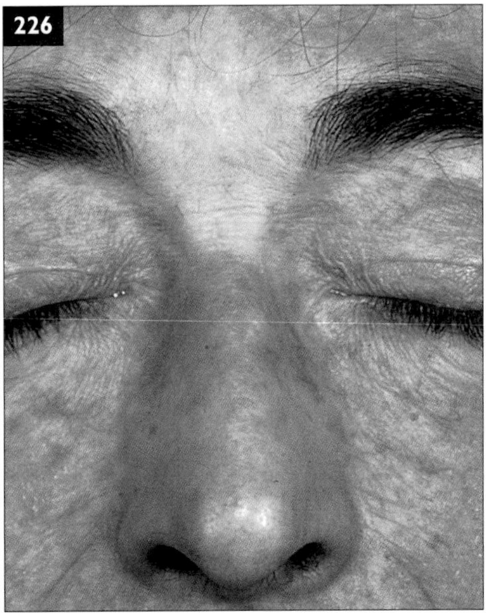

226 Dermatomyositis.

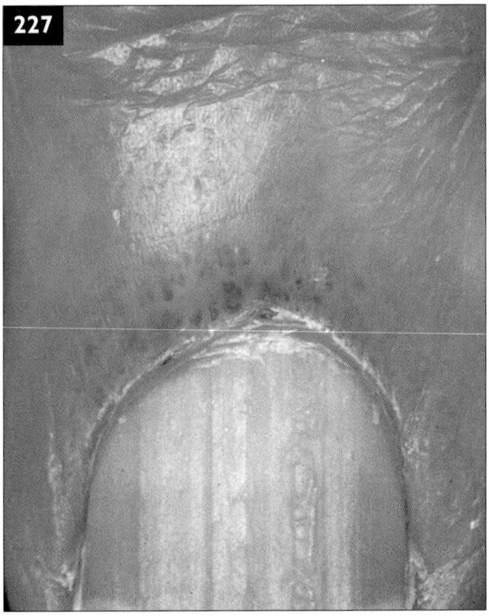

227 Dermatomyositis.

Definition and clinical features

Dermatomyositis is a multisystem disorder which causes a characteristic erythematous eruption, particularly affecting the face and hands, in association with myositis. The characteristic eruption of dermatomyositis includes a violaceous or heliotrope rash on the face with periorbital swelling (**226**). This eruption may extend in a photosensitive distribution on to the neck and upper chest. The skin over the hands shows dilated nail fold capillaries and ragged cuticles (**227**). Gottron's patches – erythematosquamous plaques – appear over the interphalangeal and metacarpophalangeal joints in association with Dowling's lines, which are similar linear lesions on the dorsal surface of the fingers over the metacarpals.

In addition to myositis involving skeletal muscle, smooth muscle may be involved, causing dysphagia and dysphonia as well as impaired intestinal motility. Pulmonary fibrosis, myocarditis and retinitis are well-recognised features. Cutaneous calcinosis is a late manifestation which is particularly prominent in the childhood variant. Livedo reticularis and cutaneous ulceration are rare.

Epidemiology

Dermatomyositis is a rare disorder with peak incidence in children under ten and in adults from the age of 40. Paediatric dermatomyositis is not associated with malignancy.

Differential diagnosis

Mixed connective tissue disease, systemic lupus erythematosus.

Investigations

The diagnosis can be confirmed by skin and muscle biopsies. Electromyography and muscle enzymes may be abnormal. Autoantibodies, including extractable nuclear antigens, should be sought. Adults should be examined and investigated for signs of an occult carcinoma.

Special points

Relapse of previously stable dermatomyositis should trigger further investigation for occult malignancy.

Discoid Lupus Erythematosus

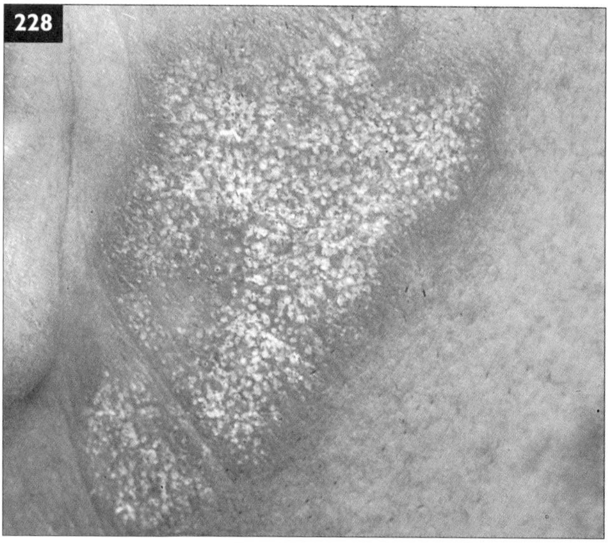

228 Discoid lupus erythematosus.

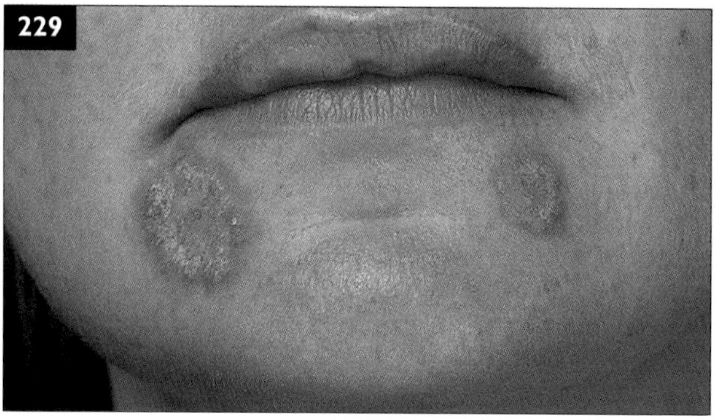

229 Discoid lupus erythematosus.

Definition and clinical features

Discoid lupus erythematosus consist of localised erythematosquamous plaques which heal with atrophy and destruction of cutaneous appendages. The plaques are commonly present on the head and neck but may also be found on the hands and occasionally in a more generalised distribution. They show erythema, scaling, follicular plugging, telangiectasia, hyper- and hypopigmentation and scarring (**228**, **229**). Plaques may be found in the scalp and a similar process may involve the vermilion border of the lips and the oral mucosa. The majority of patients do not have systemic disease.

Epidemiology

Discoid lupus erythematosus is uncommon. Sunlight may exacerbate it

Differential diagnosis

Granuloma faciale, lichen planus, lupus vulgaris, sarcoidosis and other chronic granulomatous infections.

Investigations

Diagnosis can be confirmed with a skin biopsy. A full blood count, ESR and ANA should be done to exclude the possibility of systemic involvement.

Subacute Cutaneous Lupus Erythematosus

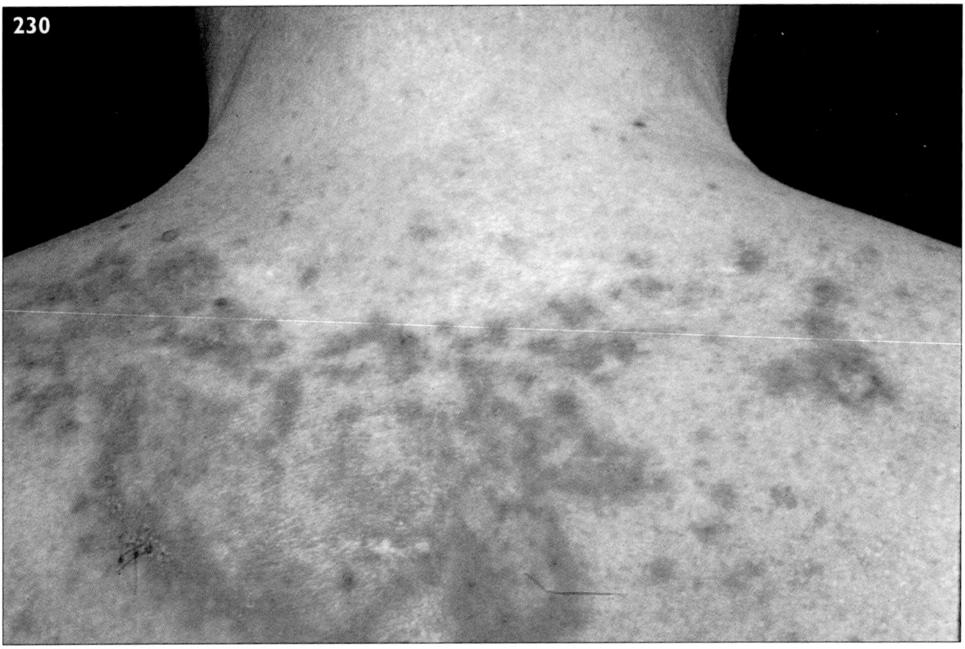
230 Subacute cutaneous lupus erythematosus.

Definition and clinical features

This disorder is characterised by a widespread erythematosquamous eruption, sometimes annular and particularly prominent on light-exposed areas, associated with photosensitivity and the presence of anti-Ro antibodies. The lesions consist of sharply demarcated, scaly, erythematous plaques in a symmetrical distribution (**230**). Lesions resolve without scarring, in contrast to discoid lupus erythematosus. Children of mothers with subacute cutaneous lupus erythematosus are at risk of congenital heart block and neonatal lupus erythematosus. Systemic involvement is frequent and should be looked for.

Differential diagnosis

Psoriasis, systemic lupus erythematosus, generalised discoid lupus erythematosus.

Investigations

Full blood count, urea and electrolytes, creatinine, liver function tests, ANA, anti-Ro, anti-La and anti-double-stranded DNA antibodies. Renal function should be assessed.

Special points

The correct diagnosis and management of patients with subacute cutaneous lupus erythematosus during pregnancy is of paramount importance to prevent congenital heart block.

Systemic Lupus Erythematosus

231
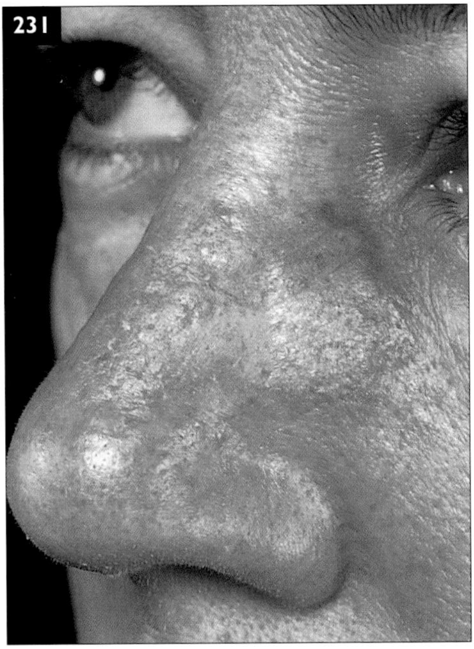

231 Systemic lupus erythematosus.

232
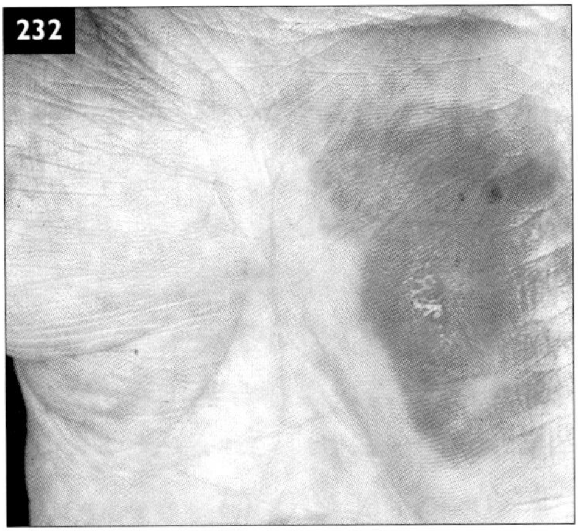

232 Systemic lupus erythematosus.

Definition and clinical features

This is a multisystem inflammatory disorder characterised by the presence of anti-double-stranded DNA antibodies and a constellation of characteristic clinical symptoms and signs.

The rash of systemic lupus erythematosus consists of erythema with or without widespread discoid papules and plaques (**231**, **232**). The classical distribution of the erythema is in a butterfly distribution over the face, but in clinical practice this is relatively uncommon. Periungual telangiectasia is a common feature, as is oral mucosal ulceration and diffuse hair fall. Photosensitivity may be marked.

Other features of acute systemic lupus erythematosus include fever, polyarthralgia, nephritis, leucopenia, serositis causing pleuritic chest pain, pericarditis, pneumonitis and encephalopathy. The skin disease is non-scarring.

Epidemiology

Systemic lupus erythematosus is an uncommon disorder.

Differential diagnosis

Mixed connective tissue disease, dermatomyositis, rosacea.

Investigations

The diagnosis can be confirmed by the finding of anti-double-stranded DNA antibodies. Drug-induced lupus is associated with these antibodies. A skin biopsy may also be helpful in confirming the diagnosis. Full blood count, ESR, urea and electrolytes, creatinine, routine urinalysis, lupus anticoagulant, anticardiolipin antibodies and coagulation screen should also be performed. Any evidence of renal involvement should be followed with an MSU, creatinine clearance and 24 hour urinary protein estimation. Infections should be carefully sought in patients with fever and acute deterioration.

Special points

Patients with systemic lupus erythematosus are at high risk of developing severe infection, in the absence of prominent physical signs, because of the immunosuppressive effect of their disease and its treatment. Patients are also prone to catastrophic thrombotic episodes in unusual sites and again a high index of suspicion is necessary for early diagnosis and treatment of problems such as sagittal sinus thrombosis, renal vein thrombosis and hepatic vein thrombosis.

Still's Disease

233

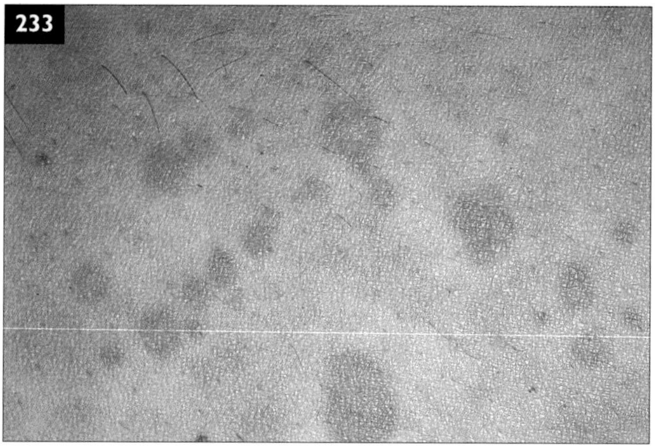

233 Still's disease.

234

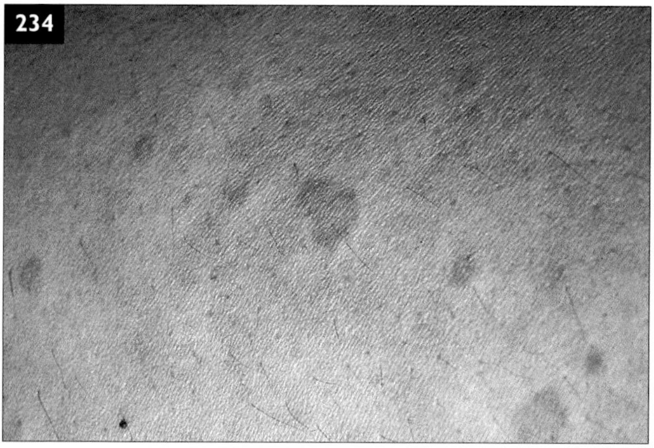

234 Still's disease.

Definition and clinical features

Still's disease is a multisystem disorder predominantly seen in childhood, consisting of an evanescent erythematous eruption, fever, arthritis, hepatitis, lymphadenopathy and splenomegaly. The rash of Still's disease consists of non-pruritic erythematous macules with central and perilesional pallor (**233**, **234**). The rash characteristically occurs synchronously with a fever in the evening and is absent in the mornings. The disorder is persistent and frequently follows a sore throat.

Differential diagnosis

Reactive erythemas, urticaria, occult infection.

Investigations

ESR is raised. Full blood count may show a neutrophilia. LFTs may show hepatitis. Urea and electrolytes are usually normal. In the event of signs of myocarditis an echocardiogram and ECG are indicated.

Special points

Careful monitoring of patients treated with non-steroidal, anti-inflammatory drugs (NSAIDs) is essential as these have been implicated in cases of fatal hepatic failure in Still's disease.

Acanthosis Nigricans

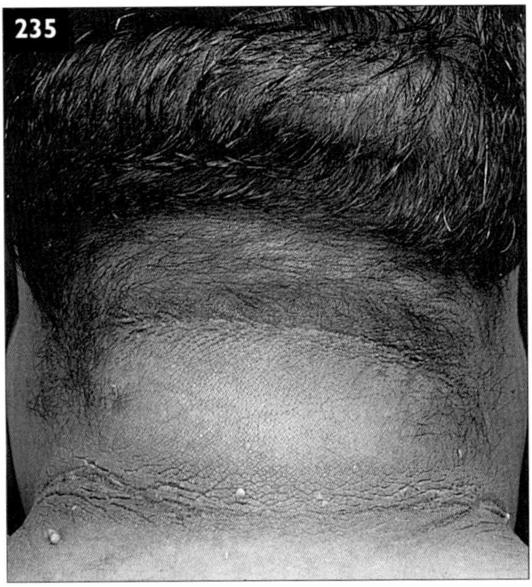

235 Acanthosis nigricans.

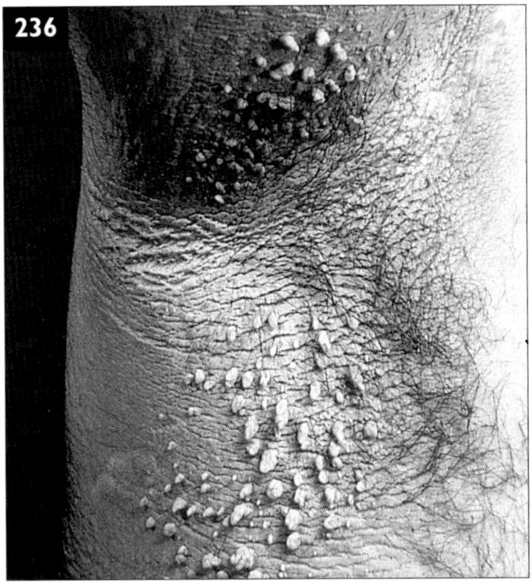

236 Acanthosis nigricans.

Definition and clinical features

Hyperpigmented, velvety plaques involving flexural sites, associated with tissue resistance to insulin. There are benign forms characterised by the insidious onset of brown, thickened papillomatous skin predominantly affecting the nape of the neck (**235**) and axillae (**236**); less commonly, the anogenital and groin regions are also involved. Features suggestive of underlying malignancy include rapid onset, extension on to extraflexural sites, involvement of mucous membranes and/or vermilion border, presence of deeply pigmented, verrucous plaques, associated palmar keratoderma and nail changes.

Epidemiology

The disorder is divided into five main subgroups according to their underlying aetiology; all share tissue resistance to insulin.

- Hereditary – benign autosomal dominant.
- Benign – caused by endocrine disorders, including acromegaly, Addison's disease, Cushing's disease, diabetes mellitus.
- Pseudoacanthosis nigricans – obese, Asian or Hispanic adults.
- Drug induced – nicotinic acid, stilboestrol.
- Malignant – especially adenocarcinoma of the gastrointestinal tract, ovary and uterus.

Differential diagnosis

Chronic, lichenified eczema, confluent and reticulate papillomatosis, lichen amyloidosis.

Investigations

Clinical differentiation between benign and malignant forms of the disorder should indicate appropriate investigation to elucidate underlying cause.

Special points

Onset of malignant acanthosis nigricans may antedate symptoms of underlying malignancy by months or years; acanthosis nigricans may resolve with successful treatment of tumour.

Porokeratoses

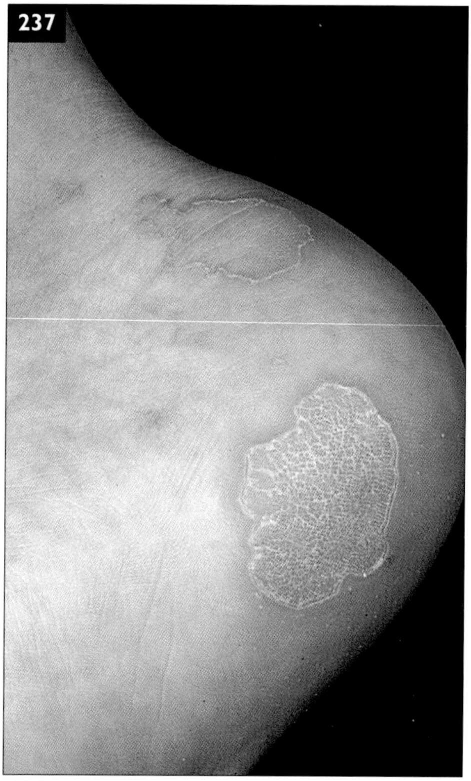

237 Porokeratosis.

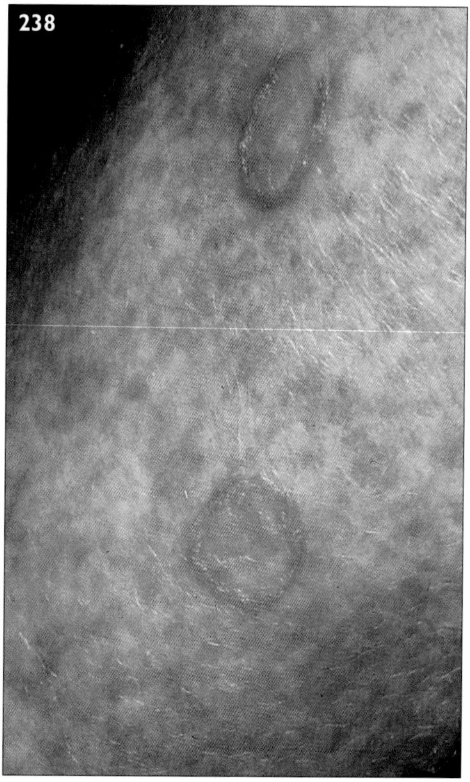

238 Porokeratosis of Mibelli.

Definition and clinical features

This is a group of dyskeratotic disorders whose histological hallmark, the cornoid lamella, gives rise to distinct clinical features. There is a discrete, annular plaque with a peripheral hyperkeratotic ridge, often with a characteristic central groove (**237**), surrounding anhidrotic, hairless, atrophic epidermis.

Five clinical subtypes are recognised:

- Porokeratosis of Mibelli refers to one (or a few) isolated plaque(s), most commonly distributed on the limbs (**238**). These begin as small papules in childhood which slowly spread centrifugally over years to reach several centimetres in diameter.
- Disseminated superficial actinic porokeratosis (DSAP) occurs during middle age and comprises multiple, small (less than 1 cm in diameter), monomorphic, flat plaques on the lower legs (**239**) and other chronically sun-exposed sites, especially in fair-skinned individuals.
- Disseminated superficial porokeratosis (also called porokeratosis plantaris, palmaris et disseminata) may be distinguished from DSAP by the presence of lesions on non-sun-exposed sites and onset in childhood. A disseminated form has also been reported following organ transplantation.
- Linear porokeratosis is always confined to one limb or side, and may occur in a zosteriform or linear configuration (**240**).
- Punctate porokeratoses are confined to the palms and soles and comprise minute, hyperkeratotic, seed-like plaques. They may be associated with porokeratosis of Mibelli or linear porokeratosis.

Porokeratoses

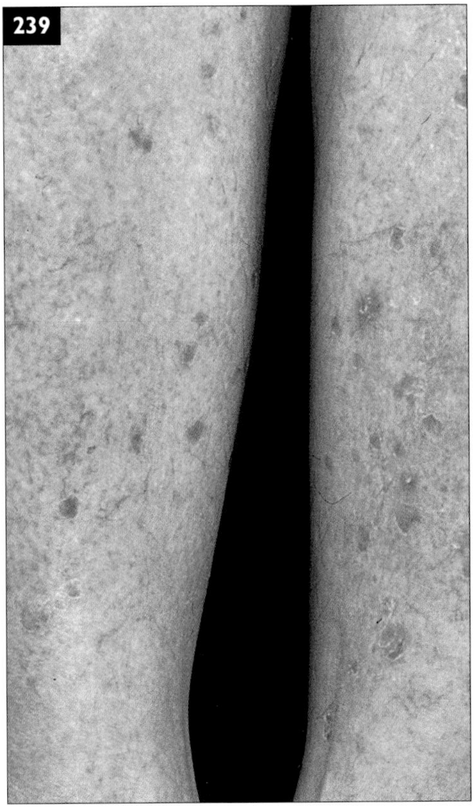

239 Disseminated superficial actinic porokeratosis (DSAP).

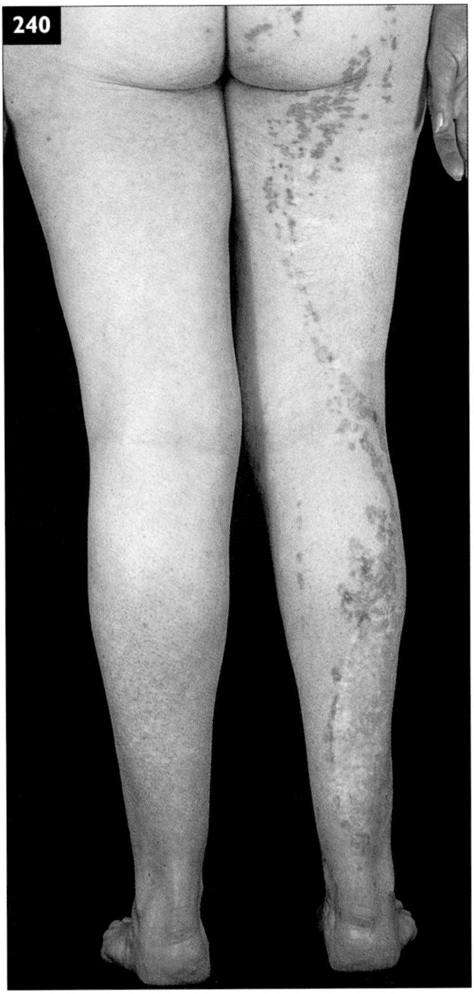

240 Linear porokeratosis.

Epidemiology

All forms of porokeratosis, with the exception of DSAP, are rare. Lesions are thought to arise from aberrant clones of keratinocytes, either inherited (usually as an autosomal dominant trait) or acquired (e.g. following sun exposure); keratinocytes demonstrate variable degrees of dysplasia and may progress to overt malignancy.

Differential diagnosis

DSAP must be distinguished from multiple actinic, stucco or seborrhoeic keratoses. Linear porokeratosis may resemble linear verrucous epidermal naevus though is easily distinguishable on histopathological examination.

Investigations

Biopsy to demonstrate the presence of the cornoid lamella – a thin column of parakeratotic cells extending through the stratum corneum, bending away from the centre of the lesion.

Special points

Squamous cell carcinoma, basal cell epithelioma and Bowen's disease may occur in porokeratosis of Mibelli.

Benign Tumours Arising from the Epidermis

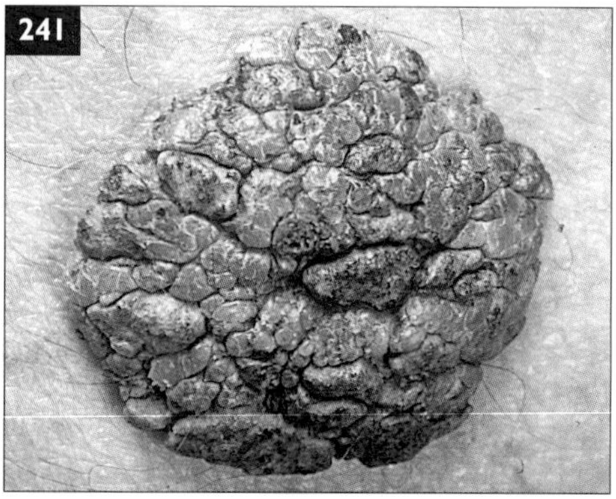

241 Verruciform seborrhoeic wart.

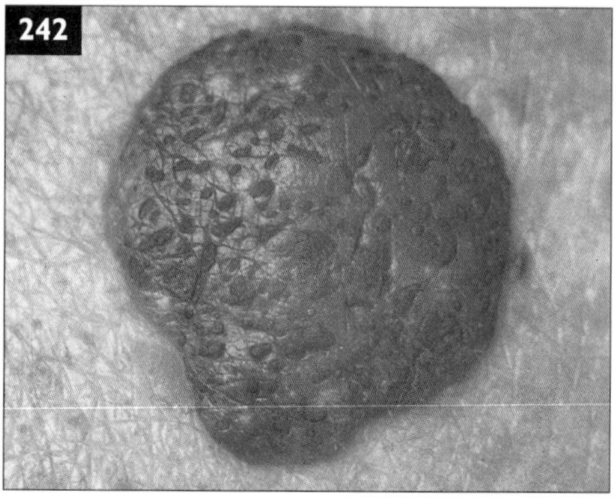

242 Smooth, dome-shaped seborrhoeic wart.

SEBORRHOEIC KERATOSIS (SEBORRHOEIC WART; SENILE WART; BASAL CELL PAPILLOMA)

Definition and clinical features

A warty, pigmented papule or plaque due to a benign proliferation of keratinocytes. These mostly arise on the trunk and face but they can occur anywhere. Clinical presentations include:

- A greasy, brown/yellow, oval-shaped-plaque with a verruciform surface, 1–2 cm in diameter, stuck on to the normal surrounding skin (**241**).
- A brown/black, dome-shaped tumour with a relatively smooth surface, punctuated with plugged follicular openings (**242**).
- A sandy brown, minimally scaly, irregular plaque (**243**).

Epidemiology

These tumours are common in individuals over 40 years old. The number of lesions tends to increase with age.

Differential diagnosis

Pale, flat, pigmented facial lesions must be differentiated from lentigo maligna. Distinction from solar keratoses, atypical melanocytic naevi and, rarely, malignant melanoma may be difficult, particularly when the clinical appearances are altered by trauma or infection.

Special points

The sudden appearance of multiple seborrhoeic keratoses has been said to be associated with underlying malignancy (sign of Leser–Trélat).

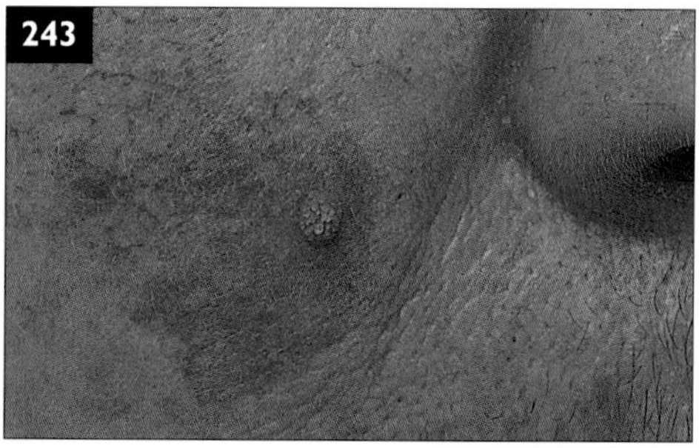

243 Irregular plaque-type seborrhoeic wart.

KERATOACANTHOMA

Definition and clinical features

A rapid proliferation of keratinocytes giving rise to a squamoproliferative nodule which resolves spontaneously. Lesions occur on sun-exposed sites, particularly on the head and upper limbs. A solitary, firm, pink or skin-coloured papule rapidly enlarges over a period of days or weeks to reach 2–4 cm in diameter. At the end of this growth phase, the lesion forms a symmetrical, dome-shaped nodule with an overlying thinned, telangiectatic epidermis and a central keratin plug (**244**, **245**). Spontaneous resolution occurs over a few months to leave a depressed scar.

Epidemiology

UV exposure is implicated in the development of keratoacanthoma though, in contrast to squamous cell carcinoma, keratoacanthomas occur predominantly in middle age, and the incidence

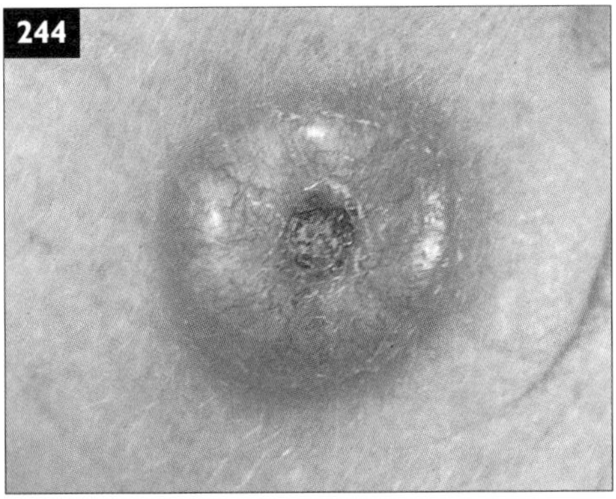

244 Keratoacanthoma – the central keratin plug.

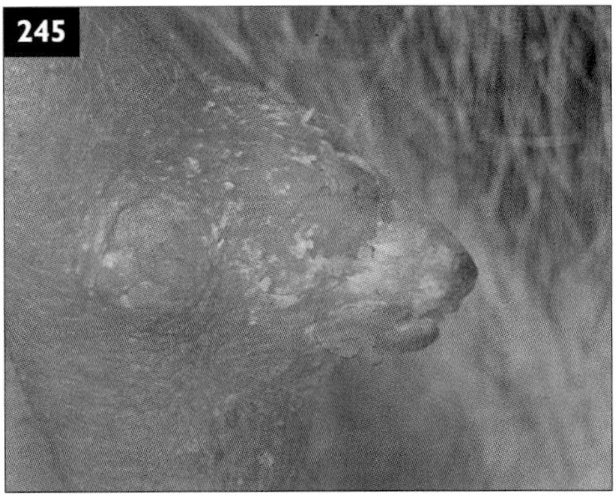

245 Keratoacanthoma.

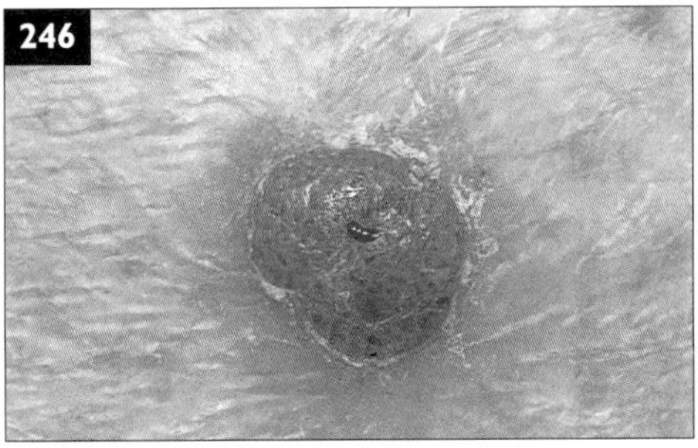

246 Clear cell acanthoma.

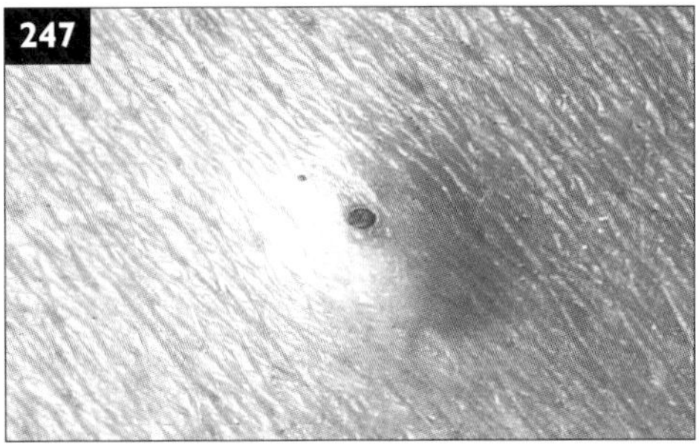

247 Epidermoid cyst.

does not increase in old age. Multiple lesions may occur in immunosuppressed individuals and those with underlying malignancy. Self-healing lesions occur in the Ferguson–Smith syndrome.

Investigation
Biopsy.

Differential diagnosis
Distinction between invasive squamous cell carcinoma and keratoacanthoma may be clinically and histologically difficult; where doubt exists, the tumour should be treated as an invasive squamous cell carcinoma.

CLEAR CELL ACANTHOMA (ACANTHOMA OF DEGOS)
Definition and clinical features
A scaly nodule on the lower leg derived from large, glycogen-containing keratinocytes. There is a solitary red (or less commonly brown), well-demarcated nodule, 0.5–2 cm in diameter, with very fine surface scale and occasional oozing (**246**).

Epidemiology
Occurs in adults of middle age or older. It is relatively uncommon.

Differential diagnosis
Dermatofibroma, pyogenic granuloma, seborrhoeic keratosis.

EPIDERMOID CYST
Definition and clinical features
A cyst containing keratin, surrounded by a lining identical in its stratification to that of epidermis. A soft, mobile, dome-shaped protuberance, varying in size from a few millimetres to several centimetres, tethered to the overlying epidermis, often with a central punctum (**247**). Commonly distributed on the head, neck, shoulders and chest. May

Benign Tumours Arising from the Epidermis

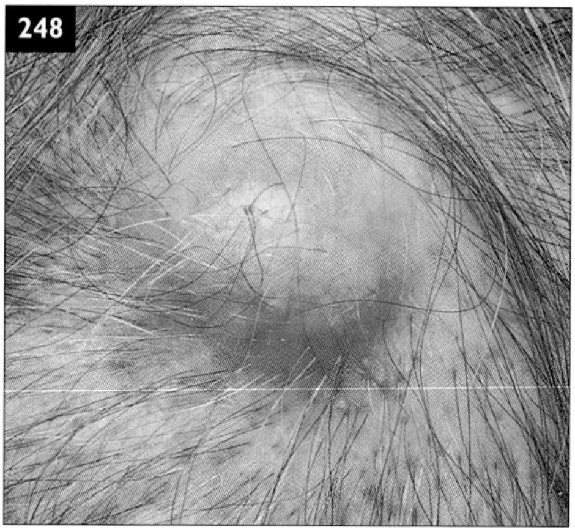

248 Tricholemmal cyst.

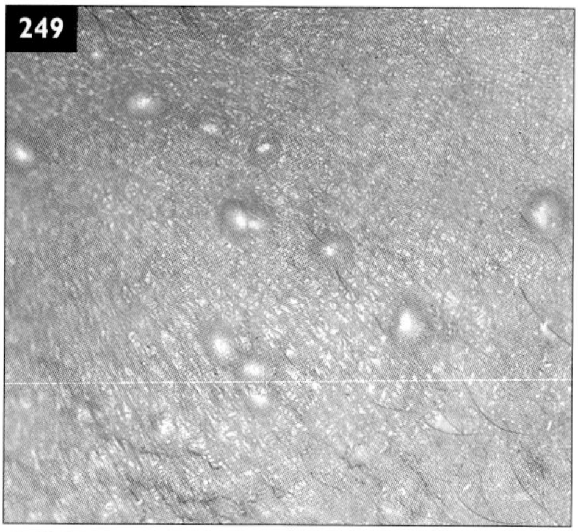

249 Milia.

become secondarily infected or spontaneously discharge white, cheesy keratinous material. May also arise following trauma, commonly on the finger.

Epidemiology
Occurs in young and middle-aged adults, often following moderate or severe acne vulgaris. Traumatic cysts arise due to implantation of a small portion of the epidermis into the dermis.

Differential diagnosis
Presence of secondary infection may rarely cause confusion with inflammatory granulomas, e.g. cutaneous leishmaniasis.

Special points
Multiple epidermoid cysts in childhood are a characteristic feature of Gardener's syndrome and the naevoid basal cell carcinoma syndrome (or Gorlin's syndrome).

TRICHOLEMMAL CYST (PILAR CYST)
Definition and clinical features
A keratin-filled cyst on the scalp surrounded by a lining resembling the external hair root sheath. A firm, mobile nodule on the scalp (**248**), which may be tender if secondarily infected.

Epidemiology
Occurs in young and middle-aged adults. Multiple cysts may be inherited as an autosomal dominant trait.

Differential diagnosis
Dermal, appendageal tumours.

MILIUM
Definition and clinical features
A small, subepidermal cyst. Multiple, small (1–2 mm in diameter), white papules are found around the eyelids and cheeks of young women (**249**). May also occur in infancy.

Epidemiology
Arises either in underdeveloped sebaceous glands or within damaged ducts of eccrine sweat glands following subepidermal bulla formation (e.g. epidermolysis bullosa, porphyria cutanea tarda, bullous pemphigoid) or skin radiotherapy.

Benign Tumours Arising from the Dermis

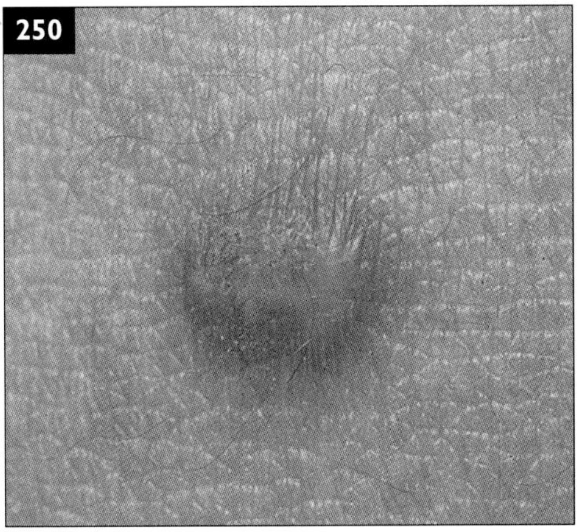

250 Dermatofibroma (histiocytoma).

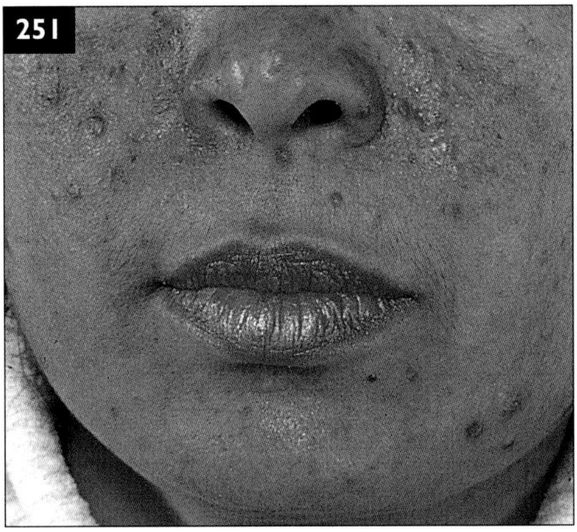

251 Angiofibromata.

DERMATOFIBROMA

Definition and clinical features

A dermal nodule comprised of an interwoven mesh of histocytes and collagen, with overlying epidermal hyperplasia. A mildly pruritic, firm nodule on the lower limbs of young adults (**250**). Palpation reveals a larger dermal component than expected on initial inspection, with puckering overlying hyperkeratotic, pigmented epidermis.

Epidemiology

Common. May represent an abnormal reaction to insect bites or other trauma, rather than a true neoplasm.

Differential diagnosis

Malignant melanoma when lesion deeply pigmented.

ANGIOFIBROMA

Definition and clinical features

A firm red papule comprised of fibrotic tissue centred around small blood vessels in the papillary dermis. Multiple smooth, red papules on the face, particularly around the nasolabial folds. Number and size increase during puberty (**251**).

Epidemiology

Multiple lesions are a pathognomonic feature of tuberous sclerosis, where misdesignated as sebaceous adenoma (adenoma sebaceum); angiofibromas are otherwise rare.

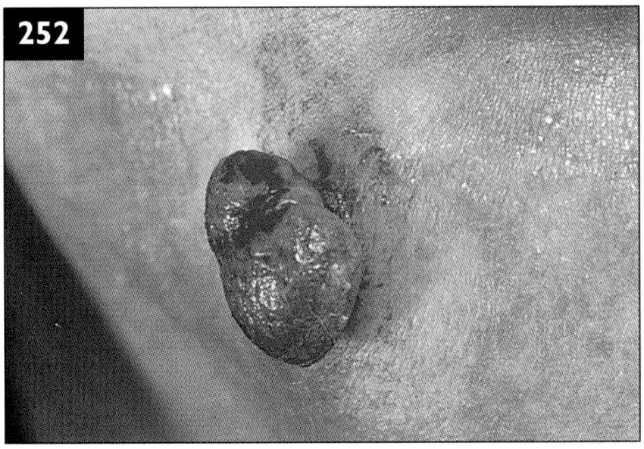

252 Pyogenic granuloma.

PYOGENIC GRANULOMA

Definition and clinical features

A rapidly expanding, painful vascular nodule that follows minor trauma, comprised of a capillary network within an oedematous stroma (**252**). Usually arises on the fingers. May recur or develop satellite lesions following excision.

Epidemiology

Common.

Differential diagnosis

Amelanotic melanoma, squamous cell carcinoma, Kaposi's sarcoma.

Investigations

Biopsy.

Benign Tumours Arising from the Dermis

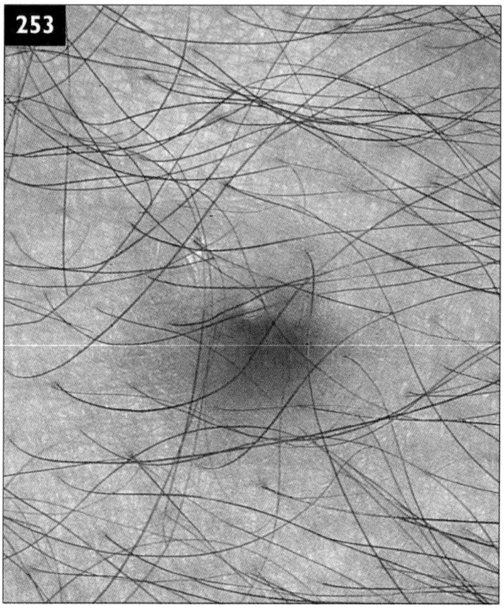

253 Glomus tumour.

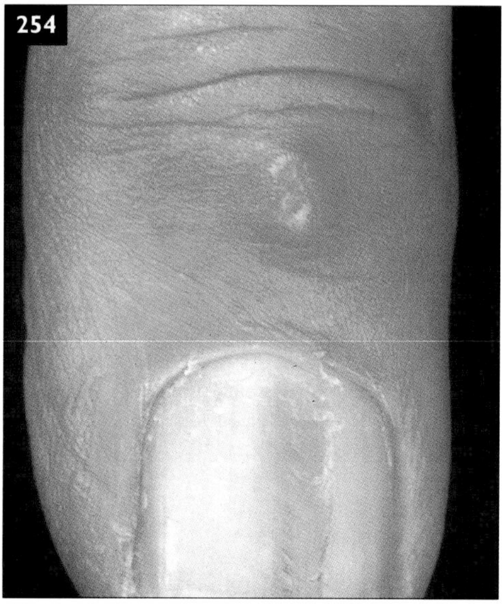

254 Myxoid cyst.

GLOMUS TUMOUR

Definition and clinical features

A painful, vascular nodule comprised of cuboidal (glomus) cells arranged around endothelial lined vascular channels. May occur either as a solitary, vascular, subungual tumour or as multiple blue/black nodules on any body site (**253**).

Epidemiology

Uncommon. Multiple type familial.

Differential diagnosis

Malignant melanoma.

Investigations

Biopsy.

Special points

Excision of solitary type invariably required because of the associated pain.

MYXOID CYST (MUCOID CYST)

Definition and clinical features

A pseudocyst, probably arising from the localised mucoid degeneration of connective tissue. A solitary, circumscribed, soft, often transparent cystic structure, up to 5–10 mm in size, which is occasionally painful. Typically found on the dorsa of the distal phalanges of the fingers or toes (**254**).

Epidemiology

More common in women.

Differential diagnosis

Ganglion.

Special points

Can be excised, or otherwise extirpated, if annoying.

Benign Tumours Arising from Skin Appendages

Virtually every cellular component of hair follicles, apocrine and eccrine sweat glands and sebaceous glands may give rise to tumour formation. Most are rare and present as nondescript, dermal papules or nodules. These lesions are therefore rarely diagnosed clinically and invariably require histological evaluation. A few of the more commonly encountered lesions will be briefly described.

HAIR FOLLICLE TUMOURS

Definition and clinical features

This is a benign tumour derived from a component of the hair follicle. Most occur on the face, and multiple lesions may be single or multiple.

Trichodiscomas and tumours of the follicular infundibulum present as multiple, smooth, superficial, skin-coloured papules. Tufts of hair occasionally emerge from tricholemmomas and are invariably present in trichofolliculomas. Trichoepitheliomas tend to centre around the nasolabial folds, have a slightly greasy appearance, and multiple lesions may be inherited as an autosomal dominant trait (epithelioma adenoides cysticum). Pilomatricoma contrasts with other hair appendage tumours in that the majority present in childhood and form hard, deep dermal nodules up to 3 cm in diameter.

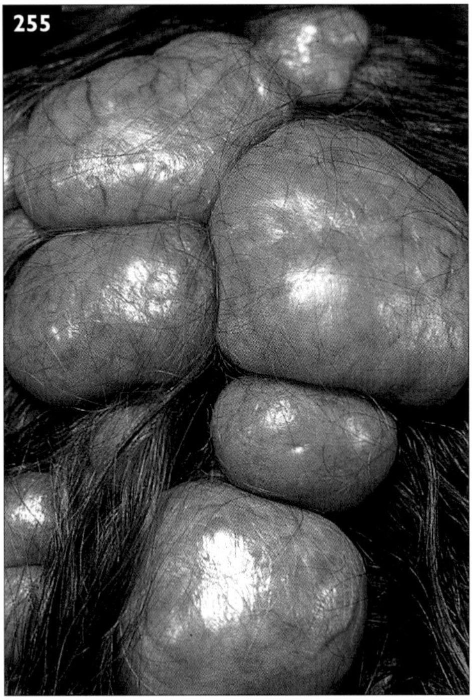

255 Cylindroma ('turban tumour').

Epidemiology

Rare. Pilomatricomas are the most commonly excised hair appendage tumour.

Differential diagnosis

Other appendageal tumours.

Investigations

Biopsy.

APOCRINE GLAND TUMOURS – CYLINDROMA (TURBAN TUMOUR)

Definition and clinical features

This is a large, dome-shaped nodule on the scalp of apocrine origin. It is a solitary, well-circumscribed, red or skin-coloured nodule a few centimetres in diameter. When left, these tumours may grow to involve much of the scalp and develop a cerebriform appearance (hence 'turban tumour') (**255**).

Epidemiology

Rare.

Differential diagnosis

Basal cell carcinoma (early lesions particularly).

Investigations

Biopsy.

Benign Tumours arising from Skin Appendages

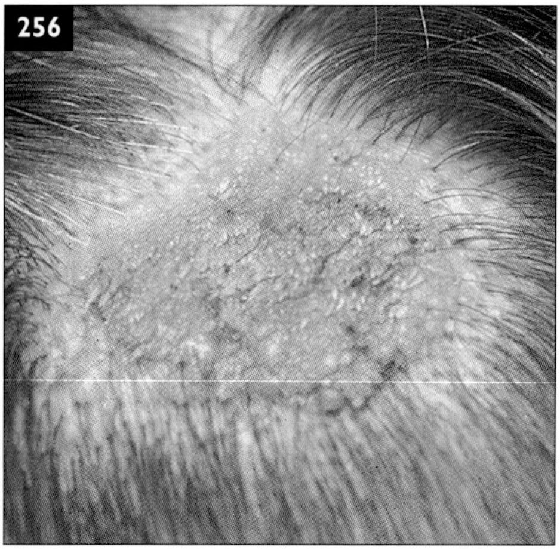

256 Sebaceous naevus.

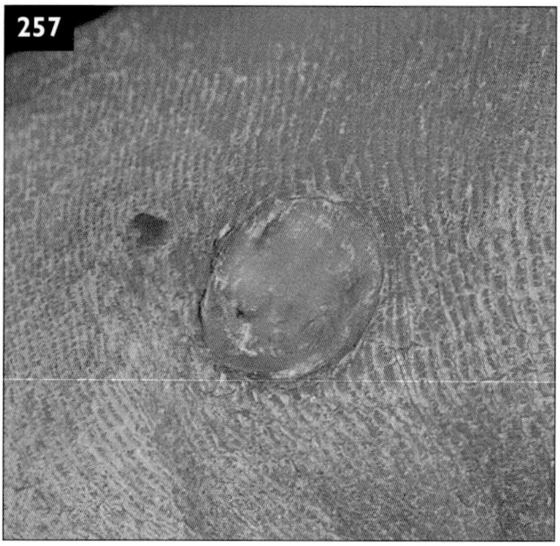

257 Eccrine poroma.

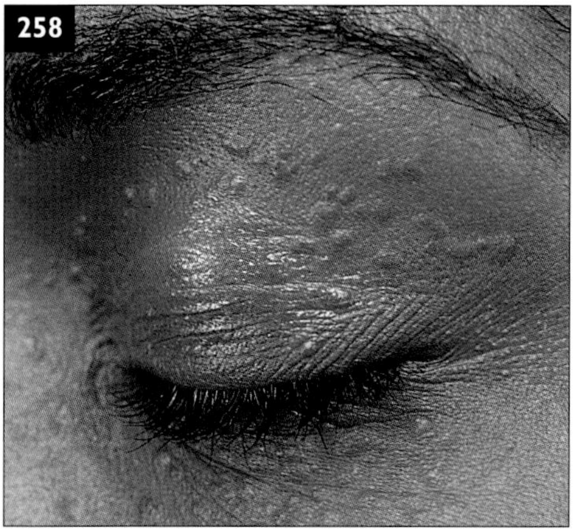

258 Syringomata.

SEBACEOUS NAEVUS (NAEVUS SEBACEUS)

Definition and clinical features

Naevus of the lobes of sebaceous glands. Presents as a congenital, elevated, soft, elastic, shiny, yellowish patch in the scalp, flat-topped and with a warty surface (**256**). May be first noticed at puberty.

Epidemiology

May develop basal cell carcinoma or a variety of benign tumours, e.g. cystadenoma papilliferum.

Differential diagnosis

Seborrhoeic wart.

Investigations

Biopsy.

Special points

Excise by early adulthood to avoid tumour development. May be associated with CNS or skeletal abnormalities.

ECCRINE SWEAT GLAND TUMOURS

Definition and clinical features

A benign tumour arising from part of the eccrine sweat gland. Eccrine poroma presents as a moist, red, nodule on the sole of the foot (**257**). Eccrine spiradenomas are painful and occur as isolated nodules on any body site. Eccrine hidradenomas form blue-black nodules. Syringomata are invariably multiple and form small (1–2 mm diameter), soft, flat papules on and around the eyelids (**258**).

Epidemiology

Rare, with the exception of syringomata, which particularly presents in young female adults.

Differential diagnosis

Syringomata may simulate plane warts or milia.

Investigations

Biopsy.

Malignant Neoplasms and their Precursors

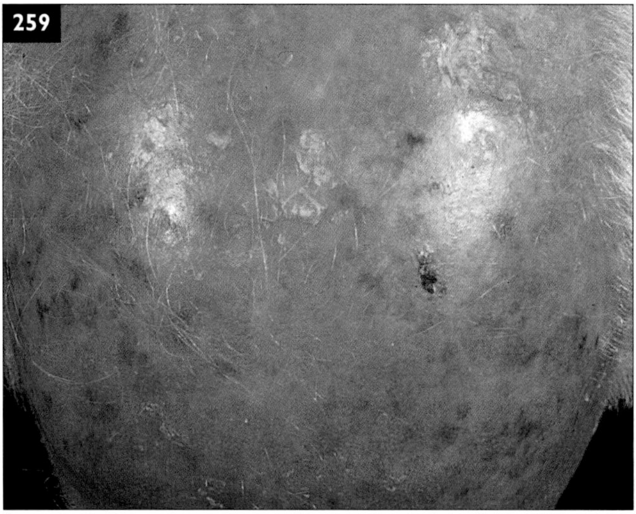

259 Solar keratoses.

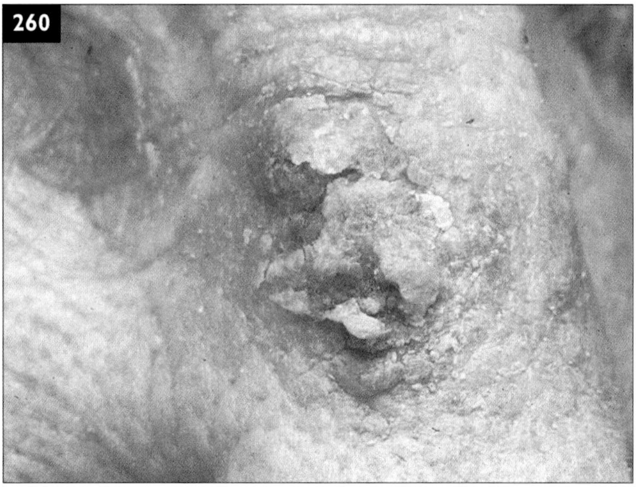

260 Solar keratosis.

SOLAR KERATOSIS (ACTINIC KERATOSIS)

Definition and clinical features

A red, scaly plaque on light-exposed skin due to dysplastic epidermal keratinocytes. It may affect the face (including lower lip), bald pate (**259**), forearms and dorsum of the hands, presenting as a red or brown plaque, 0.5–1 cm in diameter, with surface scale or crust (**260**). It may ulcerate or develop a cutaneous horn. Frequently multiple.

Epidemiology

Common, especially in fair-skinned individuals over 40 years of age with a recreational or occupational history of chronic sun exposure. Enormous numbers may occur in those chronically immunosuppressed (e.g. renal transplant recipients). Their presence is an indicator of increased risk of non-melanoma skin cancer.

Differential diagnosis

Seborrhoeic wart, viral warts, squamous cell carcinoma.

Investigations

Biopsy if diagnosis in doubt.

Malignant Neoplasms and their Precursors

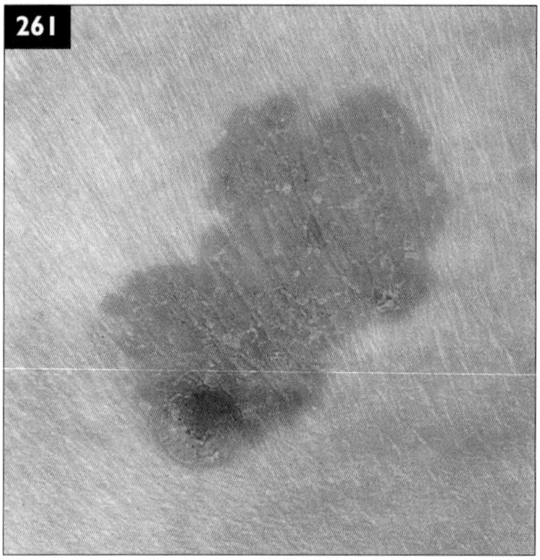

261 Bowen's disease.

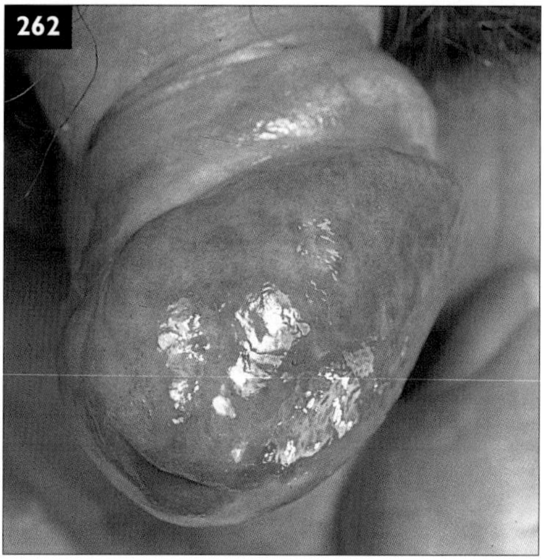

262 Erythroplasia of Queyrat.

BOWEN'S DISEASE

Definition and clinical features

A fixed, scaly, red plaque due to squamous cell carcinoma in situ. Solitary, most commonly on the trunk, 2–5 cm in diameter (**261**). May arise in uncircumcised males on the glans penis (then called erythroplasia of Queyrat) as a smooth, red, velvety plaque (**262**).

Epidemiology

Development related to UV exposure or chronic arsenic ingestion.

Differential diagnosis

Isolated plaque of psoriasis, multifocal basal cell carcinoma, actinic keratosis.

Investigations

Biopsy.

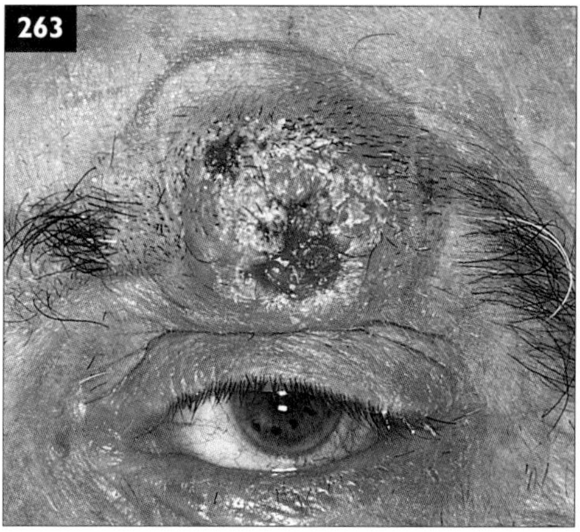

263 Squamous cell carcinoma.

SQUAMOUS CELL CARCINOMA

Definition and clinical features

A squamoproliferative lesion due to malignant, invasive, proliferation of epidermal keratinocytes. Presents as an expanding plaque or nodule with an ill-defined, indurated base, usually ulcerated, with surface scale and crust (**263**). Occurs on sun-exposed sites (face, neck, forearms, dorsum of the hands) in association with solar elastosis and multiple actinic keratoses. Local draining lymph nodes may be enlarged due to metastatic involvement.

Epidemiology

Common. More prevalent in male than females, and mostly in the elderly population. Due to chronic, excess sun exposure in fair-skinned individuals. Other aetiological factors include topical (e.g. tar, cutting oils) and systemic (e.g. arsenic) carcinogens, photochemotherapy and chronic immunosuppression. May arise at sites of long-standing radiation dermatitis, scarring (e.g. discoid lupus erythematous) or ulceration (Marjolin's ulcer). Smoking is associated with lesions on the lip (**264**).

Malignant Neoplasms and their Precursors

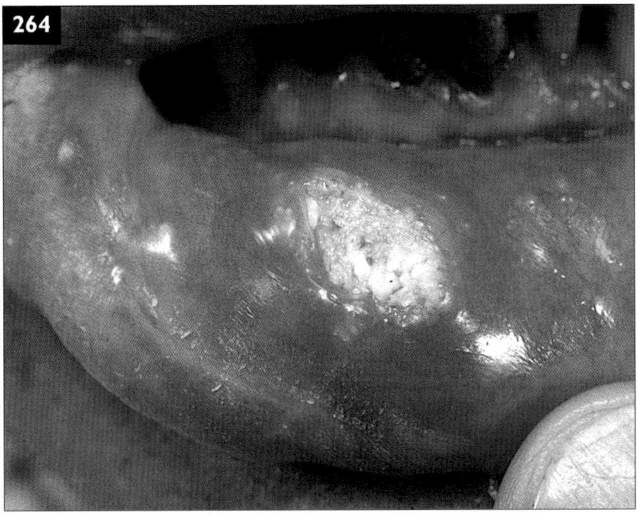

264 Squamous cell carcinoma on the lower lip.

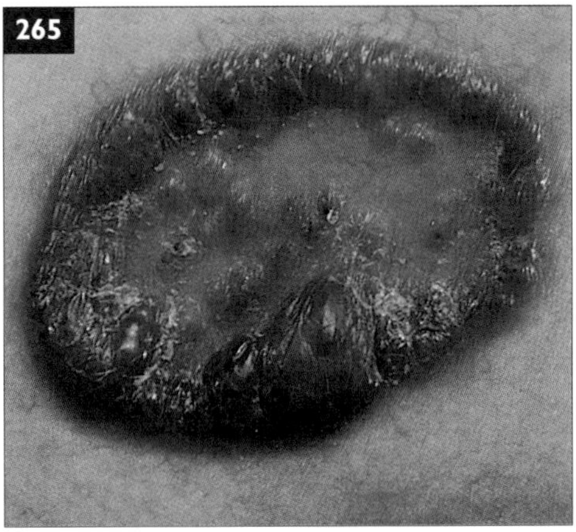

265 Pigmented basal cell carcinoma.

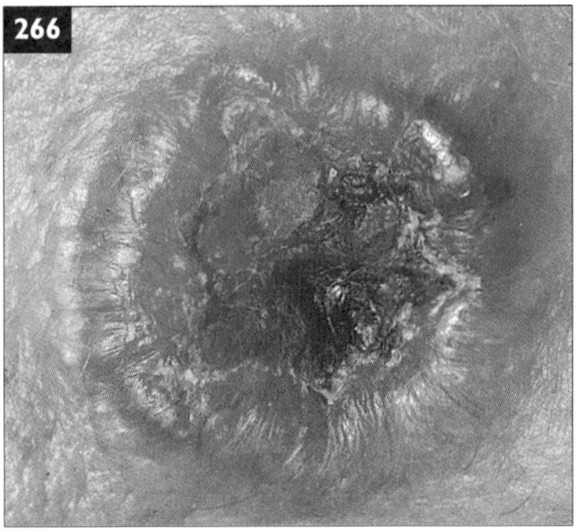

266 Basal cell carcinoma showing the 'rolled' pearly edge.

Differential diagnosis
Keratoacanthoma, proliferative solar keratosis, Bowen's disease.

Investigations
Biopsy.

Special points
Scrotal squamous cell carcinoma is practically always occupational.

BASAL CELL CARCINOMA (BASAL CELL EPITHELIOMA)

Definition and clinical features
A slow growing, locally destructive, tumour due to proliferation of basal keratinocytes.

Nodular or solid basal cell carcinoma arises on the forehead, nose or adjacent to the inner canthus of the eye. A skin-coloured, pink or pigmented (**265**), translucent nodule with surface telangiectasia; gradual enlargement leads to central ulceration and a peripheral, 'rolled' pearly edge (**266**).

Malignant Neoplasms and their Precursors

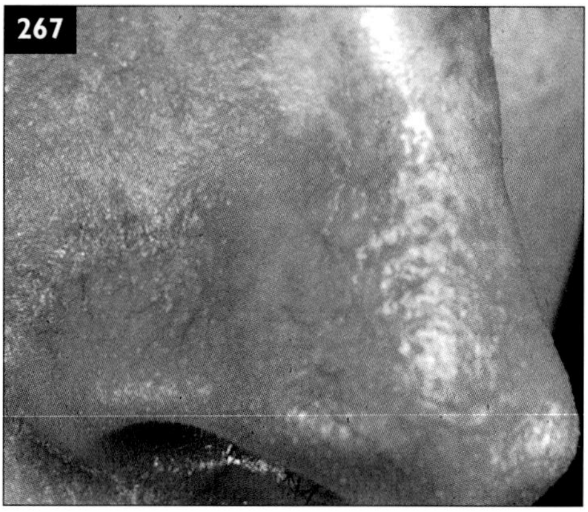

267 Morphoeic basal cell carcinoma.

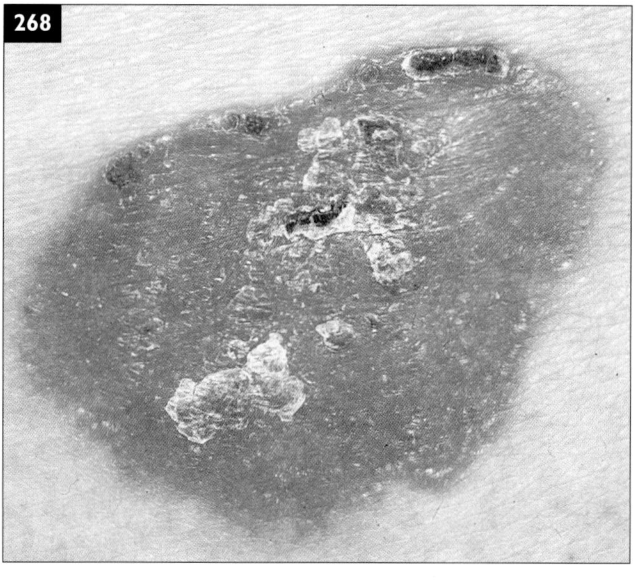

268 Superficial basal cell carcinoma.

Morphoeic basal cell carcinoma presents as a firm, indurated, skin-coloured, scar-like plaque (**267**) with ill-defined edges, commonly on the nasolabial fold or forehead.

Superficial multifocal basal cell carcinoma tends to arise on extrafacial sites as red, scaly plaques (**268**).

Epidemiology

This is the most common type of skin cancer – the ratio of basal to squamous cell carcinoma is approximately 4:1. Related to chronic, excess sun exposure in white-skinned individuals. Lesions may arise in a pre-existing naevus sebaceus or in individuals with the basal cell naevus syndrome, or following arsenic ingestion (when lesions particularly arise on extrafacial sites).

Differential diagnosis

Superficial basal cell carcinoma may mimic Bowen's disease, and morphoeic-type basal cell carcinomas may be dismissed as scar tissue. Deeply pigmented lesions should be differentiated from malignant melanoma.

Investigations

Biopsy.

Benign Melanocytic Lesions

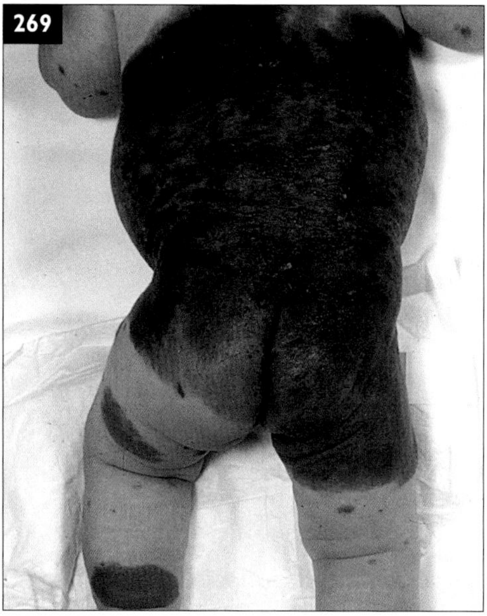

269 Giant congenital melanocytic naevus.

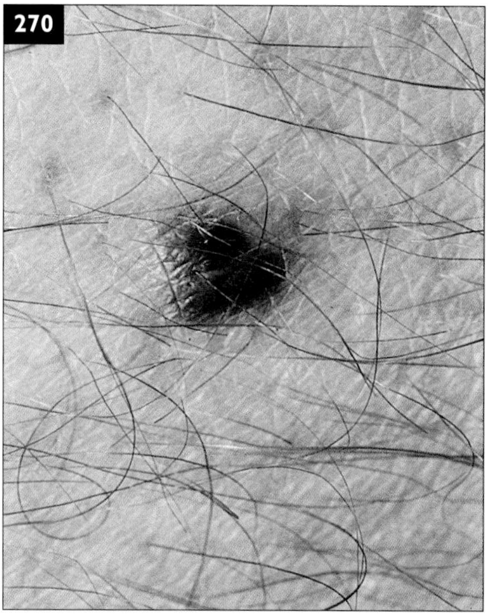

270 Blue naevus.

CONGENITAL MELANOCYTIC NAEVUS

Definition and clinical features

Pigmented naevus present at birth derived from melanocytes. Congenital naevi may be divided into small (less than 1.5 cm in diameter), medium (less than 20 cm in diameter) and giant (greater than 20 cm in diameter) (**269**). During infancy, naevi may be pale brown; increasing pigmentation and excessive terminal hair growth characterise older lesions. Giant naevi may be associated with underlying spinal defects, pigmentation of leptomeninges and numerous small congenital naevi elsewhere.

Epidemiology

The prevalence of small congenital naevi is estimated at approximately 1% of new-born infants; giant congenital naevi are rare (less than 0.002% of infants).

Differential diagnosis

Vascular and epidermal naevi.

Investigations

Biopsy if malignant change is suspected.

Special points

Giant melanocytic naevi are associated with an estimated lifetime risk of malignant transformation of approximately 5%. The risk associated with medium and small congenital naevi has not been satisfactorily established.

BLUE NAEVUS

Definition and clinical features

A deep dermal aggregate of melanocytes. An evenly pigmented bluish macule or papule (**270**) on the face, less commonly on the limbs and buttocks.

Epidemiology

This condition occurs in older children and young adults. The dermal, spindle-shaped melanocytes are thought to represent melanocytes which have failed to migrate to the epidermis during foetal life. Malignant change is rare.

Differential diagnosis

Density of pigment may cause confusion with malignant melanoma.

Benign Melanocytic Lesions

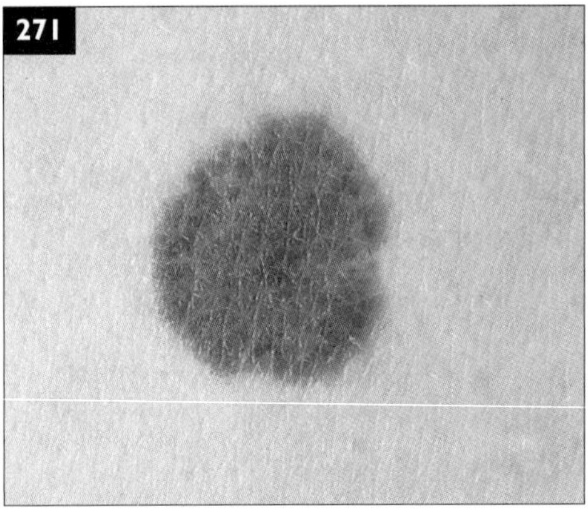

271 Junctional naevus.

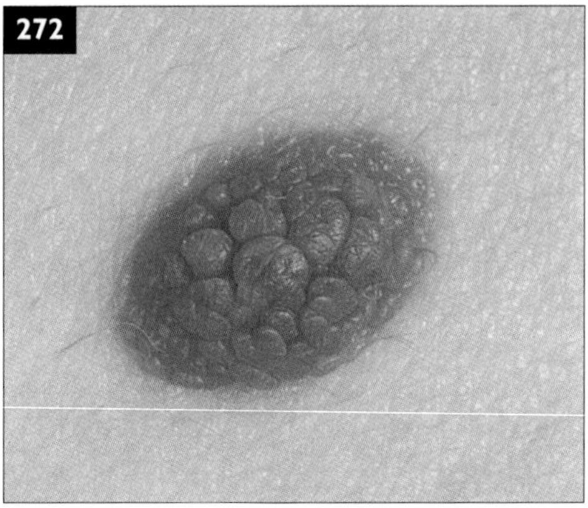

272 Compound naevus.

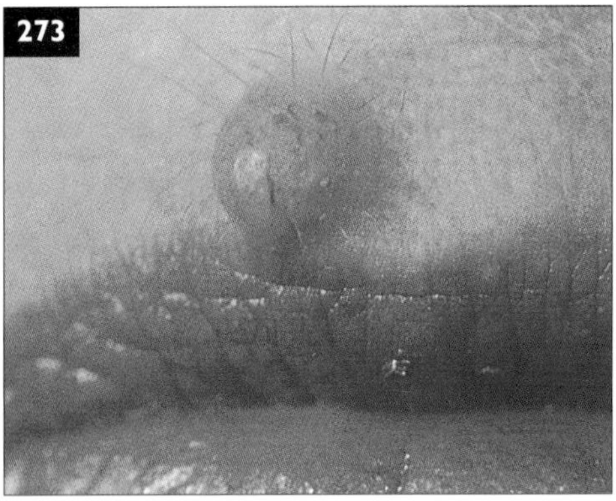

273 Intradermal naevus.

Investigations

Biopsy.

BENIGN ACQUIRED MELANOCYTIC NAEVUS

Definition and clinical features

A benign proliferation of melanocytes. Clusters of melanocytes are initially confined to the basal layer of epidermis (junctional naevus) and then migrate into dermis (compound and intradermal naevi).

Junctional naevi present as small (0.1–1 cm in diameter), dark-brown, evenly pigmented, symmetrical macules or minimally elevated papules (**271**). The majority of naevi in children are junctional and occur on any body site – those found in adults are confined to the palms, soles and genitalia. Compound naevi (where melanocytes are present in both the epidermis and the dermis) occur at any site and vary from light-brown, pigmented papules to dark-brown papillomatous and sometimes hyperkeratotic plaques (**272**). Intradermal naevi occur predominantly in the third decade, frequently on the face and may be devoid of pigment. They may be dome-shaped or papillomatous nodules, or pedunculated skin tags (**273**).

Epidemiology

Common. The frequency of naevi increases slowly during childhood and sometimes sharply at puberty. Numbers reach a plateau in the third decade and slowly disappear thereafter to become rare in old age. Numbers may increase following sun exposure, pregnancy or immunosuppression.

Differential diagnosis

Junctional and compound naevi may be confused with lentigines or seborrhoeic keratoses, respectively.

Investigations

Biopsy is required only where clinical differentiation from malignant melanoma is difficult.

Special points

Malignant change in acquired benign melanocytic naevi is extremely rare.

Benign Melanocytic Lesions

ATYPICAL MELANOCYTIC NAEVUS (DYSPLASTIC NAEVUS)

Definition and clinical features

A compound (or less commonly junctional) melanocytic naevus with atypical clinical and/or histological features (see Special points below). It is a pigmented lesion with a few or all of the following features (**274**):

- Size greater than 0.5 cm in diameter.
- Irregular, smudged border.
- Irregular pigmentation.
- Associated erythema.
- Both a papular and macular component.

Those with the so-called atypical mole syndrome (either familial or sporadic) have multiple atypical naevi distributed on non-sun-exposed sites (buttocks, genitalia, scalp, soles, dorsa of feet).

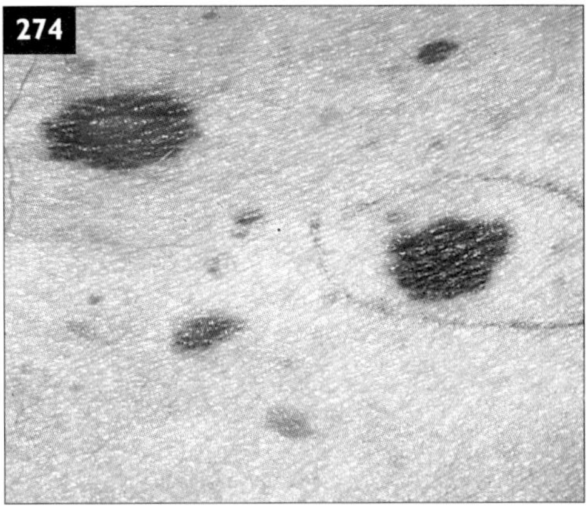

274 Atypical melanocytic (dysplastic) naevus.

Epidemiology

The atypical mole phenotype may be inherited as an autosomal dominant trait or occur sporadically. Those with the very rare familial form where first degree relatives have atypical naevi and a history of multiple malignant melanoma characteristically develop multiple primary malignant melanomas. Estimates of the prevalence of the sporadic form vary between 1 and 5% of the population. The risk of melanoma in these individuals may be increased by a factor of ten.

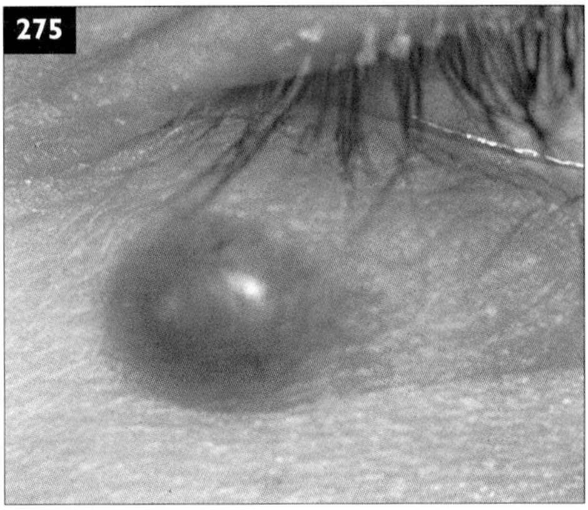

275 Juvenile melanoma.

Investigations

Biopsy may demonstrate cytological melanocytic atypia, architectural atypia (bridging of rete ridges, lentiginous melanocytic hyperplasia) and host response (lymphocytic infiltrate, lamellar fibrosis).

Special points

The definition of an atypical naevus may or may not include histological features of atypia. Epidemiological studies examining associated risks of malignant melanoma are based, in general, on clinical, rather than histological, features of atypia. Clinical atypia may be present in the absence of histological atypia, and vice versa.

SPINDLE AND EPITHELIOID NAEVUS (SPITZ NAEVUS; JUVENILE MELANOMA)

Definition and clinical features

A benign melanocytic tumour clinically and histopathologically distinct from common acquired melanocytic naevi. The majority occur in children as a discrete, red-brown or pink papule on the face (**275**). The dorsum of the hand is an additional site in adults. The initial papule may increase rapidly to reach 1–2 cm in diameter but thereafter remains static.

Epidemiology

Probably represents 1% of all childhood naevi although its true prevalence is difficult to ascertain.

Differential diagnosis

Malignant melanoma, benign melanocytic naevus, juvenile xanthogranuloma.

Benign Melanocytic Lesions

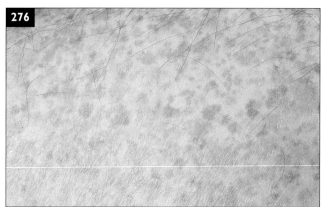

276 Freckles.

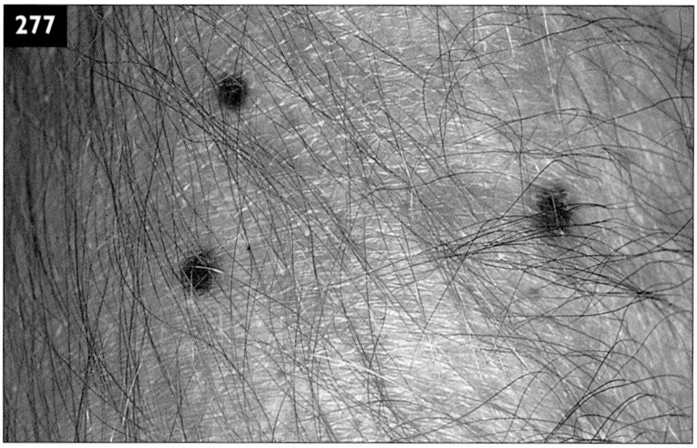

277 Lentigines.

Investigations

Lesions in adults should be excised.

FRECKLES (EPHELIDES)

Definition and clinical features

Pale brown macules, less than 3 mm in diameter, due to the UV-induced production of melanin by a normal number of basal melanocytes. They are multiple and distributed on sun-exposed sites (**276**). Prominent during the summer particularly following UV exposure; virtually disappear in the winter.

Epidemiology

Common, especially in children and individuals with Type I or II skin.

Differential diagnosis

Lentigo.

LENTIGO

Definition and clinical features

Symmetrical brown macule due to a linear increase in the number of melanocytes within the basal layer of the epidermis (**277**). Lentigines may occur at any site on the skin, conjunctivae and mucocutaneous junctions. In contrast to freckles, lentigines are unaffected by sunlight. Pigmentation may be increased by pregnancy and in Addison's disease.

Epidemiology

Lentigo is common. Multiple lentigines may rarely be a manifestation of Peutz–Jeghers disease (particularly when distributed on the lips, buccal mucosae and acral sites), centrofacial lentiginosis (associated with cardiac abnormalities) and the LEOPARD syndrome (i.e. lentigines, ECG abnormalities, ocular hypertelorism, pulmonary

Benign Melanocytic Lesions

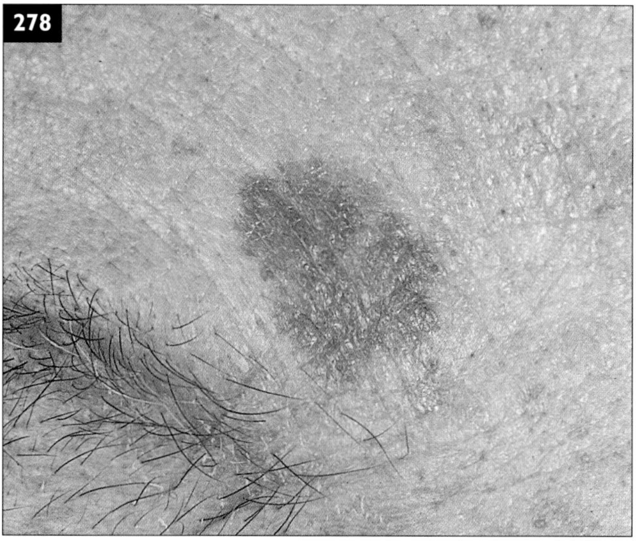

278 Solar lentigo.

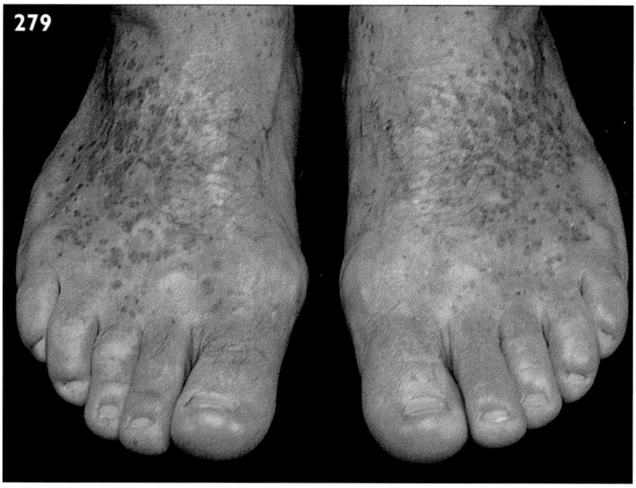

279 Multiple solar lentigines from PUVA therapy.

stenosis, abnormal genitalia, retarded growth, deafness).

Differential diagnosis

Freckle, junctional melanocytic naevus.

SOLAR LENTIGO (LENTIGO SENILIS; ACTINIC LENTIGO)

Definition and clinical features

An irregular brown macule that appears on either acute or chronic sun exposure due to a linear increase in the numbers of melanocytes in the basal layer of the epidermis. It appears on sun-exposed sites following either acute, severe sunburn in young adults or chronic UV exposure in elderly individuals (liver or age spots) (**278**). Multiple solar lentigines may result from PUVA therapy (**279**) or excessive sunbed use.

Epidemiology

Common.

Malignant Melanoma

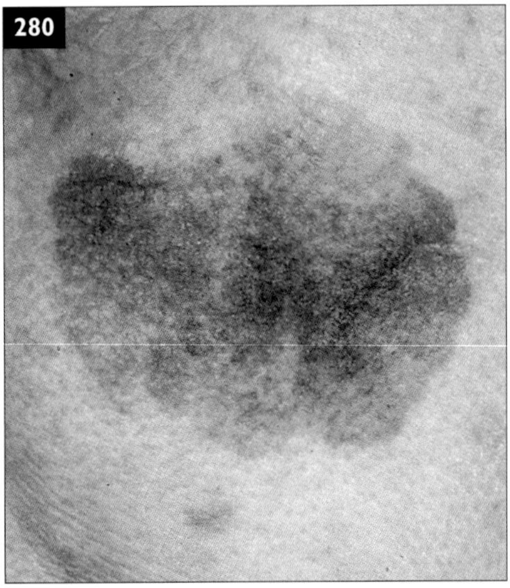
280 Lentigo maligna.

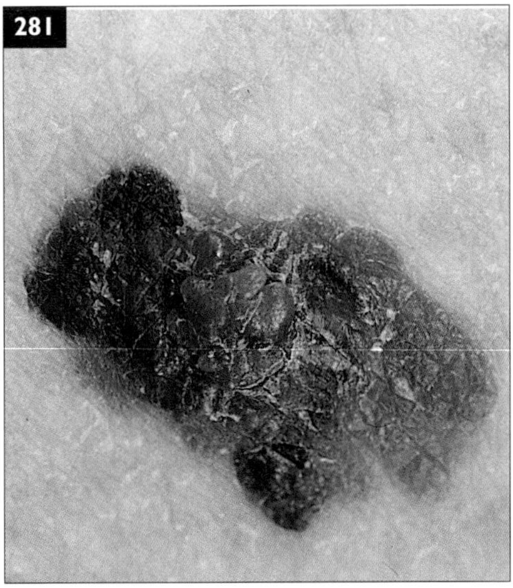
281 Superficial spreading melanoma.

Definition and clinical features

A malignant proliferation of melanocytes. Features more commonly seen in malignant than in benign melanocytic lesions include a diameter greater than 1 cm, increasing size, variation in pigment, irregular edge, presence of inflammation, crusting or bleeding, altered sensation or itch. Four main clinical subtypes are recognised:

- Lentigo maligna – an irregularly pigmented macule, slowly enlarging over many years, commonly on the cheek or temple of an elderly person (**280**). Development of a more rapidly growing, deeply pigmented papule or nodule indicates dermal invasion by malignant melanocytes (lentigo maligna melanoma).
- Superficial spreading melanoma – a macule or papule, usually greater than 0.5 cm in diameter at presentation, with variable pigmentation from pale brown to blue-black, an irregular edge, and surface oozing or crusting (**281**).
- Nodular melanoma – a rapidly enlarging, frequently ulcerated, blue-black nodule (**282**).
- Acral lentiginous melanoma – an irregularly pigmented macule on the sole of the foot or palm of the hand (**283**). Subungual or periungual melanoma (a variant of acral lentiginous melanoma) occurs either as a linear pigmented streak in the nail or an isolated nail dystrophy, accompanied by pigmentation of the proximal nail fold (Hutchinson's sign) (**284**).

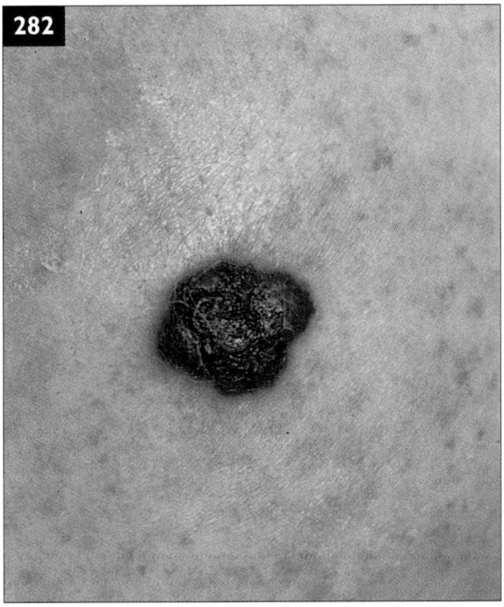
282 Nodular melanoma

Malignant Melanoma

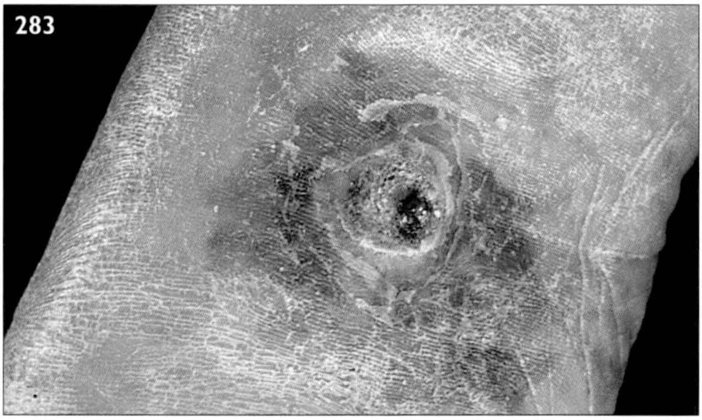

283 Acral lentiginous melanoma.

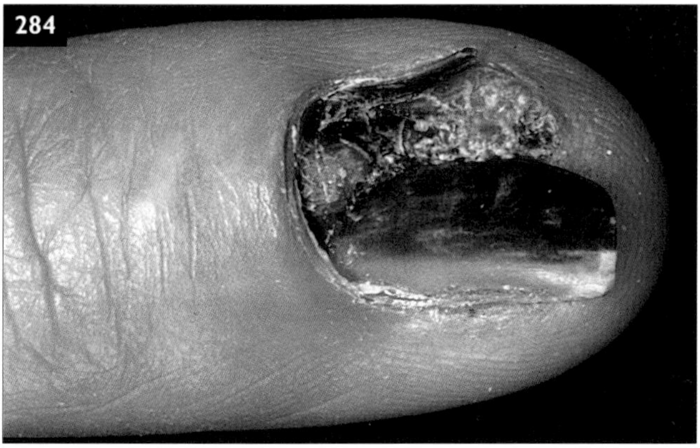

284 Subungual melanoma.

Epidemiology

Incidence of (and mortality from) melanoma is increasing: the highest figures recorded are in white-skinned individuals in Australia and New Zealand. UV exposure is a major aetiological factor, particularly short, intense, exposure resulting in sunburn, and during childhood. Lentigo maligna contrasts with this pattern, where total cumulative exposure appears to be more relevant. Phenotypic risk factors include fair skin, red or blonde hair, blue eyes, inability to tan, freckles, lentigines, large numbers of benign melanocytic naevi and the presence of atypical naevi.

Melanoma is more common in women than men. It most frequently involves the lower leg in women, and the back in men.

Differential diagnosis

Melanoma must be distinguished from benign pigmented or vascular lesions. Particular difficulty may arise in differentiating lentigo maligna from simple lentigo, seborrhoeic keratosis or pigmented solar keratosis; or differentiating nodular melanoma from a vascular tumour or pyogenic granuloma; or differentiating subungual melanoma from fungal infection or subungual haematoma.

Investigations

Excision or biopsy.

Special points

Any change in a pre-existing pigmented lesion should alert the clinician to the possibility of malignant melanoma. Prognosis is significantly related to the Breslow thickness (the depth of dermal invasion by malignant melanocytes from the granular cell layer) and therefore early diagnosis is crucial.

Cutaneous Lymphoproliferative Disorders

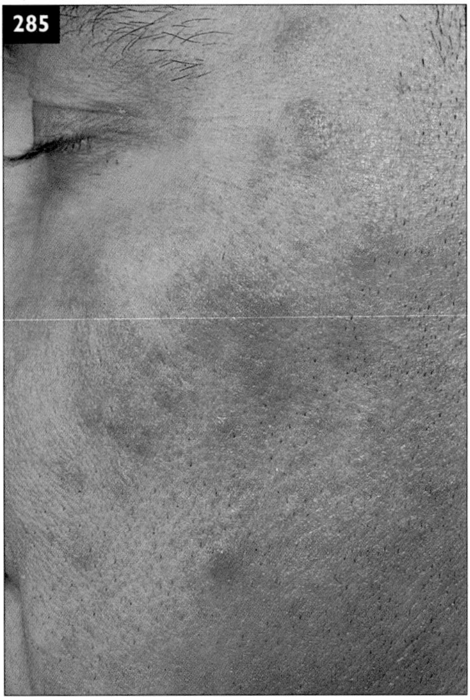

285 Benign lymphocytic infiltrate of Jessner–Kanof.

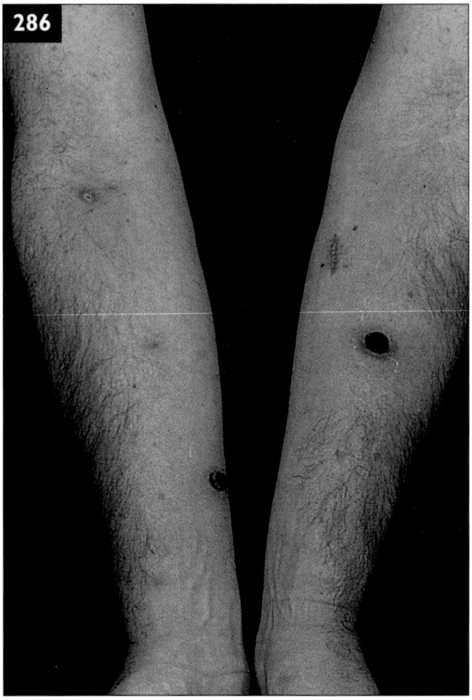

286 Lymphomatoid papulosis.

BENIGN LYMPHOCYTIC INFILTRATE OF JESSNER–KANOF

Definition and clinical features

A chronic, benign disorder of unknown cause, characterised by multiple, smooth, cherry-pink papules on the head and neck (**285**). Lesions may coalesce and are non-scarring. Histology shows a perivascular, lymphocytic infiltrate in the superficial and mid-dermis, with a normal overlying epidermis. Treatment with potent topical or intralesional corticosteroids or antimalarial drugs may be tried, but the condition often proves resistant to therapy.

Epidemiology

Usually affects adults, and is more common in males. Familial cases have been reported.

Investigations

Histology usually helps support the diagnosis, although there is much overlap with other diseases characterised by dermal lymphocytic infiltrates. Direct immunofluorescence and serum autoimmune profile are negative and can help exclude lupus erythematosus.

Differential diagnosis

Lupus erythematosus, pseudolymphoma and malignant lymphocytic infiltrates such as chronic lymphocytic leukaemia and lymphoma.

LYMPHOMATOID PAPULOSIS

Definition and clinical features

A benign lymphoproliferative disorder characterised by recurrent, scaly papules which heal with scars. There are recurrent, well-circumscribed, red-brown indurated papules with a collarette of scale, of variable size, up to 2 cm in diameter, which may heal spontaneously to leave depigmented, atrophic scars. Distributed predominantly on the inner flexural aspects of the limbs (**286**).

Epidemiology

Rare. Approximately 5% of patients go on to develop systemic lymphoma.

Cutaneous Lymphoproliferative Disorders

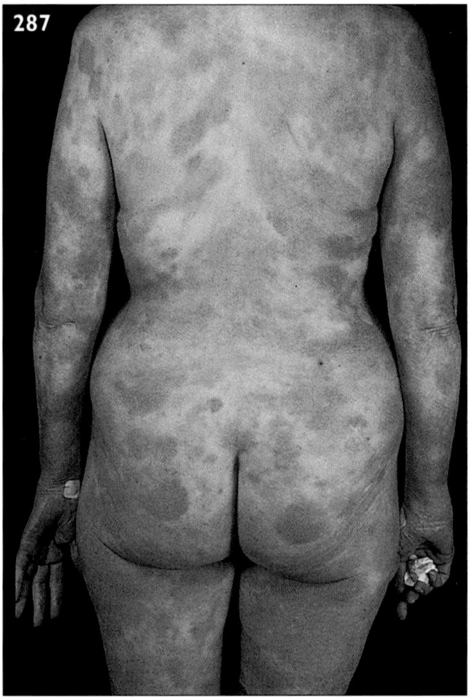

287 Plaque stage mycosis fungoides.

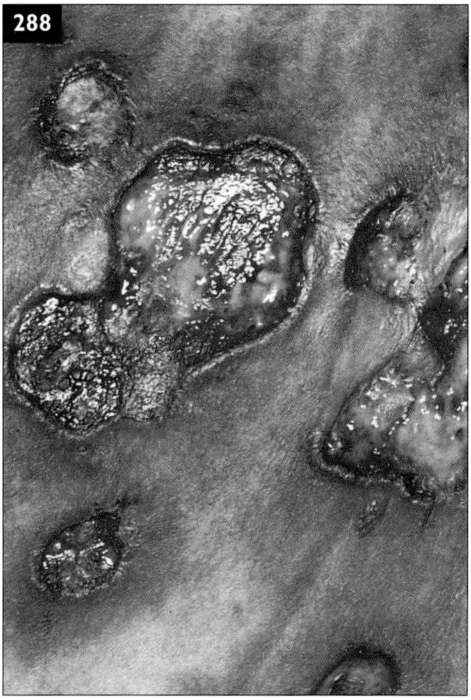

288 Tumour stage mycosis fungoides.

Differential diagnosis
Pityriasis lichenoides chronica, cutaneous B cell lymphoma.

Investigations
Biopsy.

MYCOSIS FUNGOIDES
Definition and clinical features
A low grade, cutaneous T cell lymphoma which gives rise to a chronic, scaly dermatosis, and rarely lymph node and systemic involvement. Cutaneous involvement may manifest as patch, plaque and tumour stage disease. Initially presents as asymptomatic or slightly itchy chronic, scaly, erythematous patches, of variable size. These may be distributed anywhere but occur especially on the trunk and buttocks (**287**). The majority of patients do not progress beyond this stage. Patches may develop into infiltrated, purplish-red plaques and, rarely, ulcerating plaques or nodules (tumour stage) (**288**). All three stages may occur concurrently.

Involvement of the scalp may lead to alopecia. Peripheral lymphadenopathy and, rarely, hepatosplenomegaly and systemic lymphomatous infiltration may develop.

Epidemiology
Rare. Affects males more than females, predominantly in the sixth and seventh decades. Due to clonal proliferation of T helper cells; proposed aetiological factors include HTLV1 infection and an abnormal response to chronic antigenic stimulation.

Differential diagnosis
Eczema, psoriasis and chronic superficial scaly dermatitis.

Investigations
Biopsy. Radiological and haematological investigation to exclude systemic involvement where extensive plaque or tumour stage disease is present. T cell receptor gene rearrangement studies may identify early skin or lymph node involvement.

Cutaneous Lymphoproliferative Disorders

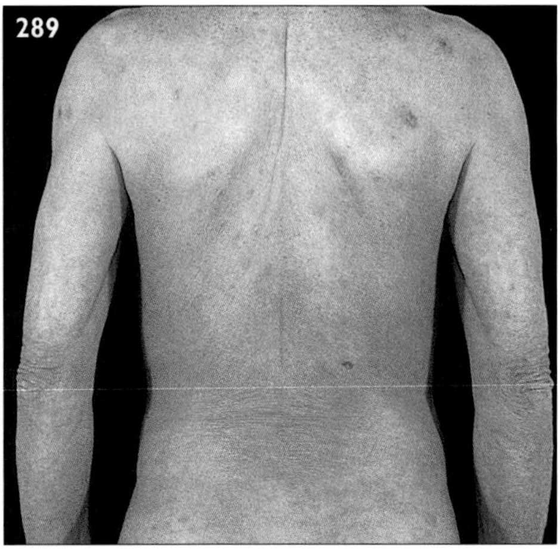

289 Erythroderma in Sézary syndrome.

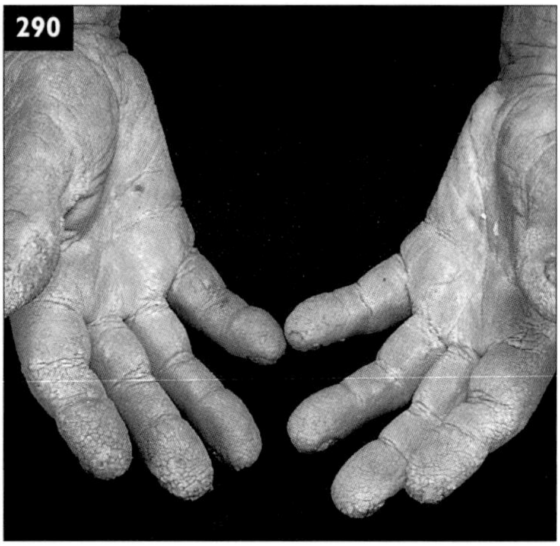

290 Keratoderma in Sézary syndrome.

SÉZARY SYNDROME

Definition and clinical features

T cell leukaemia giving rise to erythroderma (**289**), lymphadenopathy, pruritus and circulating atypical lymphocytes (Sézary cells). Also lymphadenopathy, hepatomegaly, alopecia, nail dystrophy and keratoderma (**290**).

Epidemiology

Rare. Occurs in males more often than females and usually presents in the sixth and seventh decades. Putative aetiological agents include environmental toxins (e.g. pesticides, solvents) and HTLV1 infection.

Differential diagnosis

Other causes of erythroderma.

Investigations

Biopsy of skin and lymph node. Blood film for Sézary cells.

CUTANEOUS B CELL LYMPHOMA

Definition and clinical features

A malignant proliferation of B lymphocytes within the skin that presents as multiple, smooth, red-purple, indurated plaques and nodules of variable size, on the head and neck (**291**). May heal spontaneously.

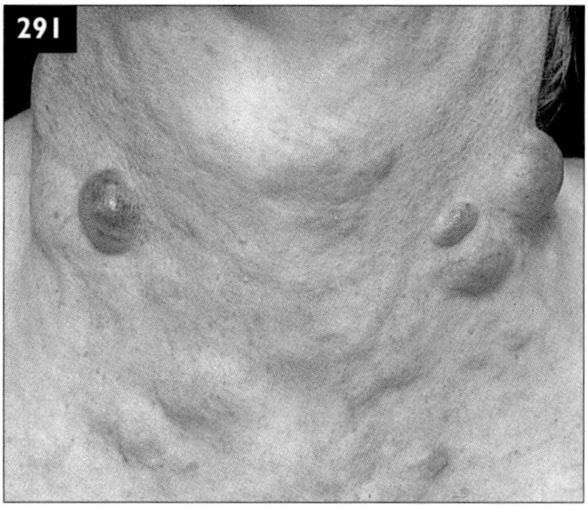

291 Cutaneous B cell lymphoma.

Epidemiology

Rare. Most have an excellent prognosis, in contrast to B cell lymphomas occurring at extracutaneous sites.

Differential diagnosis

Benign lymphocytic infiltrates.

Investigations

Biopsy.

Blisters – Introduction

292

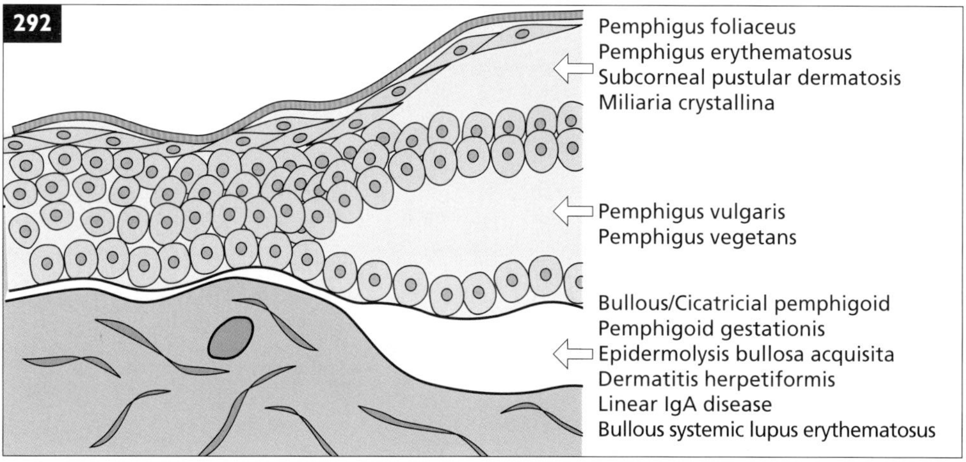

292 Level of cleavage of blister in the bullous skin diseases.

Blistering may be a feature of a wide range of skin diseases. The autoimmune bullous diseases are a rare group of disorders characterised by blistering and erosions of the skin and/or mucous membranes. The morphology of the blister depends on the level of the split within the skin (**292**). Subcorneal (beneath the stratum corneum) and intraepidermal blisters (within the prickle cell layer) rupture easily, whereas subepidermal ones (between the dermis and epidermis) are less fragile.

Immunofluorescence (IF) techniques are the mainstay of diagnosis and classification of bullous diseases. In pemphigus, pemphigoid, dermatitis herpetiformis and linear IgA bullous dermatosis the findings are specific for the particular disease (*Table 1*). Direct IF of the skin or mucosal surface demonstrates where immunoglobulins, components of complement (C3) and fibrinogen have been deposited. Indirect IF of the serum detects circulating autoantibodies. Split skin techniques, which artificially cleave the lamina lucida of the basement membrane zone (BMZ), improve the sensitivity of indirect IF and aid diagnosis of subepidermal bullous diseases.

Blisters – Introduction

Disease	Direct	Indirect
Pemphigus		
foliaceus	Intercellular IgG	Intercellular IgG
vulgaris	When disease is active,C3 is present	
vegetans		
erythematosus	Mixed IF pattern with intercellular IgG/C3 associated with granular BMZ	Intercellular IgG
Pemphigoid		
bullous	Linear BMZ IgG/C3	Anti-BMZ IgG. The binding on split skin is to the roof
cicatricial		
Pemphigoid gestationis	Linear BMZ C3	Complement binding and anti-BMZ IgG. The binding on split skin is to the roof
Epidermolysis bullosa skin acquisita	Linear BMZ IgG	Anti-BMZ IgG. The binding on split is to the base
Linear IgA bullous dermatosis (LAD and CBDC)	Linear BMZ IgA	Anti-BMZ IgA. The binding on split skin is usually to the roof
Dermatitis herpetiformis	Granular deposits of IgA in the dermal papillae	No circulating antibodies to BMZ or dermal papillae components * IgA endomysial antibodies
Discoid lupus erythematosus	Granular BMZ IgM band (lupus band) in lesional skin; uninvolved skin is negative	
Systemic lupus erythematosus	Granular BMZ IgM band (lupus band) in both lesional and uninvolved skin	

* This is a specific marker for the presence of underlying gluten-sensitive enteropathy

Table 1 Immunofluorescence findings.

Subcorneal Blisters

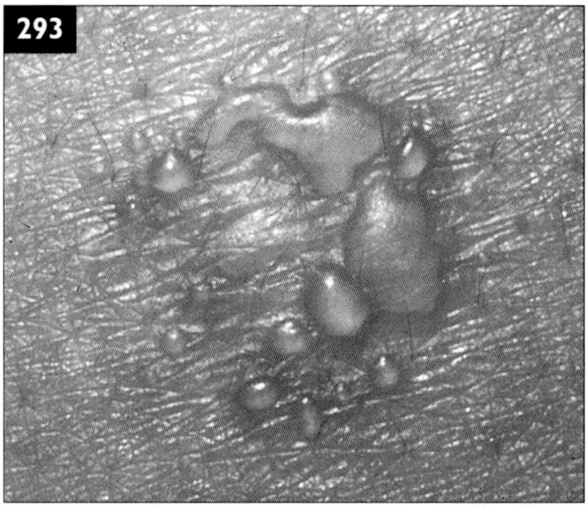

293 Miliaria crystallina.

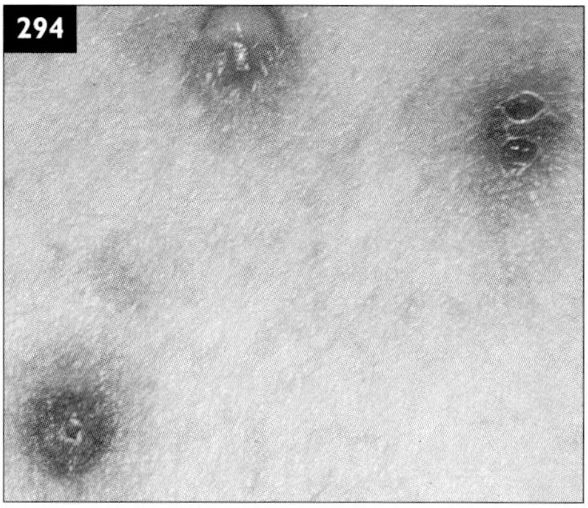

294 Subcorneal pustular dermatosis.

MILIARIA CRYSTALLINA

Definition and clinical features

Miliaria crystallina follows the superficial obstruction of sweat ducts, leading to the development of subcorneal vesicles. The proposed mechanism is that sweat accumulates under the stratum corneum leading to the appearance of vesicles without underlying erythema. Clear thin-walled vesicles about 1–2 mm in diameter develop on non-inflamed skin (**293**). Lesions occur in crops, especially on the trunk, and are asymptomatic. In persistent febrile illnesses, recurrent crops may occur. The vesicles rupture easily and are followed by a superficial brawny desquamation. Lesions may become secondarily infected with bacteria.

Epidemiology

Miliaria crystallina is often seen in febrile illnesses associated with profuse sweating. It may also occur after heavy exertion.

Special points

A cool water compress and proper ventilation are all that is necessary to treat this self-limiting process.

SUBCORNEAL PUSTULAR DERMATOSIS

Definition and clinical features

Subcorneal pustular dermatosis is also called Sneddon–Wilkinson disease. It is a chronic, benign, relapsing, pustular eruption which has a distinctive histology with subcorneal blisters containing neutrophils. The individual lesion is either pustular from the start or pustules appear after a very transient vesicular stage. The pustule is flaccid, turbid and often oval rather than circular (**294**). Some may demonstrate a level of pus with clear fluid above. Pustules can dry up within a few days resulting in superficial scale and crusting. They form groups and produce a spreading edge. The eruption occurs mainly in the groins, axillary, submammary areas and flexor aspects of the limbs. The face is not usually involved.

Epidemiology

The average age of onset is 40–50 years although it may occur in children. The male to female ratio is 1:4.

Differential diagnosis

Impetigo, pemphigus foliaceus, dermatitis herpetiformis, chronic bullous disease of childhood, eosinophilic spongiosis, erythema multiforme and pustular psoriasis must all be considered.

Investigations

Histology shows numerous neutrophils in a subcorneal blister.

Special points

IgA pemphigus may present with similar clinical features, and shows intercellular IgA in the upper epidermis on direct IF.

Intraepidermal Blisters

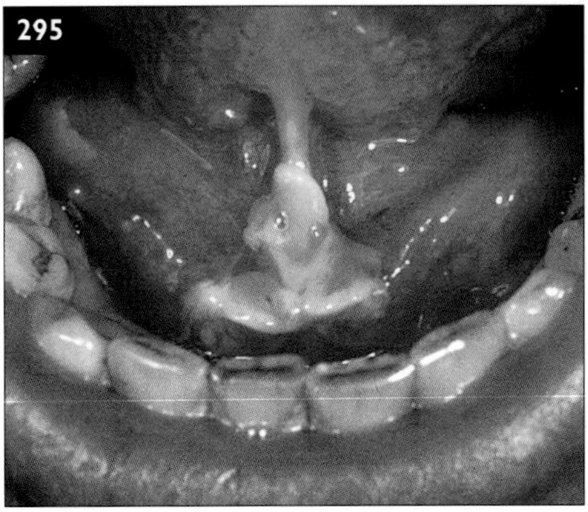

295 Oral pemphigus vulgaris.

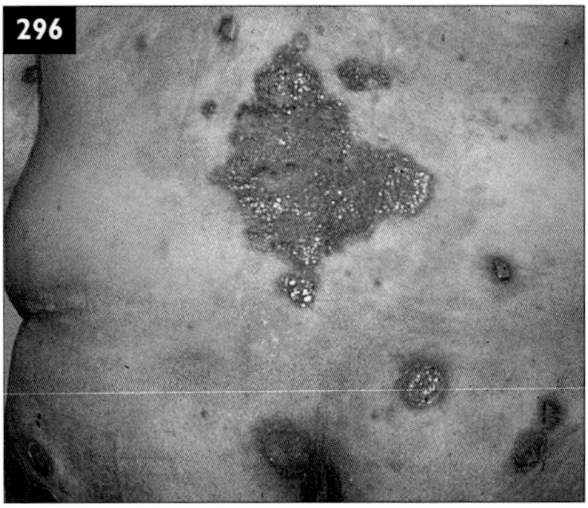

296 Pemphigus vulgaris.

PEMPHIGUS

Definition and clinical features

Pemphigus is an uncommon autoimmune bullous dermatosis caused by a circulating IgG autoantibody directed against epidermal antigens. There are several forms of pemphigus, which differ in their geographical distribution, clinical presentation, histology and target antigens. Pemphigus vulgaris and pemphigus foliaceus are the two main forms, and the rarer variants include pemphigus vegetans, pemphigus erythematosus and pemphigus herpetiformis. Pemphigus mediated by IgA antibodies has been described under a variety of names but is often termed IgA pemphigus (see above).

The disease affects the skin and mucous membranes. Widespread flaccid blisters develop which rapidly rupture forming generalised erosions and crusts, often with secondary bacterial infection. The blisters are not haemorrhagic. Shearing stresses on normal skin may cause a new lesion to form (Nikolsky's sign). The oral cavity is the commonest mucous membrane affected and in one-third of cases the mouth is affected prior to the skin (**295**). Pemphigus vulgaris is the commonest type, in which blisters and erosions predominate (**296**). In pemphigus foliaceus, widespread very superficial blisters rupture, leaving predominantly erosions and crusts (**297**). There is no mucosal involvement. Pemphigus vegetans is a more localised form in which heaped-up or cauliflower-like lesions are present, especially in flexural sites such as the groins and axillae (**298**). Pemphigus erythematosus (also called Senear–Usher disease) probably represents pemphigus occurring together with lupus erythematosus. Paraneoplastic pemphigus has been described in patients with underlying malignancy. Transient neonatal disease may occur in the offspring of mothers with pemphigus, due to transplacental transfer of IgG autoantibodies.

Epidemiology

Pemphigus is a disease of all ages and shows marked racial and geographical variation. The commonest age of onset is in the fifth and sixth decades. Pemphigus vulgaris tends to be common in Jews and in India. Pemphigus foliaceus is endemic in Brazil, where it affects all age groups, and is thought to be initiated by an insect-borne trigger. Drug-induced cases may also occur.

Differential diagnosis

Other immunobullous disorders, impetigo and seborrhoeic eczema (pemphigus foliaceus).

Investigations

Biopsy shows intraepidermal blisters high in the epidermis in pemphigus foliaceus and suprabasal in pemphigus vulgaris. Acantholysis of the epidermal cells is seen in both forms. Direct IF of uninvolved skin shows characteristic intercellular epidermal deposits of IgG and C3. Around 90% of patients also have circulating autoantibodies. Western blotting of serum helps distinguish the different types.

Intraepidermal Blisters

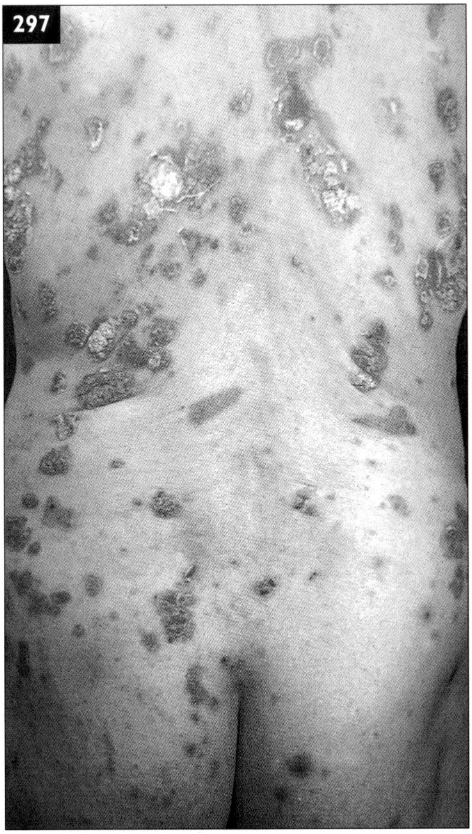

297 Pemphigus foliaceus.

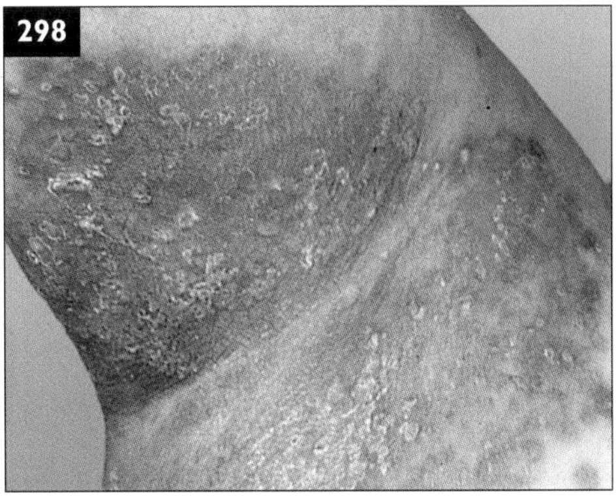

298 Pemphigus vegetans.

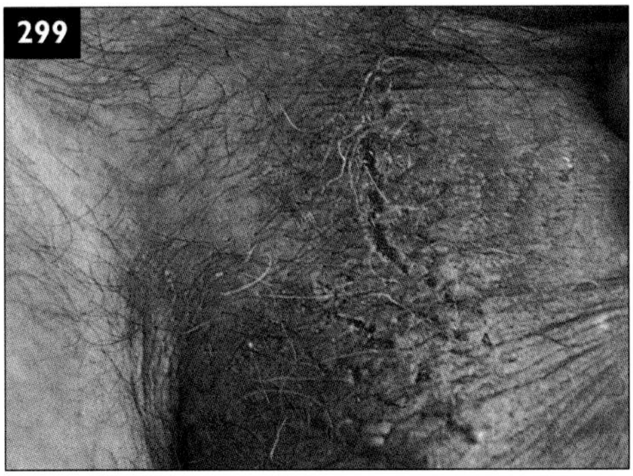

299 Hailey–Hailey disease.

Special points

The titre of circulating autoantibody often correlates with disease activity.

HAILEY–HAILEY DISEASE (BENIGN FAMILIAL CHRONIC PEMPHIGUS)

Definition and clinical features

Hailey–Hailey disease is a rare autosomal dominant genodermatosis, characterised by defective keratinocyte adhesion, and has been mapped to chromosome 3 (*cf.* Darier's disease – chromosome 12). Small blisters develop in the intertriginous areas, such as the axillae, groins and submammary regions. The neck may also be involved. The blisters easily rupture resulting in erythematous eroded areas on which crusts form. A typical feature is small linear fissures in the affected skin (**299**).

Epidemiology

The disease usually presents in early or middle adult life and both sexes are equally affected.

Differential diagnosis

Seborrhoeic eczema, psoriasis, fungal and especially candidal infections.

Investigations

Skin biopsy shows separation of suprabasal keratinocytes (acantholysis) leading to splits, lacunae and blisters. Dyskeratosis and acanthosis may also occur. Direct and indirect IF are negative.

Special points

Secondary bacterial, candidal or herpes simplex infection can cause exacerbations.

Subepidermal Blisters

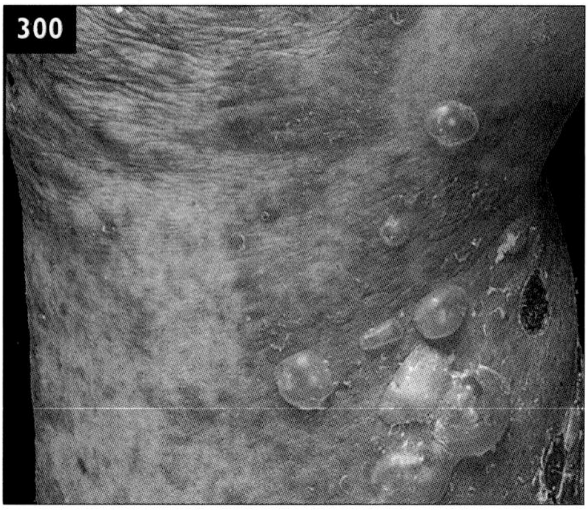

300 Bullous pemphigoid.

BULLOUS PEMPHIGOID

Definition and clinical features

Bullous pemphigoid is a chronic autoimmune condition in which subepidermal blisters develop due to a circulating IgG autoantibody directed against the dermoepidermal junction of the BMZ. Tense blisters develop on erythematous urticarial areas, especially on the flexural aspects of the limbs (**300**). The lesions may be very itchy and the blisters may become large and remain intact for days; sometimes they become haemorrhagic. The face and scalp are not usually affected. The mucous membranes are involved in about 50% of cases. Nikolsky's sign is negative (see under Pemphigus).

Epidemiology

Bullous pemphigoid is predominantly a disease of the elderly. Females are more commonly affected than males. There is no racial or geographical predilection.

Differential diagnosis

Other immunobullous diseases, bullous systemic lupus erythematosus and erythema multiforme. Drugs may induce or trigger pemphigoid.

Investigations

Biopsy shows subepidermal blisters often with an infiltrate of eosinophils. Direct IF of uninvolved skin demonstrates linear deposition of IgG and C3 along the BMZ. Indirect IF demonstrates circulating autoantibodies, which bind to the roof of salt-split skin.

Special points

The titre of circulating autoantibody does not correlate with disease activity. Although such an association was previously suggested, there appears to be no increased risk of malignancy in these patients when compared to age- and sex-matched controls.

CICATRICIAL PEMPHIGOID (BENIGN MUCOUS MEMBRANE PEMPHIGOID)

Definition and clinical features

Cicatricial pemphigoid (also called benign mucous membrane pemphigoid) primarily causes chronic erosion and ulceration of the mucous membranes, but may also affect the skin. The oral mucosa is usually involved. There is a localised ocular variant. Other sites of involvement include the upper respiratory tract, oesophagus and anogenital mucosa, where scarring may result in strictures. Conjunctival involvement may lead to blindness (**301**).

Epidemiology

This disease is less common than bullous pemphigoid. It mainly occurs in middle-aged and elderly people with a female to male ratio of 1.5:1. There does not appear to be any racial or geographical predilection.

Differential diagnosis

Principally from the other subepidermal blistering diseases and erosive lichen planus.

Investigations

Skin biopsy shows subepidermal blistering with eosinophils and neutrophils. There may be dermal scarring. Direct IF of the buccal mucosa is positive in most patients. Circulating autoantibodies may be present in low titre.

Special points

Multidisciplinary management may be indicated.

PEMPHIGOID GESTATIONIS

Definition and clinical features

Pemphigoid gestationis is a rare, acquired bullous disorder associated with pregnancy or the post-partum period. It has occasionally been reported with trophoblastic tumours. It characteristically begins in the second or third trimester. Blisters develop on urticated areas initially around the

Subepidermal Blisters

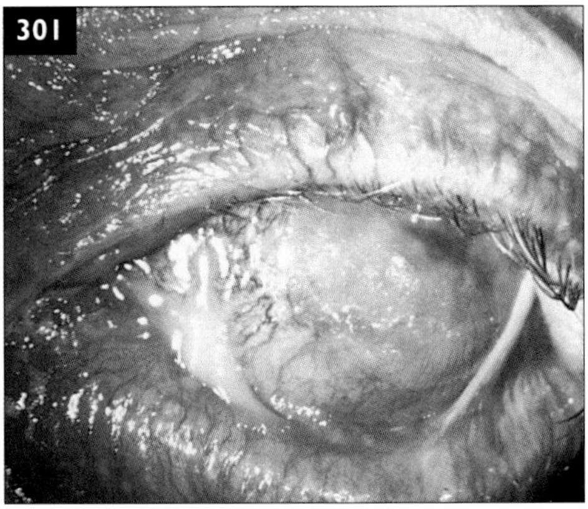

301 Cicatricial pemphigoid.

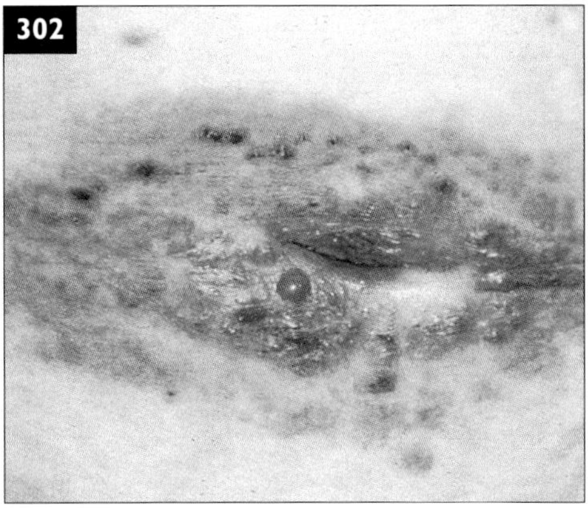

302 Pemphigoid gestationis.

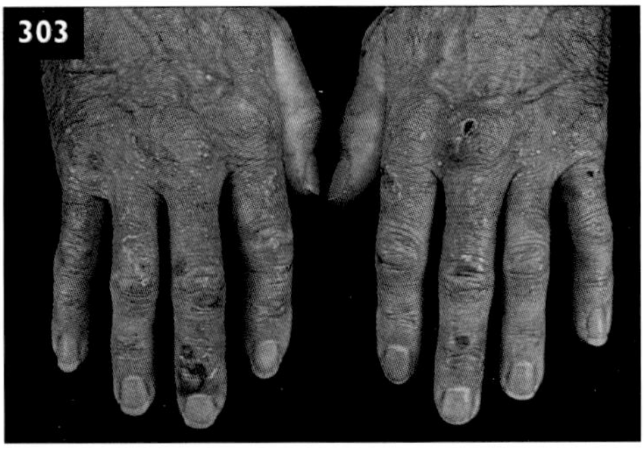

303 Epidermolysis bullosa acquisita.

umbilicus (**302**) and may spread to involve the rest of the body, especially the hands and feet (usually sparing the face and mucosal areas).

Differential diagnosis

Especially in the pre-bullous phase, polymorphic eruption of pregnancy and eczema.

Investigations

Biopsy shows subepidermal blisters. All patients have complement binding activity at the BMZ as shown on direct and indirect IF, and about 50% have circulating autoantibodies.

Special points

Pemphigoid gestationis may occur in subsequent pregnancies, often with increased severity. Transient blistering may occur in the neonate due to the transplacental passage of the autoantibody.

EPIDERMOLYSIS BULLOSA ACQUISITA

Definition and clinical features

Epidermolysis bullosa acquisita (EBA) is one of the rarest immunobullous diseases. The classic form is characterised by acquired fragility, blistering and erosion of the skin and mucosa. Lesions heal with scarring and milia (**303**). An inflammatory bullous-pemphigoid-like variant is also recognised.

Epidemiology

The approximate incidence in Europe is 1 per 5 million per annum.

Differential diagnosis

Porphyria cutanea tarda as well as other blistering disorders.

Investigations

Biopsy usually shows a non-inflammatory subepidermal bulla. The inflammatory variant may have a neutrophilic infiltrate. Circulating IgG BMZ antibodies bind to the dermal side of the salt-split skin. Direct IF is indistinguishable from that of bullous pemphigoid.

Special points

There is an association with inflammatory bowel disease and underlying malignancy The target antigen has been identified as collagen VII of anchoring fibrilla.

Subepidermal Blisters

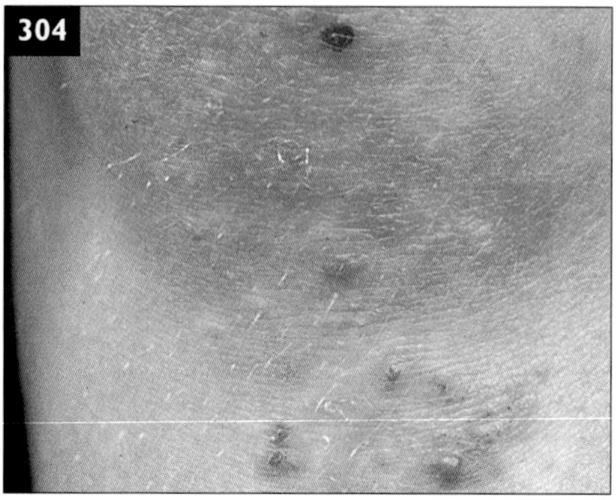

304 Dermatitis herpetiformis.

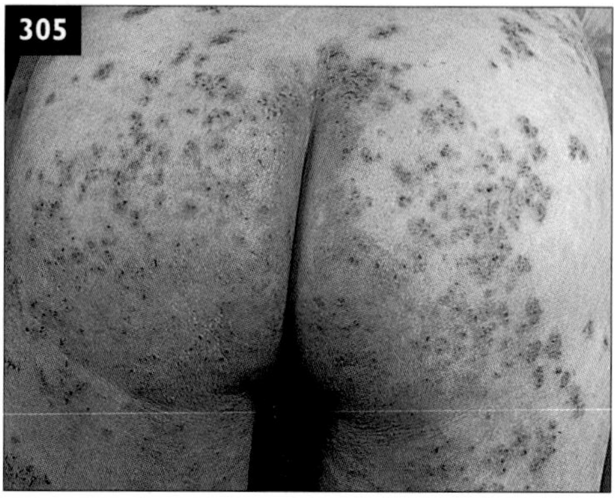

305 Dermatitis herpetiformis.

DERMATITIS HERPETIFORMIS

Definition and clinical features

Dermatitis herpetiformis is an acquired autoimmune disorder with subepidermal blister formation. Grouped papules and vesicles are symmetrically distributed on the extensor aspects of the elbows, knees (**304**), buttocks (**305**), shoulders and scalp and are intensely pruritic. Mucosal involvement is usually minor and asymptomatic. It is associated with gluten-sensitive enteropathy, though this is usually subclinical.

Epidemiology

Dermatitis herpetiformis is essentially a European disease. It most often presents in young adults but any age may be affected. Both adenoviral infection and heavy exposure to cereals have been proposed as triggers.

Differential diagnosis

Other pruritic dermatoses, such as eczema.

Investigations

Biopsy of intact blister and surrounding urticarial skin shows subepidermal blister and papillary microabscesses at the tips of the dermal papillae which are full of neutrophils. The characteristic direct IF feature of normal, uninvolved skin is the presence of granular deposits of IgA in the upper papillary dermis. There are no circulating antibodies to the BMZ or dermal papillae. However, 80% have endomysial antibodies which is a specific marker for the presence of underlying gluten-sensitive enteropathy. Most have an abnormal mucosa on small intestinal biopsy with partial or subtotal villous atrophy on histological examination.

Special points

The eruption responds slowly to the removal of gluten from the diet. Dermatitis herpetiformis is associated with an increased incidence of lymphoma especially affecting the gastrointestinal tract. There is a very high incidence of HLA B8 and DR3, and association with autoimmune disorders such as thyroid disease and pernicious anaemia.

LINEAR IGA DISEASE

Definition and clinical features

Linear IgA disease is a rare, acquired subepidermal blistering disease which has been defined on the basis of its unique immunopathological finding of linear deposits of IgA along the cutaneous basement membrane. It encompasses a clinically heterogeneous group of patients divided into 2 main forms, linear IgA of adults (LAD) and chronic bullous disease of childhood (CBDC).

Clinically it resembles dermatitis herpetiformis but some lesions develop on the trunk and limbs similar to bullous pemphigoid (**306**). The trunk and limbs are almost always involved. However, in young children the perineum is a characteristic site (**307**). Mucosal involvement can be prominent and associated with scarring.

Subepidermal Blisters

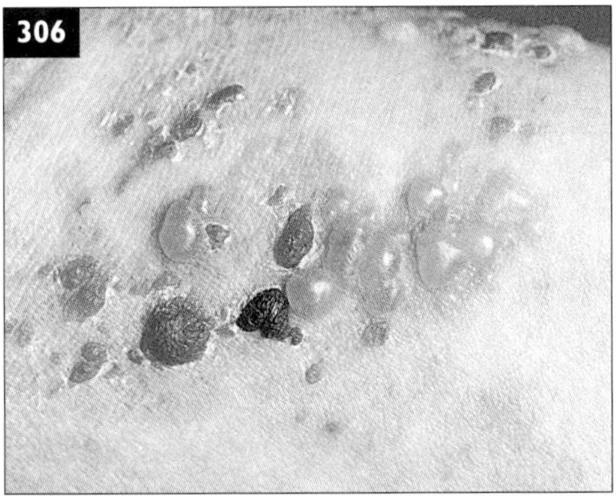

306 Linear IgA disease of adults.

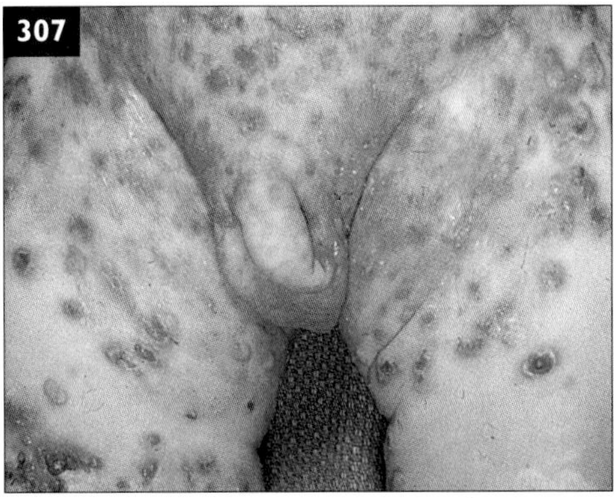

307 Chronic bullous disease of childhood.

Epidemiology
Linear IgA disease is less common in the west than either bullous pemphigoid or dermatitis herpetiformis. LAD may present throughout adult life with peaks at 30 and 65 years. The onset of CBDC is usually in the pre-school years.

Differential diagnosis
Bullous impetigo, erythema multiforme and other immunobullous diseases.

Investigations
Histology shows a subepidermal blister with eosinophils and neutrophils. Direct IF shows linear IgA deposition at the BMZ. Around 20% of LAD patients have circulating autoantibodies compared to 75% of CBDC patients.

Special points
Unlike dermatitis herpetiformis there is no associated gluten-sensitive enteropathy.

BULLOUS SYSTEMIC LUPUS ERYTHEMATOSUS

Definition and clinical features
This is defined by its clinical, pathological and immunopathological features, which include a diagnosis of systemic lupus erythematosus (SLE; by criteria of the American Rheumatism Association), a chronic widespread blistering eruption on either sun- or non-sun-exposed skin, subepidermal blistering with a neutrophil-rich infiltrate in the upper dermis, and immune deposits at the BMZ.

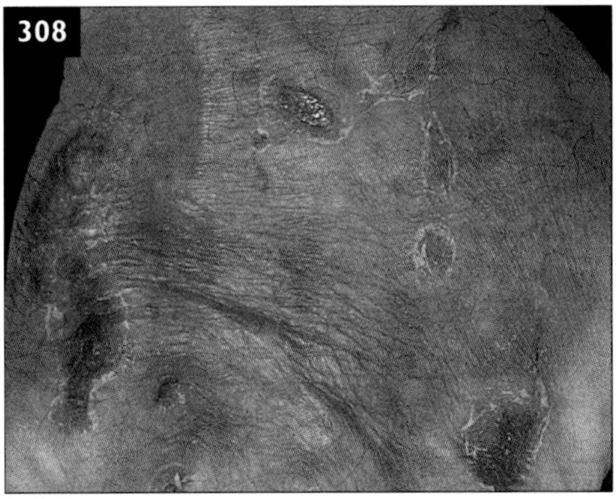

308 Bullous systemic lupus erythematosus.

Blisters do not arise within specific LE lesions but, as in the primary blistering diseases, arise *de novo* on clinically normal-appearing skin. The clinical features of this eruption are not diagnostic. Primary lesions include vesicles, bullae and maculopapular erythema. Blisters are usually tense and not easily ruptured but when they do they can leave erosions and crust (**308**). Pruritus may be severe. Involvement of the oral mucous membranes occurs in about a third of patients. Most patients do not have other cutaneous manifestations of SLE.

Epidemiology
It is a rare, specific manifestation of SLE. The onset is usually in young adults. The age, sex

Subepidermal Blisters

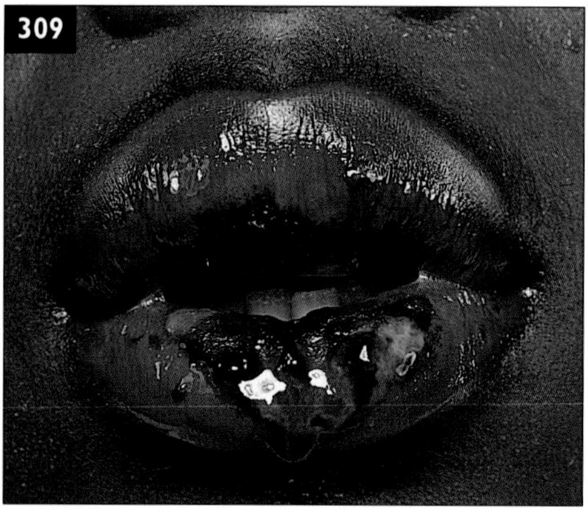

309 Erythema multiforme (Stevens–Johnson syndrome).

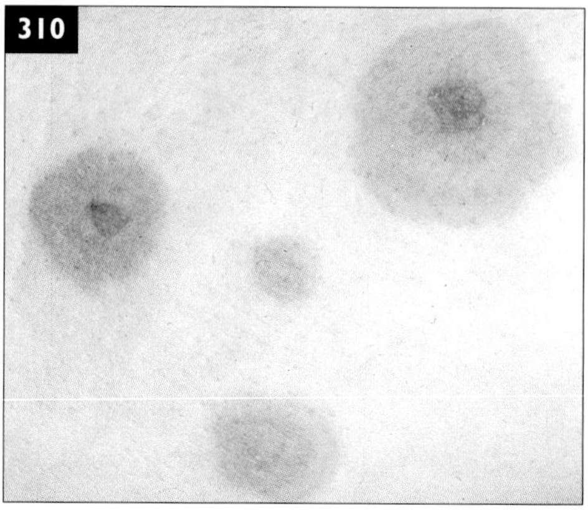

310 Erythema multiforme.

and racial distribution appears to be the same as in SLE in general, i.e. 75% of patients are female and 70% are black.

Differential diagnosis

Coexistence of SLE and bullous pemphigoid or other immunobullous diseases.

Investigations

Histology of skin biopsy shows subepidermal blister formation with a neutrophil-rich infiltrate in the upper dermis. Direct and indirect IF demonstrate IgG anti-BMZ antibodies that are indistinguishable from those found in EBA.

Special points

Bullous eruption of SLE is often associated with more severe forms of SLE. This correlates with a high incidence of clinically significant glomerulonephritis.

BULLOUS ERYTHEMA MULTIFORME

Definition and clinical features

Erythema multiforme is characterised by acute, self-limiting but often recurrent episodes of erythematous maculopapular lesions which may develop into classical target or iris lesions or may blister.

The lesions are typically distributed symmetrically on the extremities, especially on the dorsum of the hands and extensor aspects of the forearms and legs. The frequency of mucosal involvement varies widely between 2% and 60% and affects organs such as the mouth (**309**), eyes, pharynx, oesophagus, genitalia and anus. Severe cases (called Stevens–Johnson syndrome) may develop significant complications such as visual impairment secondary to keratitis with conjunctival scarring. Tense bullae clear or haemorrhagic arise in the centre of target lesions and are usually less than 1 cm in diameter (**310**).

Epidemiology

Erythema multiforme occurs at all ages but mainly in young adults with a peak incidence in the third decade. A history of recent recurrence of herpes simplex, other infectious diseases and drug exposure should be sought.

Differential diagnosis

Toxic epidermolysis necrolysis, drug-induced eruption, Sweet's syndrome, cutaneous vasculitis and immunobullous diseases should all be considered.

Investigations

Histology of a bullous lesion demonstrates a subepidermal blister with overlying vacuolation of the epidermis.

Special points

Long-term prophylactic antiviral therapy may be of benefit in recurrent disease.

Inherited Forms of Epidermolysis Bullosa

311

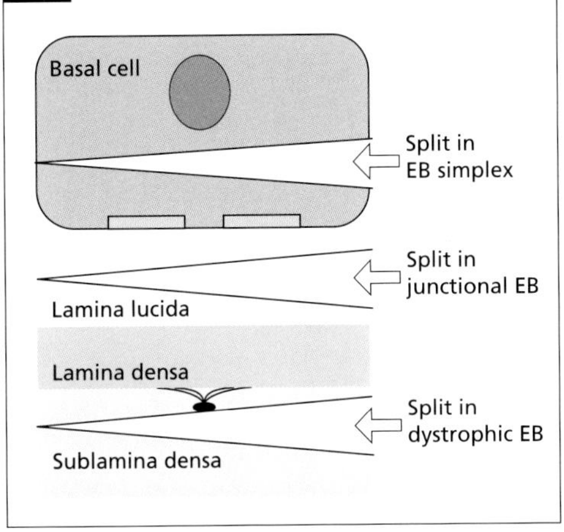

311 Level of split in inherited forms of epidermolysis bullosa.

312

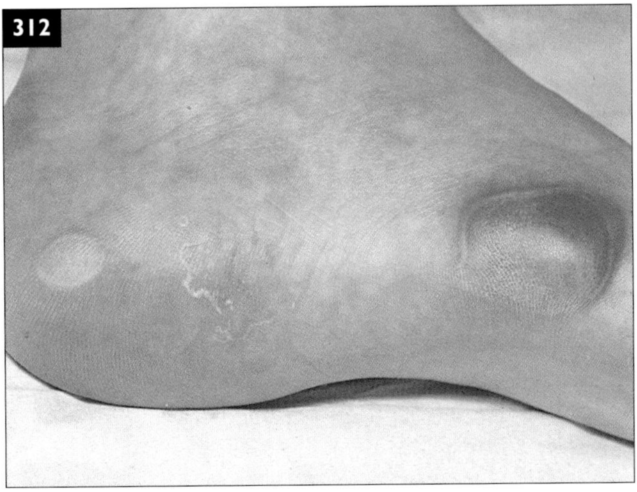

312 Weber–Cockayne disease.

There are three major forms of inherited epidermolysis bullosa which are determined according to the level in the skin within which blisters spontaneously develop. These are called simplex, junctional and dystrophic (**311**).

EPIDERMOLYSIS BULLOSA SIMPLEX

Epidermolysis bullosa simplex (or EB simplex) is the commonest form. It is usually inherited as an autosomal dominant condition, although occasionally X-linked; autosomal recessive cases have been reported. Several variants of EB simplex exist, the most common of which is Weber–Cockayne disease with localised involvement of the palms and soles (**312**). The more generalised variants include Köbner and Dowling–Meara. Trauma-induced blisters heal without scarring and tend to be worse in warm weather. In the generalised forms grouped blisters develop, especially on the trunk, with marked keratoderma on the palms and soles.

In general, in EB simplex, there is no significant extracutaneous involvement or nail abnormalities.

Inherited Forms of Epidermolysis Bullosa

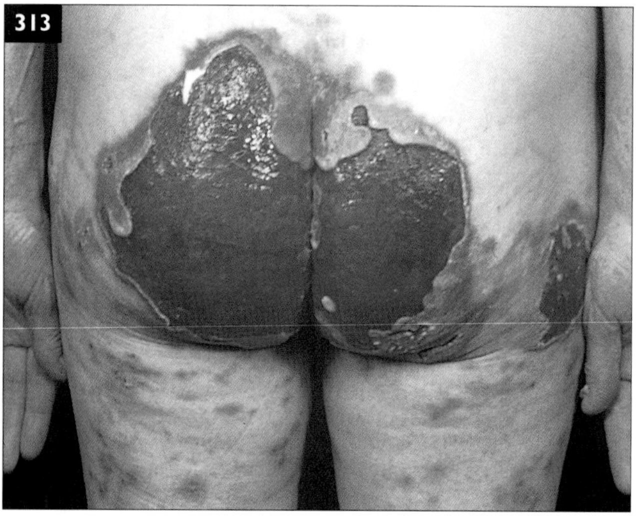

313 Junctional epidermolysis bullosa.

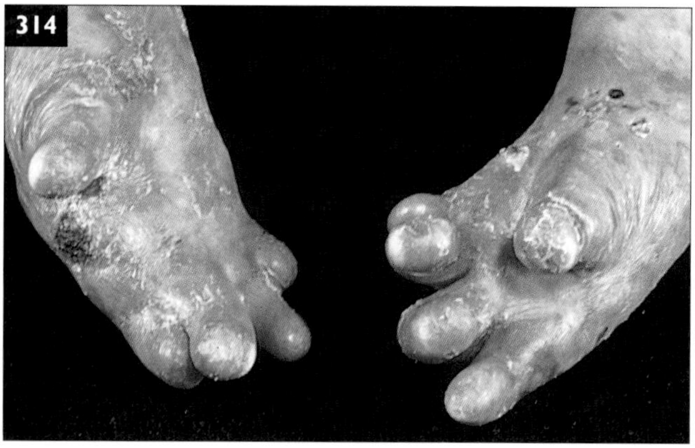

314 Dystrophic epidermolysis bullosa.

JUNCTIONAL EPIDERMOLYSIS BULLOSA

Junctional epidermolysis bullosa (or junctional EB) is inherited as an autosomal recessive condition. There are several phenotypic variants that differ in extent and severity of disease involvement, extracutaneous involvement and the presence or absence of excessive granulation tissue. These include Herlitz (usually lethal), generalised, localised (**313**), inverse and progressive. At birth, large erosions develop around the mouth and anus which are slow to heal. Blisters and erosions heal with atrophic scars. Nails are abnormal or absent and scarring alopecia of the scalp may occur. Also, there is characteristic pitting of the tooth enamel.

DYSTROPHIC EPIDERMOLYSIS BULLOSA

There are two main variants of dystrophic epidermolysis bullosa (or dystrophic EB), autosomal dominant (DDEB) and autosomal recessive (RDEB). Those with the autosomal dominant variant usually have milder disease. Both show widespread blistering with scarring and milia formation. Scarring alopecia may occur and the nails and teeth may be absent or abnormal. In RDEB there is fusion of the skin between the digits of the fingers and toes with web formation resulting in mitten deformities (**314**). There is extensive mucous membrane involvement, which may lead to oesophageal and anal strictures. Other

Blistering in Lichen Planus

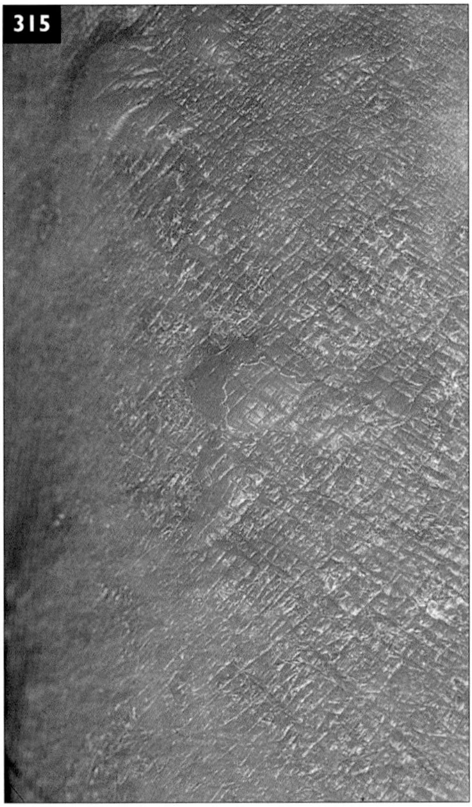

315 Blistering in lichen planus.

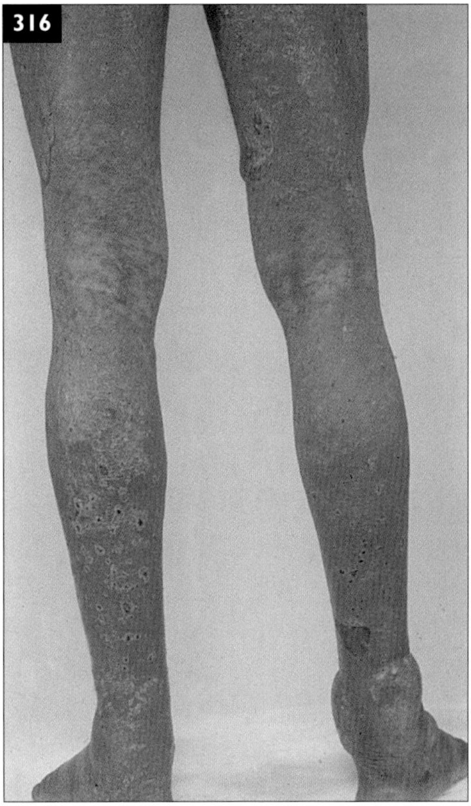

316 Blistering in lichen planus pemphigoides.

complications include anaemia, growth retardation and squamous cell carcinomas in areas of repeated blistering and scarring.

Definition and clinical features

Blistering is an uncommon feature of lichen planus, and tends to occur within typical lesions on the lower legs (bullous lichen planus) (**315**), The gross blistering is thought to be secondary to severe liquefaction degeneration of basal keratinocytes, which causes formation of subepidermal splits. Blistering also occurs in lichen planus pemphigoides (LPP), a rare disorder that shares clinicopathological features with bullous pemphigoid and lichen planus (**316**). It is speculated that antibasement membrane zone antibodies arise in LPP secondary to damage to the basal keratinocytes. Blistering in LPP is not confined to lichenoid lesions and may occur in apparently normal skin. Systemic corticosteroids and immunosuppressant therapy may be needed for disease control in LPP.

Epidemiology

LPP usually affects a younger age group than classic bullous pemphigoid, and tends to be less severe

Differential diagnosis

Other immunobullous disorders, bullous systemic lupus erythematosus, bullous drug reaction.

Investigations

Histology of lesional skin may show a mixed infiltrate in LPP with subepidermal blistering, and direct IMF and indirect IMF are positive, with identical features to bullous pemphigoid.

Structural Abnormalities of Blood Vessels

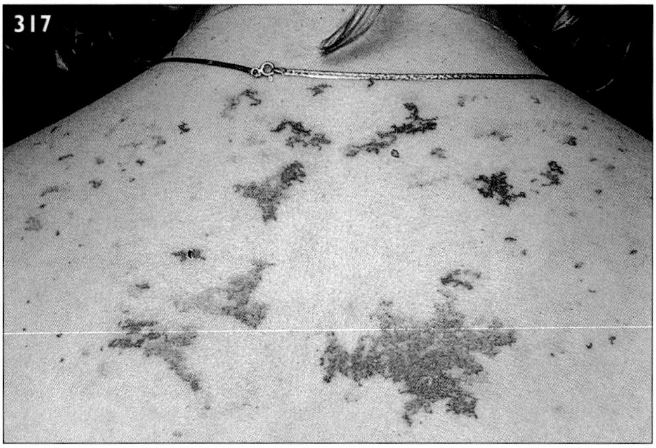

317 Telangiectatic naevus.

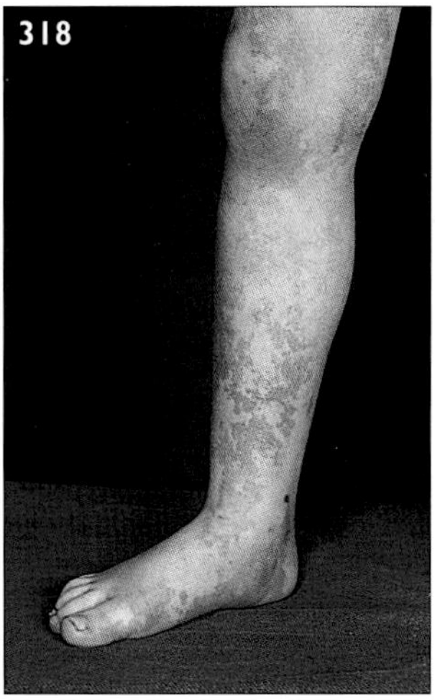

318 Angioma serpiginosum.

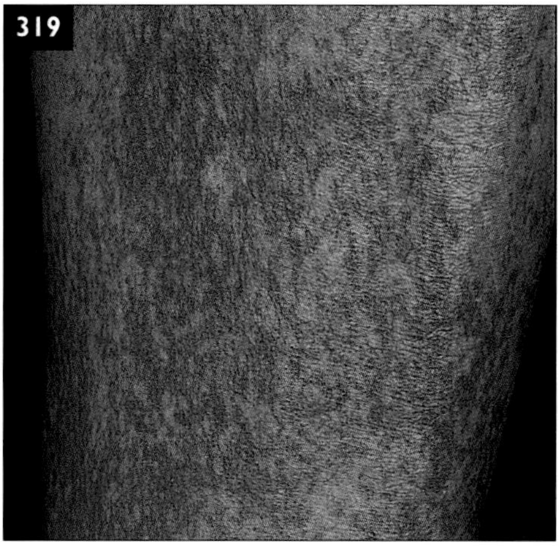

319 Essential telangiectasia.

There is a wide variety of vascular abnormalities, both congenital and acquired, that are manifest as alterations in the distribution of blood vessels in the skin.

TELANGIECTASIA

Definition and clinical features

This is a permanent dilatation of capillaries and small venules. The visible vessels, on both the skin and mucosae, manifest as red lines and dots that fade on pressure. Telangiectasia can be isolated or grouped, giving rise to differing clinical patterns. They are classified as primary, of unknown origin, or secondary, when other dermatological conditions or external factors have damaged the vessels.

Primary telangiectasia can be present at birth as part of a vascular naevus (**317**) or may appear in childhood or adult life (angioma serpiginosum (**318**), essential telangiectasia (**319**)). Vascular abnormalities may be a sign of more serious problems such as ataxia telangiectasia, Osler–Weber–Rendu syndrome (hereditary haemorrhagic telangiectasia) (**320**) or CREST syndrome (**321**).

Spider naevi (**322**) are telangiectasia formed from a central feeding vessel with a star of surrounding vessels. They are a common finding

Structural Abnormalities of Blood Vessels

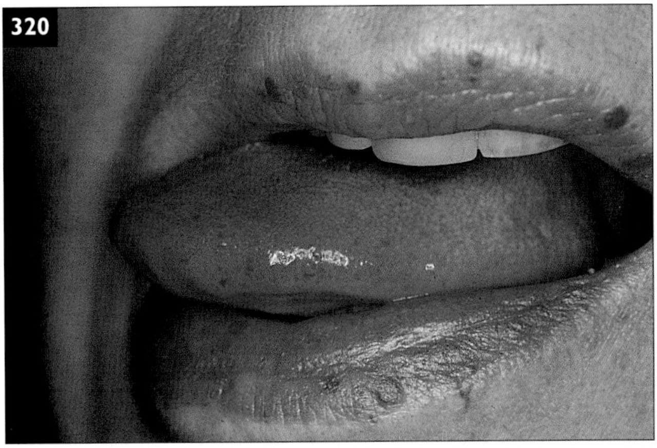

320 Haemorrhagic telangiectasia.

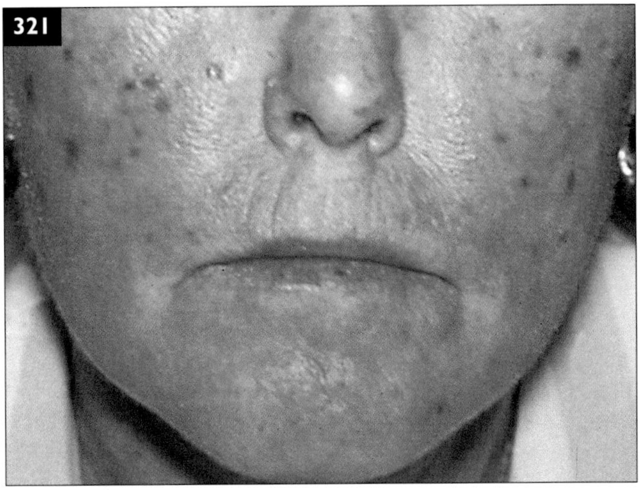

321 CREST syndrome.

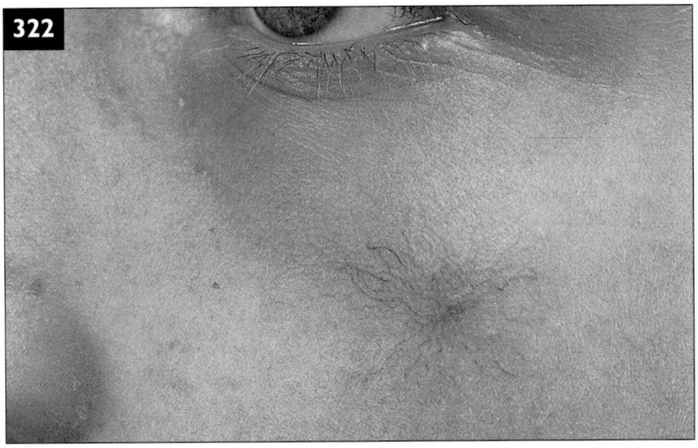

322 Spider naevus.

Structural Abnormalities of Blood Vessels

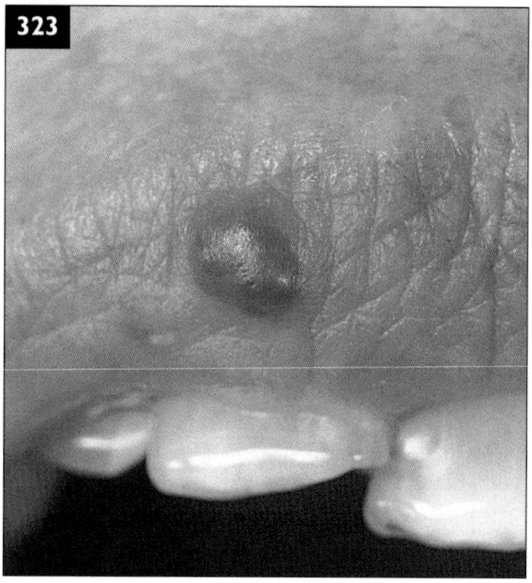

323 Venous lake.

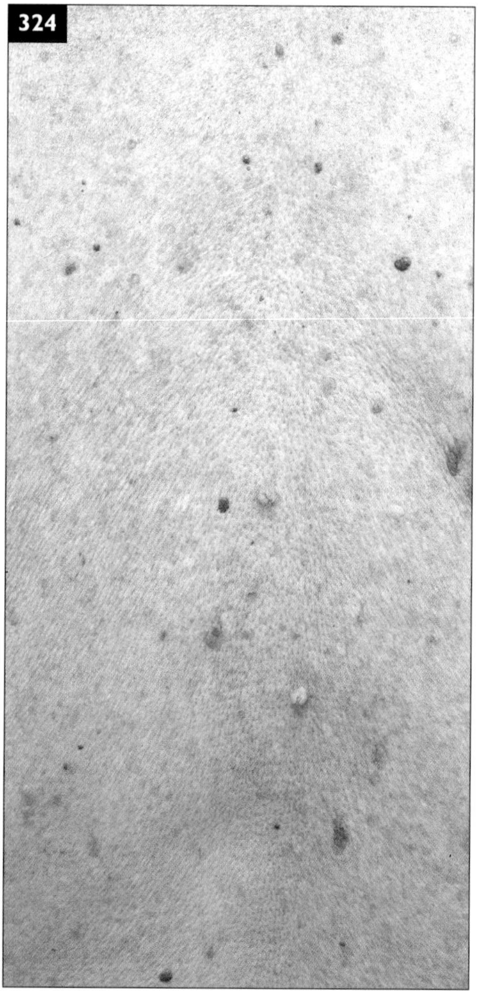

324 Campbell de Morgan spots.

in childhood and pregnancy and may regress spontaneously. Spider naevi may be numerous in patients with liver disease.

Venous lakes (**323**) are flat or papular, blanchable, blue-red lesions, seen in the elderly, often on the lips.

Epidemiology

Some types of primary telangiectasia are hereditary. Secondary lesions occur as a result of damage to blood vessels or their surrounding structures by a very wide range of causes, including exposure to solar and ionising radiation, dermatoses (e.g. rosacea, connective tissue disorders, mastocytosis) and venous stasis.

Differential diagnosis

Purpura can be distinguished because it is not blanched by pressure.

Investigations

Depends on the type of lesion and focuses on finding the underlying cause and extent of the abnormality.

ANGIOKERATOMATA

Definition and clinical features

Dilated and distorted vessels with overlying hyperkeratosis. They occur as solitary lesions, plaques or may be part of multisystem disease. Solitary angiokeratomata are dark-red, warty lesions. The common Campbell de Morgan or cherry spot (**324**) is a brighter red and shows less keratosis but is similar histologically. Angiokeratoma circumscriptum (**325**) are warty vascular plaques present at birth or in early childhood. Angiokeratoma of Mibelli (**326**) usually occur on the fingers and toes of girls in later childhood. Scrotal angiokeratomata (**327**) are multiple, small dark-red papules (see p. 212). In angiokeratoma corporis diffusum (Anderson–Fabry's disease)

Structural Abnormalities of Blood Vessels

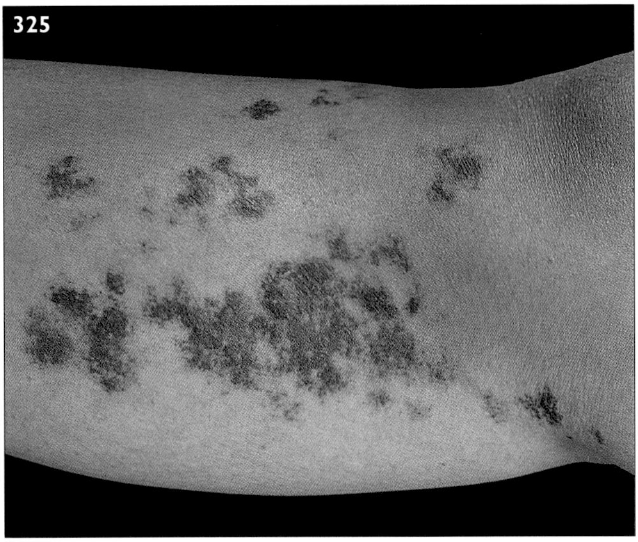

325 Angiokeratoma circumscriptum.

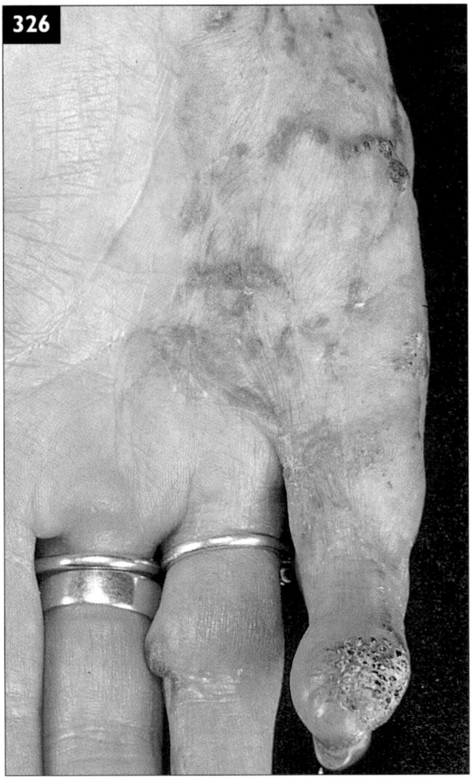

326 Angiokeratoma of Mibelli.

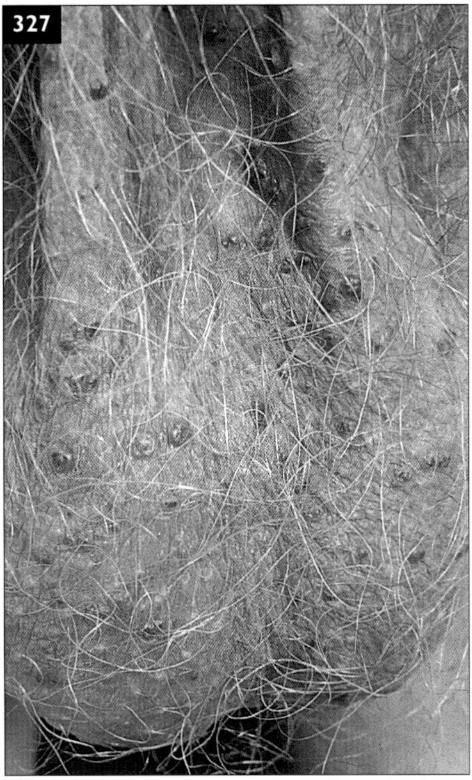

327 Scrotal angiokeratomata.

Structural Abnormalities of Blood Vessels

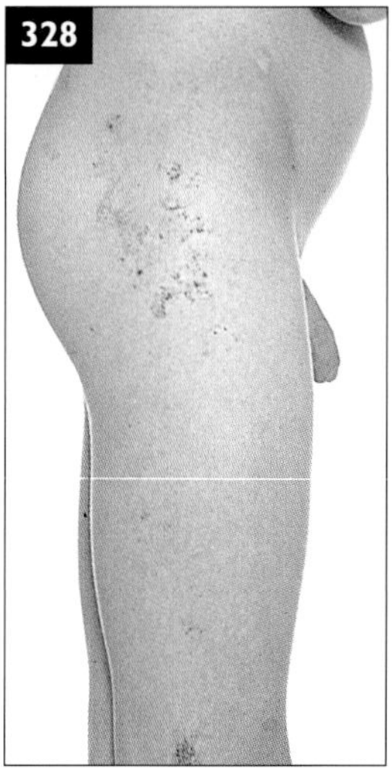

328 Angiokeratoma corporis diffusum (Anderson–Fabry's disease).

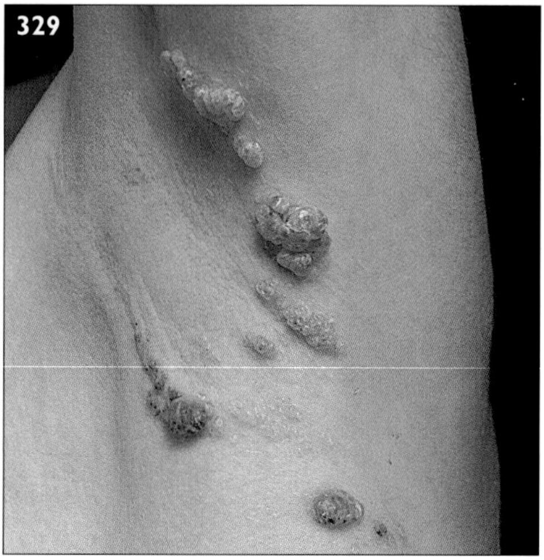

329 Lymphangioma circumscriptum.

(**328**) scattered cutaneous lesions are associated with hypertension, renal failure, ocular changes and digital pain.

Epidemiology
Angiokeratoma corporis diffusum is an inherited disorder of sphingolipid metabolism.

Differential diagnosis
Solitary lesions can, when very dark, be mistaken for malignant melanoma. Multiple lesions can be confused with vasculitis.

Investigations
Angiokeratoma corporis diffusum is diagnosed by demonstrating an enzyme deficiency, usually α-galactosidase A.

LYMPHANGIOMA; LYMPHANGIECTASIA

Definition and clinical features
Dilatation of lymphatics resulting in fluid-filled blebs. Lymphangioma circumscriptum (**329**) is seen as a patch or band of blister-like lesions, filled with a mixture of blood and lymph. Lesions can be present at birth, usually on the trunk or proximal limbs, or may appear in childhood or early adult life. The surface may be warty with the lesions possibly extending into deep dermis and fat. Lymphangiectases (**330**) are lymphatics that are dilated because of obstruction by a wide variety of inflammatory and neoplastic processes.

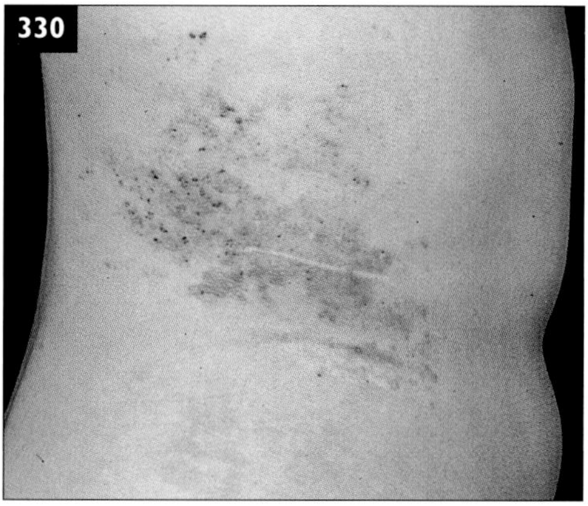

330 Lymphangiectases.

Epidemiology
Lymphangiomata are uncommon and have an equal sex distribution.

Differential diagnosis
Keratotic lesions can be confused with angiokeratomata and verrucous haemangiomata.

Special points
If surgical treatment of lymphangioma circumscriptum is to be curative it must be realised that the underlying defect is deep in the dermis.

Structural Abnormalities of Blood Vessels

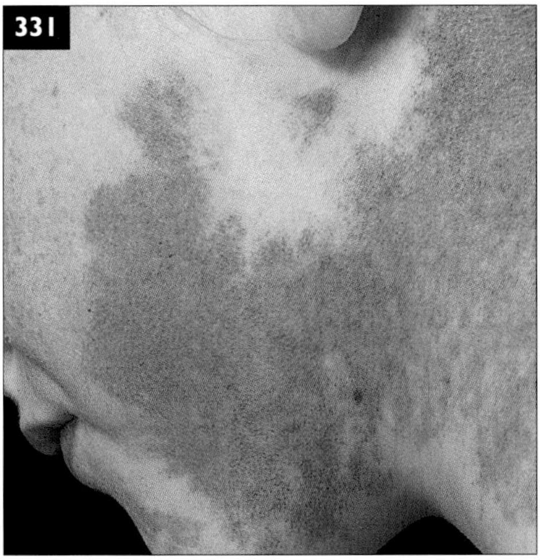

331 Portwine stain.

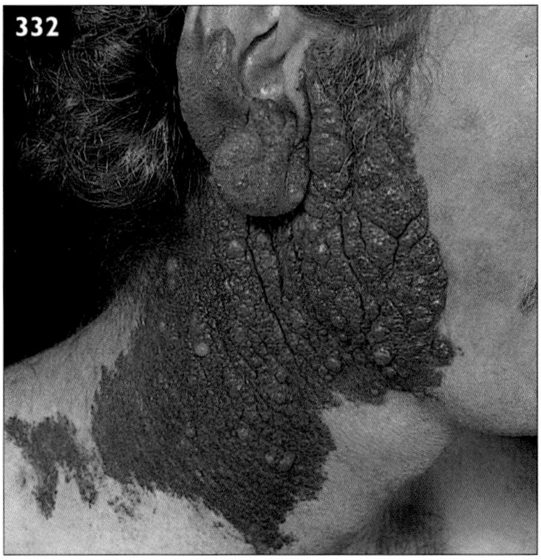

332 Thickened and darkened portwine stain.

PORTWINE STAIN (NAEVUS FLAMMEUS)

Definition and clinical features

A vascular birth mark that is less common but of more significance than the salmon patch (see p. 150). It is a red patch, usually unilateral, often affecting the face (**331**). Lesions are present but flat at birth, and thicken and darken with age (**332**).

The vascular abnormality is not always confined to the skin. Meningeal involvement, often manifest by epilepsy, may be associated with a facial portwine stain: the Sturge–Weber syndrome. Glaucoma also occurs. Numerous other syndromes are described in which portwine stains are associated with other abnormalities. Lesions can be complicated by arteriovenous malformations (**333**). High pressure vascular shunts result in rapid growth of the lesion and destruction of tissue locally.

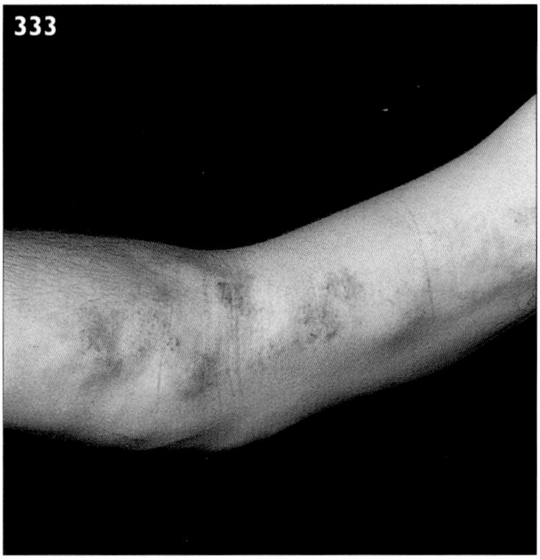

333 Arteriovenous malformation.

Epidemiology

There is evidence that the underlying defect is in the neural control of the blood vessels. The cause is unknown and lesions are usually sporadic with equal sex incidence.

Differential diagnosis

Deep haemangiomata can be distinguished by their rapid growth, although the presence of arteriovenous malformations can made the distinction difficult.

Investigations

Uncomplicated lesions do not need investigation.

Special points

Social and psychological problems are associated with facial portwine stains. Advances in laser technology are resulting in better results with less scarring. Cosmetic camouflage can improve quality of life but is less successful for raised lesions.

Structural Abnormalities of Blood Vessels

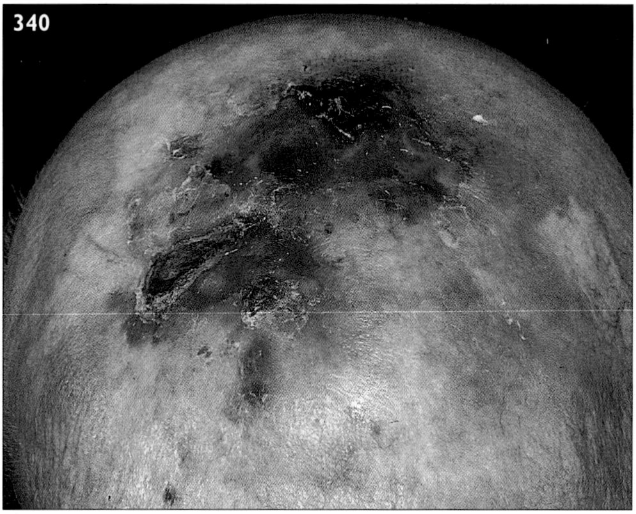

340 Angiosarcoma.

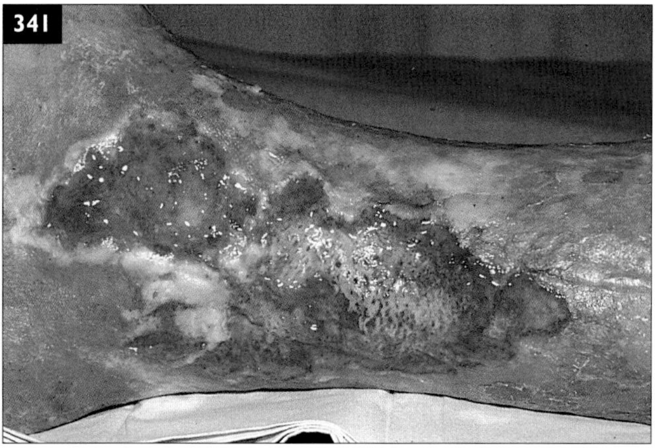

341 Varicose ulcer.

ANGIOSARCOMA

Definition and clinical features

A rare, aggressive, malignant tumour of blood vessels. The initial change is a bruise-like discoloration, typically on the scalp. Thickening and development of dark-red nodules can affect a wide area (**340**). Metastases and death are usual.

Lymphangiosarcoma of Stewart and Treves is a similar change seen in the lymphoedematous arm after mastectomy.

Epidemiology

Most cases are in the elderly though deep angiosarcomas have been reported in children.

Differential diagnosis

Early signs are subtle and may be mistaken for bruising or erysipelas.

Investigations

Histology shows disorganised vessels with plump endothelial cells.

Special points

Prognosis is poor. Treatment includes wide excision and radiotherapy.

Structural Abnormalities of Blood Vessels

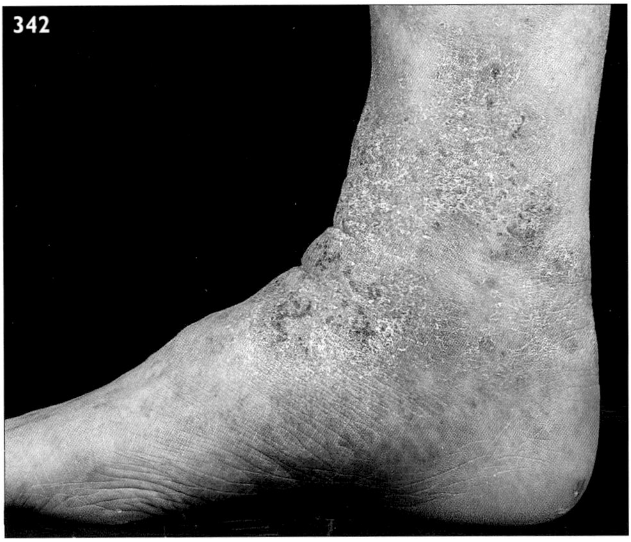

342 Varicose eczema.

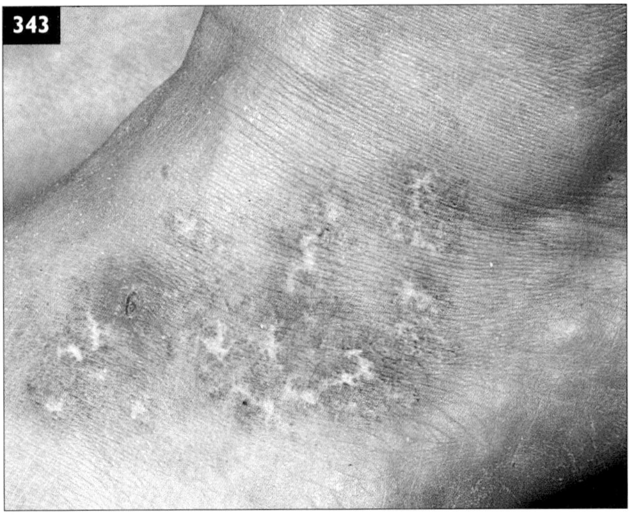

343 Atrophie blanche.

ULCERATION OF THE LEG

Definition and clinical features

There are many causes for ulceration of the lower leg. In industrialised nations the most common ulcers are those due to chronic venous insufficiency as a result of varicose veins and/or post-thrombotic damage. Ischaemic ulcers, secondary to atherosclerosis, and diabetic ulcers are also major causes of morbidity.

Varicose ulcers usually affect the medial side of the lower leg (**341**) but may become circumferential. The surrounding skin will often show the changes of varicose eczema (**342**) with thickening and pigmentation of the skin and dry, rough, red areas of eczema. The limb is often oedematous and there may be areas of atrophie blanche (**343**), seen as firm white plaques with telangiectasia.

Structural Abnormalities of Blood Vessels

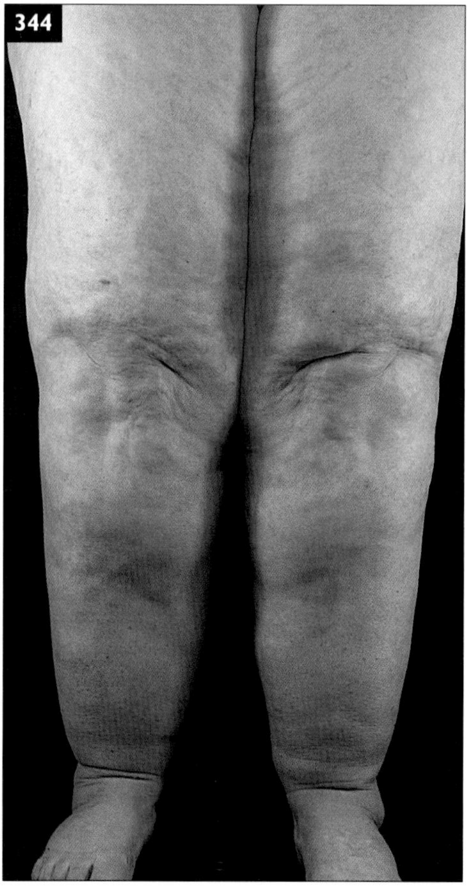

344 Lymphoedema.

Lymphoedema (**344**), either congenital or acquired, can predispose to chronic ulceration.

Arterial ulcers are often small but painful. They are often acral or over bony prominences (**345**).

Diabetic ulcers vary in appearance depending on the degree of large or small vessel damage, and the presence of neuropathy.

Epidemiology

Ulcers are a major cause of morbidity, particularly in elderly women. Venous ulcers are relatively rare in the Third World.

Differential diagnosis

Distinguishing venous and arterial ulcers is essential. Ulcers are also seen in sickle cell anaemia, pyoderma gangrenosum, vasculitis and other rarer conditions. Malignant change (**346**) can both mimic and complicate venous ulcers.

Investigations

Ankle or brachial Doppler pressure index to exclude significant arterial impairment. Contact dermatitis from medicaments is a common complication for which patch testing may be helpful.

Special points

A wide range of dressings and medications is available for the treatment of ulcers. The mainstay of treatment for varicose ulcers remains adequate compression bandaging. Healing of arterial ulcers is difficult unless vascular–surgical intervention improves the circulation.

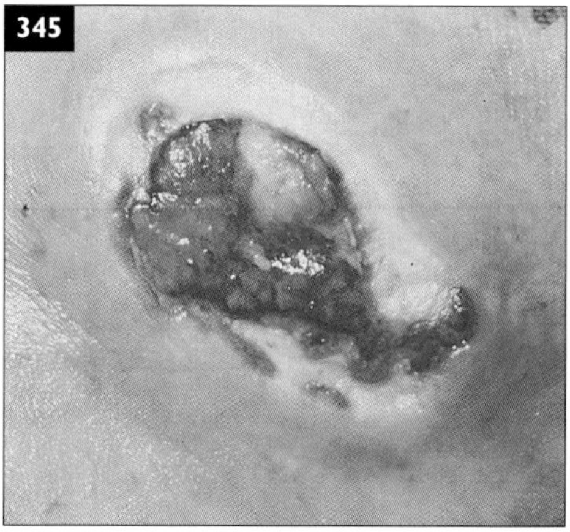

345 Arterial ulcer on the ankle.

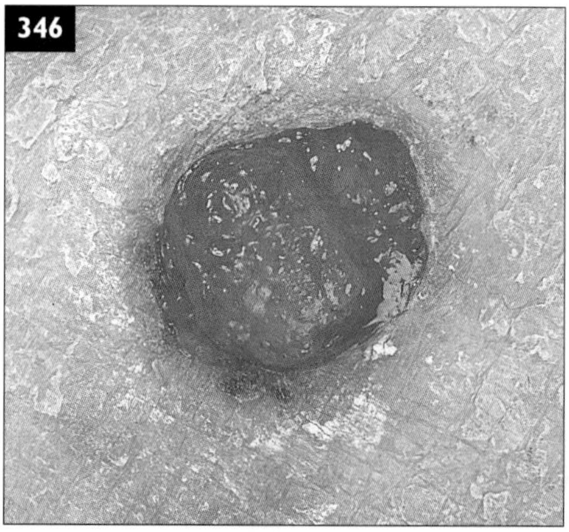

346 Malignant ulcer (BCE).

Inflammatory Disorders Affecting Blood Vessels

Inflammation of blood vessels is seen, histologically, in many dermatological conditions. The terminology is complex as the clinical appearance varies depending on the size of the damaged vessel and the type and degree of damage. When blood vessels show histological evidence of structural damage the term vasculitis is used.

CAPILLARITIS

Definition and clinical features

A group of conditions characterised by a purpuric eruption, caused by inflammation of the capillaries. It presents as bright red, 'cayenne pepper' spots (**347**) usually affecting the legs. Old lesions become brown, as haemosiderin is deposited. The clinical pattern varies, with lichenoid and annular subtypes.

Epidemiology

Uncommon. May be an incidental finding in low-grade, asymptomatic cases.

Differential diagnosis

Many conditions show purpura on the lower legs, particularly in the presence of coagulation defects.

Investigations

In most cases no cause is found.

VASCULITIS

Definition and clinical features

Inflammation and damage to blood vessels, thought to be caused by immune complexes. Clinical manifestations depend on the size of the vessels involved. Organs other than the skin may be affected.

Palpable purpura is the characteristic sign of small vessel damage (**348**).

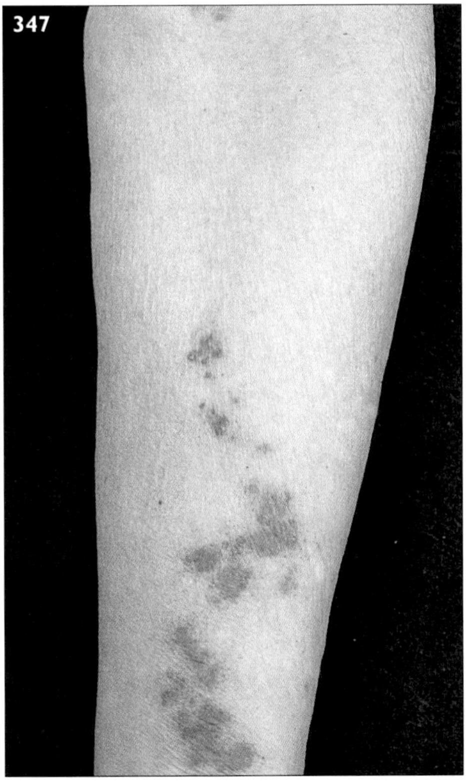

347 Capillaritis.

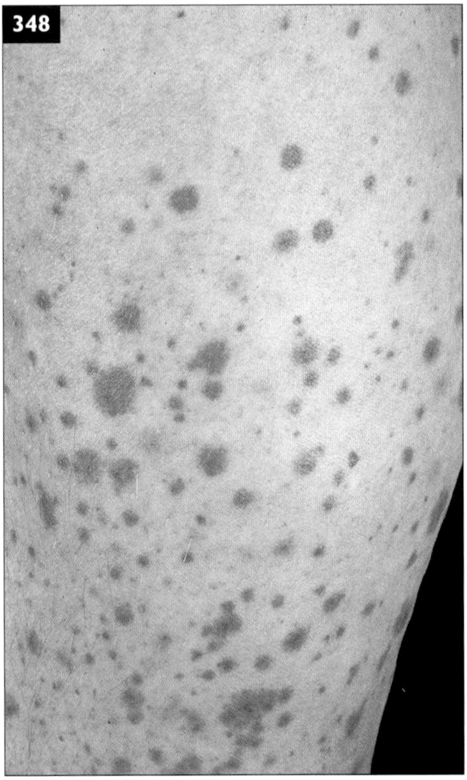

348 Palpable purpura in vasculitis.

Inflammatory Disorders Affecting Blood Vessels

Other signs include erythematous swelling known as urticarial vasculitis (**349**) and ulceration of the skin (**350**). In most forms of vasculitis, gravitational effects result in the lower legs being most severely affected.

In Henoch–Schönlein purpura, the eruption initially affects the lower legs and buttocks of children and is associated with arthritis, renal involvement and abdominal pain (**351**).

Nodular vasculitis (**352**) and panniculitis (**353**) result from the involvement of deeper vessels leading to painful red or bruise-like lumps which heal to leave discoloured areas or depressed scars. Erythema nodosum (**354**) is a form of panniculitis predominantly affecting the shins, and associated with infections or systemic diseases.

Polyarteritis nodosa (**355**) affects small and medium-sized arteries, resulting in nodules in the skin and livedo reticularis, often with multisystem involvement.

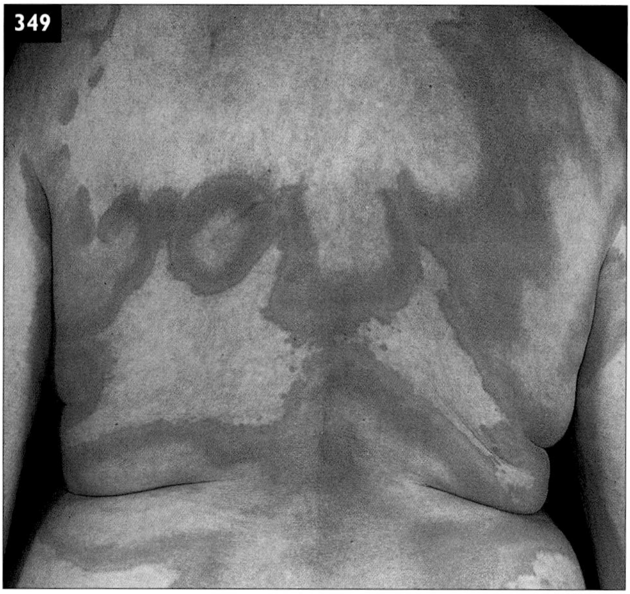

349 Urticarial vasculitis.

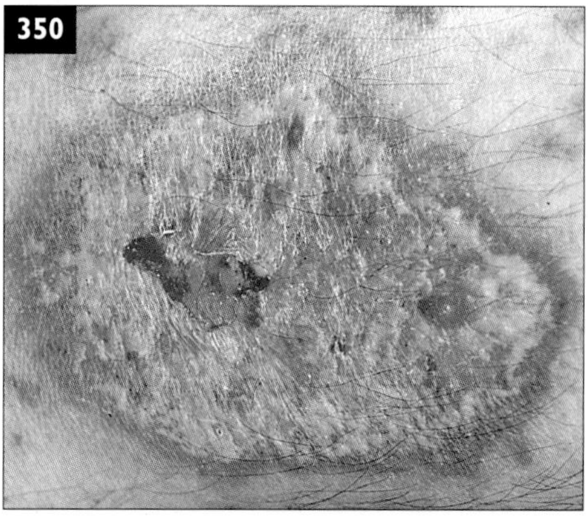

350 Vasculitic ulceration of the skin.

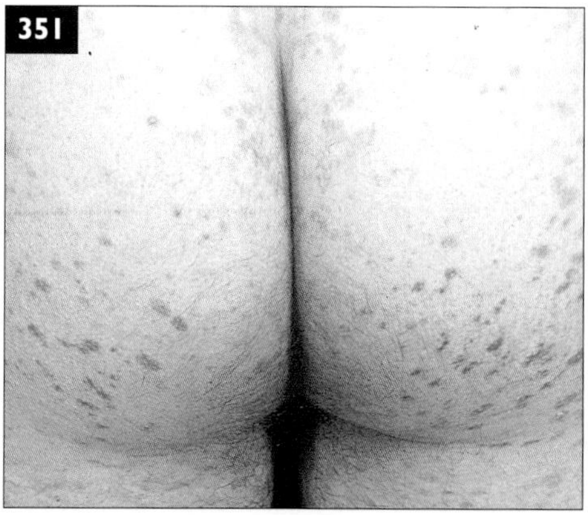

351 Henoch–Schönlein purpura.

Inflammatory Disorders Affecting Blood Vessels

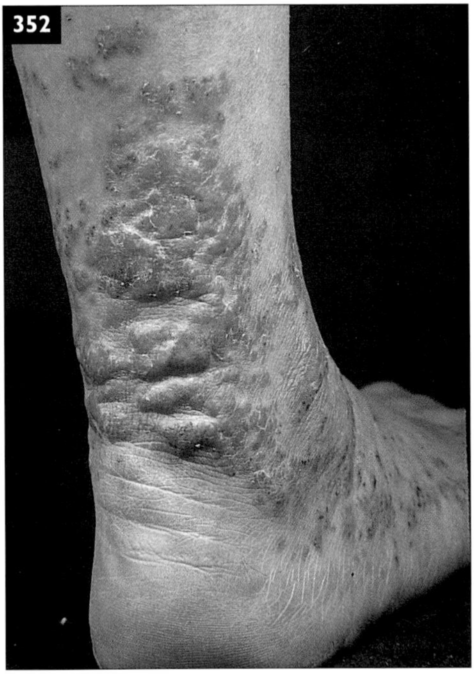

352 Nodular vasculitis.

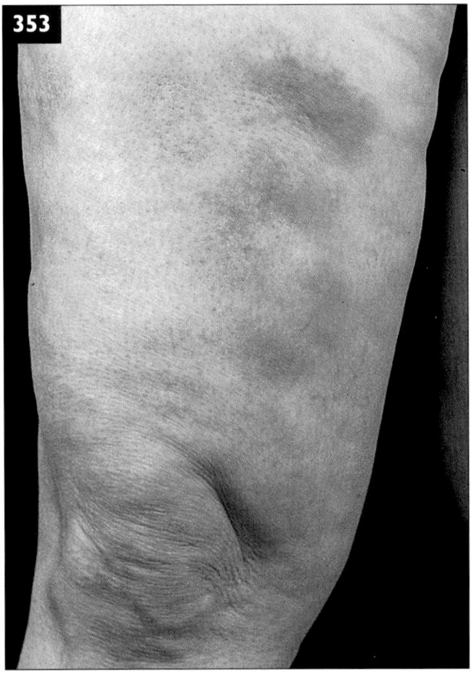

353 Panniculitis.

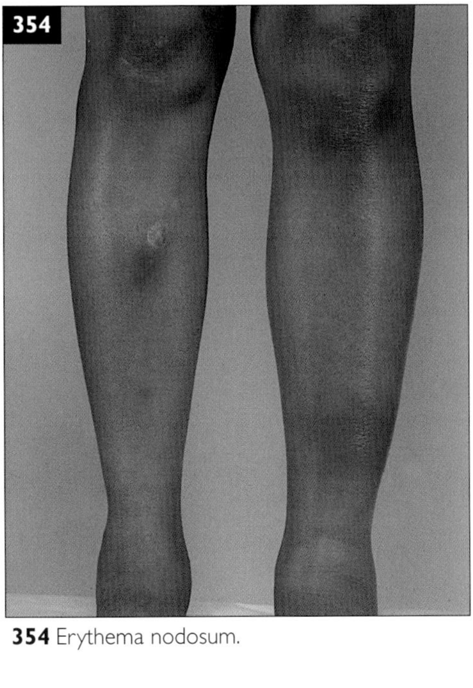

354 Erythema nodosum.

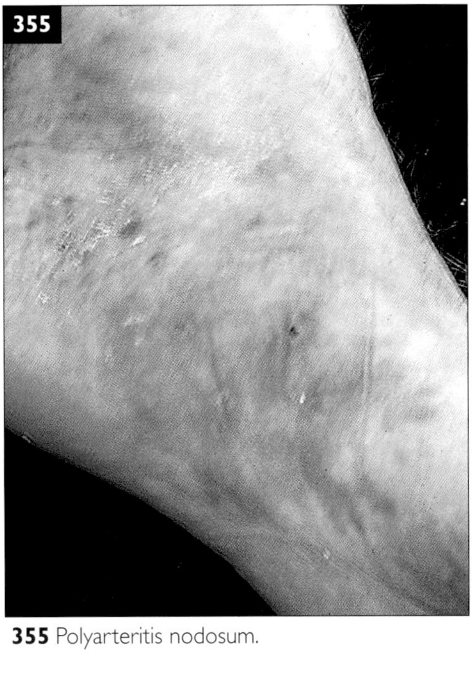

355 Polyarteritis nodosum.

Inflammatory Disorders Affecting Blood Vessels

Wegener's granulomatosis (**356**) is a form of vasculitis in which granulomas are seen histologically. It affects the upper and lower respiratory tracts and the kidneys, but can affect other systems. In the skin it produces a range of signs, from purpura to pyoderma-like ulceration.

Epidemiology
All ages can be affected. Henoch–Schönlein purpura is usually seen in children and may follow streptococcal infection. Vasculitis has a wide variety of causes including drugs, infections, connective tissue diseases and neoplasia.

Differential diagnosis
Causes of purpura such as coagulopathies. Nodular vasculitis and panniculitis can be confused with atypical infections.

Investigations
Histology may be needed to confirm the clinical diagnosis of vasculitis. Further investigations aim to determine the extent of systemic involvement and the underlying cause.

Special points
Treatment depends on the severity of skin eruption, involvement of other organs, and the underlying cause.

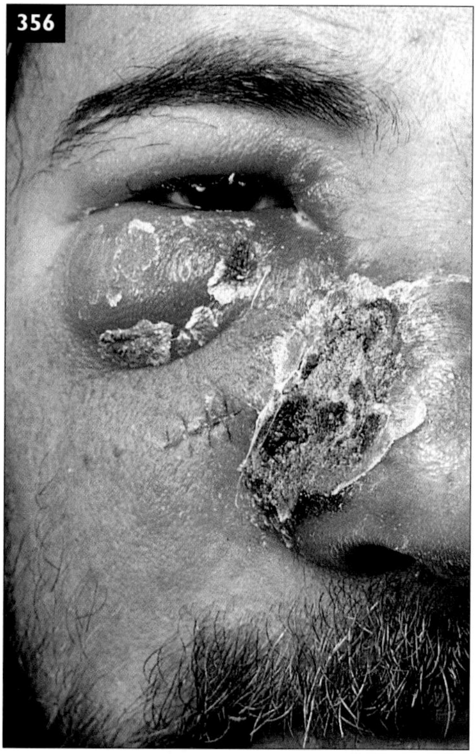

356 Wegener's granulomatosis.

LIVEDO RETICULARIS
Definition and clinical features
Purple mottling of the skin, in a net-like pattern, resulting from a disturbance of dermal circulation. The area affected depends on the cause. Physiological livedo is usually seen over the thighs and calves. Relative cyanosis is seen in an irregular network (**357**).

Epidemiology
Physiological livedo is more common in children and is seen as a response to cold. A wide range of conditions cause livedo. These can be grouped into: disorders of the vessel wall, including vasculitis; structural abnormalities of the vasculature; increased viscosity of the blood; microemboli; and unknown.

Differential diagnosis
Erythema ab igne – the reticulate discoloration of the skin from excessive heat exposure.

Investigations
To establish the underlying cause.

ERYTHEMA MULTIFORME
Definition and clinical features
Inflammation of the skin and mucosa with characteristic target lesions. This condition presents as rings of erythema, often with central blisters, known as target lesions (**358**). The eruption is most severe on the hands and feet but can become widespread. Mouth ulcers, conjunctivitis and genital ulcers may also occur (**359**). Attacks may be recurrent (see also bullous erythema multiforme, p. 140).

Epidemiology
The most common trigger is herpes simplex virus infection but drugs and other infections can also precipitate attacks.

Differential diagnosis
Typical target lesions are characteristic.

Investigations
To establish a precipitating factor.

Inflammatory Disorders Affecting Blood Vessels

357
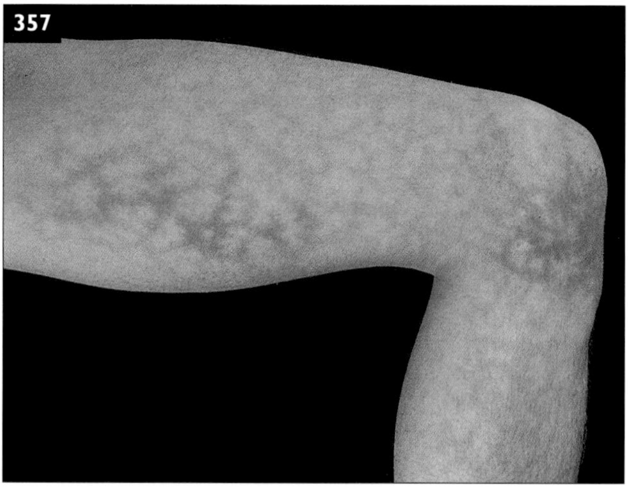

357 Livedo reticularis.

358
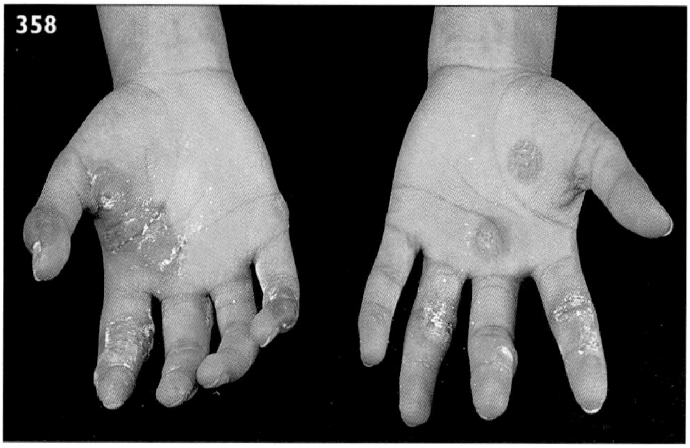

358 Erythema multiforme.

359
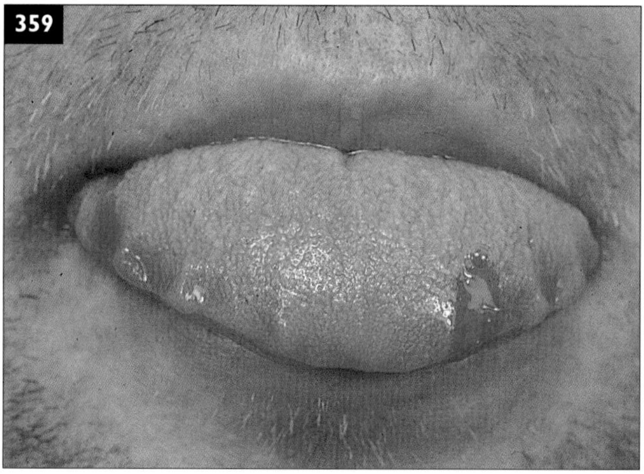

359 Erythema multiforme on the tongue.

Inflammatory Disorders Affecting Blood Vessels

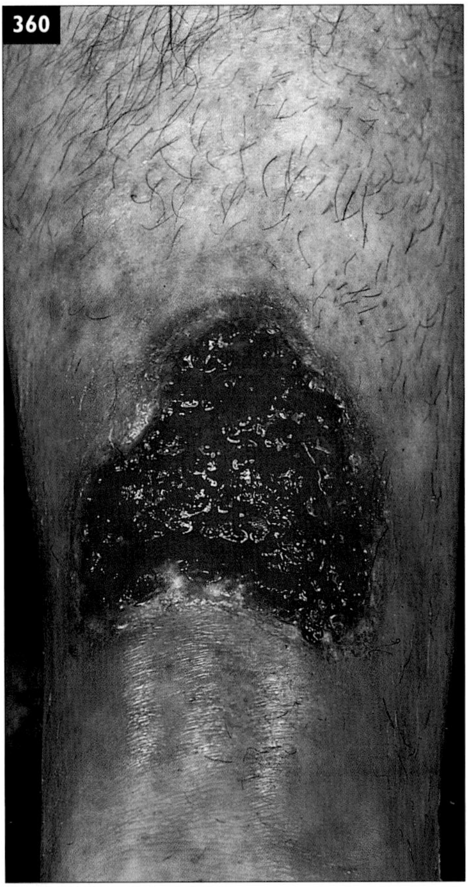

360 Pyoderma gangrenosum – ulceration.

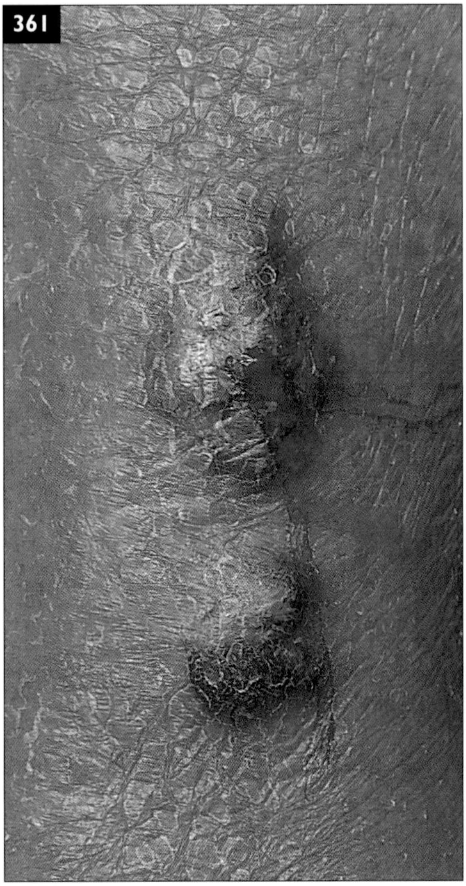

361 Pyoderma gangrenosum – bullae.

PYODERMA GANGRENOSUM

Definition and clinical features

Inflammatory necrosis of the skin of unknown cause, associated with a variety of inflammatory and haematological conditions. The lower leg is most frequently affected but the lesions can affect any site. Painful red–blue nodules develop central ulceration, spreading rapidly with ragged blue–black undermined edges (**360**). Variants include superficial lesions – pustules and vesicles. Larger haemorrhagic bullae also occur (**361**). Patients are often unwell with general malaise and fever.

Epidemiology

An uncommon condition associated with inflammatory bowel disease, rheumatoid and seronegative arthritis, monoclonal gammopathy and haematological malignancy. The bullous variant is most commonly seen with the latter.

Differential diagnosis

Other forms of leg ulceration. Unusual and atypical infections, vasculitis and disorder of coagulation.

Investigations

Histology will show a neutrophilic infiltrate and sometimes vasculitis, but may be non-specific. Microscopy and culture of skin biopsy. Investigation of underlying cause.

Special points

Systemic corticosteroids are needed for rapidly advancing or widespread disease.

General Definition of the Ichthyoses

Ichthyosis (from ichthys, Greek for fish) describes dry, rough skin with persistent scaling which may resemble fish scale. It is a disorder of keratinisation and differs from other scaly skin diseases such as eczema and psoriasis by being diffuse, uniform and generally fixed in pattern. Mucosal surfaces are spared and hair, nails and teeth are rarely affected. The inherited ichthyoses are a heterogeneous group comprising primary ichthyotic diseases and several ichthyosiform syndromes. Acquired ichthyosis may occur as a result of malabsorption, chronic hepatic or renal disease, hypothyroidism, sarcoidosis, leprosy, HIV disease, lymphoma and other malignancies.

Recessive X-Linked Ichthyosis

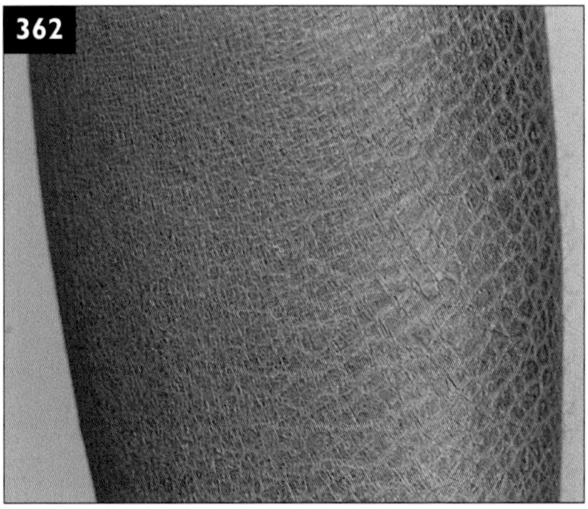

362 Recessive X-linked ichthyosis.

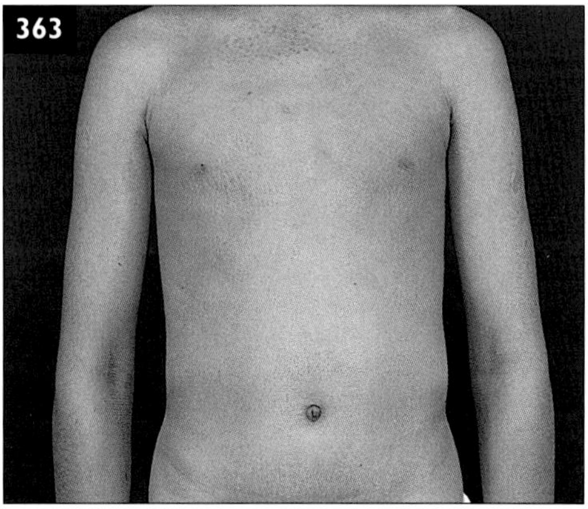

363 Recessive X-linked ichthyosis.

Definition and clinical features

Scaling is generally evident within the first month of life and increases throughout childhood, stabilising in the teens with little subsequent change. The scale typically is polygonal, adherent and light brown in colour (**362**). It affects the extensor surfaces of the upper arms, the outer thighs and around the lower legs. The neck, abdomen (**363**) and pre-auricular facial skin are also commonly affected. The palms and soles are spared. In most patients scaling improves in the summer months.

Epidemiology

Recessive X-linked ichthyosis affects male offspring of unaffected carrier mothers. It has a world-wide distribution with an incidence of 1 in 6000 in the UK. Important extracutaneous manifestations occur.

Investigations

Biopsy of affected skin shows hyperkeratosis and a variable granular cell layer. Steroid (cholesterol) sulfatase deficiency can be demonstrated in fibroblast and leucocyte cultures. Raised serum cholesterol sulphate can be detected on a serum lipoprotein electrophoresis strip, a simple and cheap screening test. Serum cholesterol levels are normal.

Special points

Placental steroid sulfatase deficiency coexists and may lead to prolonged and complicated labour, putting the infant at risk. An increased incidence of testicular maldescent, cryptorchidism and testicular cancer has been reported. Kallman's syndrome is the association of recessive X-linked ichthyosis with hypogonadotropic hypogonadism, anosmia and a variety of neurological defects. Corneal opacities occur in up to 50% of patients and 24% of female carriers.

The underlying metabolic defect is steroid sulfatase (SS) deficiency and the SS gene has been identified on the short arm of the X chromosome at the Xp 22.3 locus.

Lamellar Ichthyosis

364

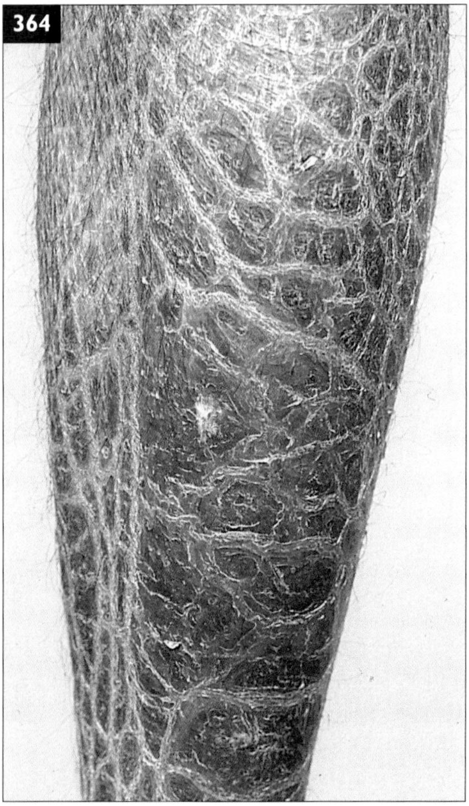

364 Lamellar ichthyosis.

Definition and clinical features

Most affected infants present as collodion babies. Typically, a mild erythroderma with thick, plate-like, pigmented, adherent scale (**364**) over most of the skin ensues but mild variants occur. Additional problems include pruritus, hypohidrosis, ectropion and crumpled pinnae.

Epidemiology

Lamellar ichthyosis is a severe, autosomal, recessive ichthyosis with an incidence of approximately 1 in 600 000. An even rarer autosomal dominant variant has been reported.

Investigations

Light microscopy of the skin shows variable parakeratosis but massive orthohyperkeratosis; the remainder of the epidermis may be of normal thickness.

Ichthyosis Vulgaris

Definition and clinical features
Scaling is usually obvious from 2 months onwards but may be delayed until childhood. The scale is white, flaky and semi-adherent. It is most pronounced on the extensor surfaces of the arms (**365**) and lower legs and characteristically spares the flexures. The trunk, especially the abdominal wall, perioral skin and the pinnae may also be involved. Palmoplantar hyperlinearity and keratosis pilaris are common associated features of both ichthyosis vulgaris and atopic eczema. Pruritus and cosmetic disability in isolated ichthyosis vulgaris are minimal. The condition shows seasonal variation in most patients, improving in warm and sunny weather. Many patients improve in later life.

Epidemiology
Ichthyosis vulgaris is the commonest inherited ichthyosis affecting roughly 1 in 250 people. It is an autosomal dominant disorder. Up to 50% of those with ichthyosis vulgaris also show features of atopic eczema.

Differential diagnosis
Acquired ichthyosis, severe xerosis and recessive X-linked ichthyosis.

Investigations
Family history to exclude other inherited ichthyoses. Histology of affected skin typically shows mild hyperkeratosis and a diminished or absent granular layer. Electron microscopy reveals scanty and fragmented keratohyaline granules in the granular cells.

Special points
May vary in severity between and within generations.

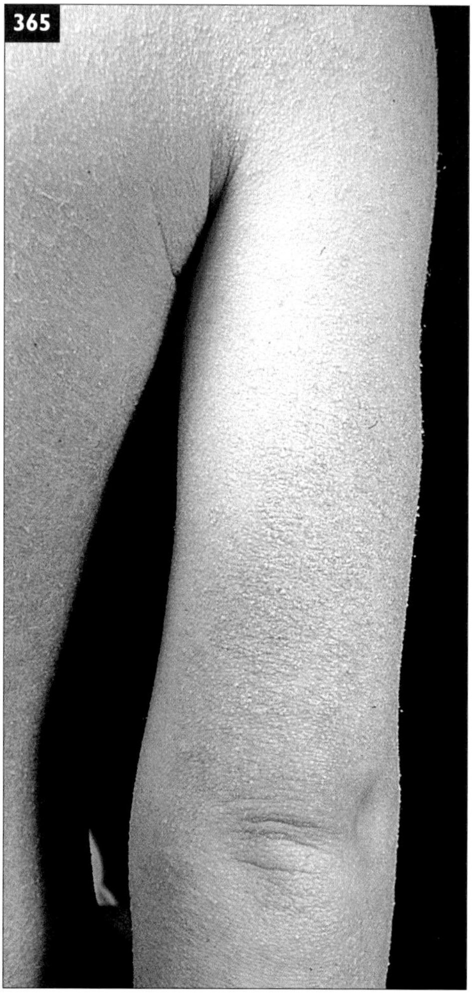

365 Ichthyosis vulgaris.

Non-Bullous Ichthyosiform Erythroderma

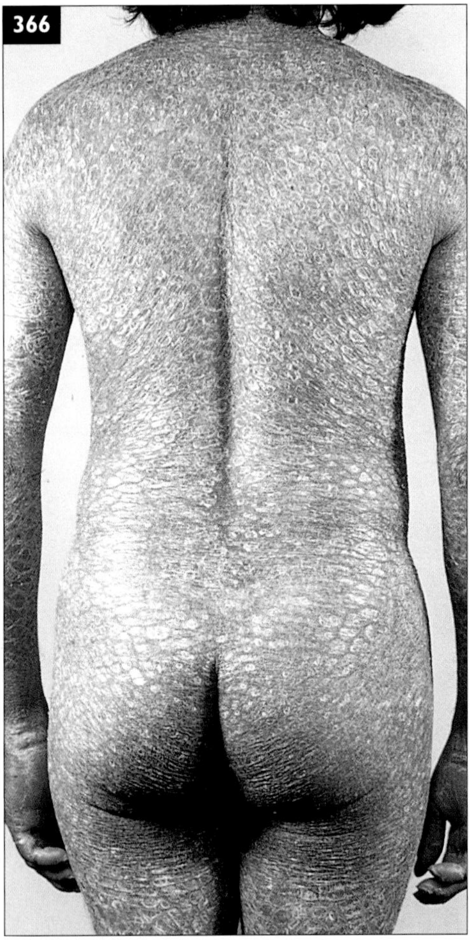

366 Non-bullous ichthyosiform erythroderma.

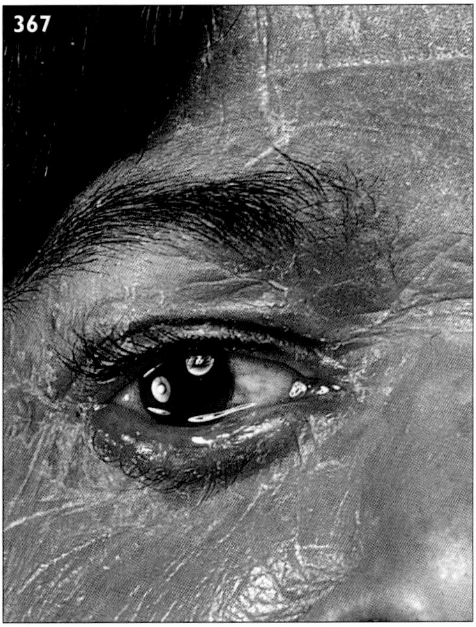

367 Ectropion in non-bullous ichthyosiform erythroderma.

Definition and clinical features

Over 90% of cases present at birth with a collodion membrane, a yellow, shiny, tight film which resembles a sausage skin. Ectropion and constricting bands may occur and the membrane sheds over a period of weeks, revealing a generalised scaly erythroderma. Scaling can affect all areas (**366**) including the scalp, ears, face, flexures, palms and soles and is white, light, superficial and semi-adherent. Scalp involvement often causes tinea amiantacea and may lead to patchy cicatricial alopecia. Ectropion (**367**), which generally improves, digital constriction and a nail dystrophy are features of severe disease. In most patients, sweating is absent or reduced.

Epidemiology

This is a rare and usually severe autosomal recessive inflammatory ichthyosis with an incidence of 1 in 300 000 (referred to as erythrodermic lamellar ichthyosis in the German literature).

Investigations

Light microscopy of the skin reveals hyperkeratosis, mild parakeratosis and acanthosis, and a mild dermal lymphocytic infiltrate. The molecular defect has not been identified and prenatal diagnosis is limited to a foetal skin biopsy at 20–22 weeks to detect premature keratinisation.

Bullous Ichthyosiform Erythroderma

368

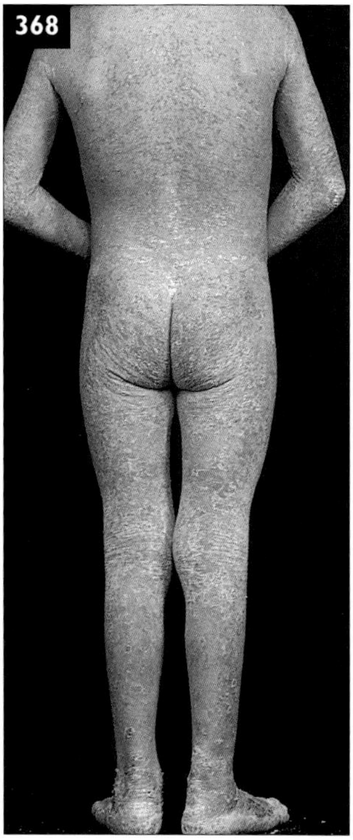

368 Bullous ichthyosiform erythroderma.

369

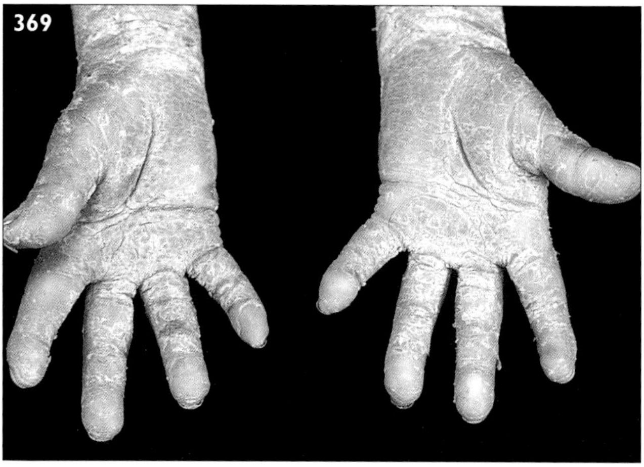

369 Palmar hyperkeratosis in bullous ichthyosiform erythroderma.

Definition and clinical features

Extensive, flaccid blistering, peeling and skin fragility are apparent at birth and severe infection, dehydration and malnutrition often led to death in the past. Blistering and erythroderma diminish in childhood as the characteristic grey, waxy scale increases. Linear hyperkeratosis is most prominent in the flexures, scalp, anterior neck, abdominal wall and infragluteal folds (**368**). Erosions and recurring skin infections occur and an embarrassing body odour is a troublesome complication. Palmoplantar hyperkeratosis develops in many patients (**369**). A naevoid pattern of scaling may occur. This condition tends to improve with age.

Epidemiology

A rare, autosomal dominant ichthyosis with many cases apparently due to new mutations. The incidence is less than 1 in 100 000 and it is, in certain countries, referred to as epidermolytic hyperkeratosis.

Investigations

Skin biopsy shows marked acanthosis and hyperkeratosis. Granular layer keratinocytes contain multiple perinuclear vacuoles and large, clumped keratohyaline granules, and, in a bullous lesion, a split and oedema are seen in the granular layer (the hallmarks of epidermolytic hyperkeratosis). Electron microscopy reveals clumped keratin filaments around granular keratinocyte nuclei and immunoelectron microscopy, using keratin monoclonal antibodies, indicates a primary genetic defect in keratins 1 or 10.

Special points

At least half of the cases have no family history of the disease and are due to new keratin mutations. Genetic mosaicism, however, may produce focal keratotic lesions in a parent with a subsequent 50% risk in their offspring. Prenatal diagnosis relies on ultrastructural examination of a skin biopsy at around 20 weeks gestation.

Ichthyosiform Syndromes

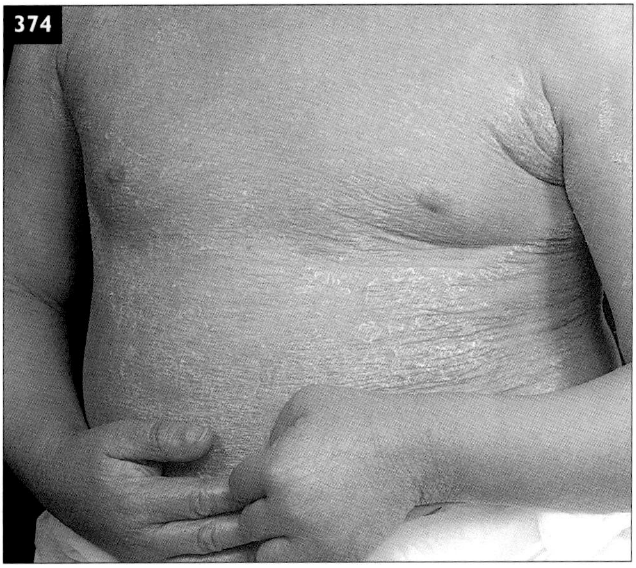

374 Neutral lipid storage disease (Chanarin–Dorfman syndrome).

presence of lipid droplets in the lower epidermis. The underlying metabolic defect is impaired oxidation of phytanic acid, a long chain branched fatty acid derived from plant chlorophyll, due to a deficiency of phytanic acid oxidase.

IBIDS (TRICHOTHIODYSTROPHY OR TAY'S SYNDROME)

This is an acronym for ichthyosis, brittle hair, impaired intelligence, decreased fertility and short stature. Photosensitivity is a feature in some patients (hence PIBIDS). This autosomal recessive group of disorders is presumed to be due to one or more DNA repair defects.

Hair microscopy shows pili torti and trichoschisis (transverse fractures) with alternating light and dark bands (tiger tail) under polarising light. The sulfur-containing amino acids of hair, cystine and proline are reduced.

CONRADI–HÜNERMANN SYNDROME

This is an X-linked dominant ichthyosis (females only affected) causing a distinctive mosaic pattern ichthyosis which improves with age. It is associated with a transient chondrodysplasia punctata and focal cataracts. Features in adult life include mosaic follicular atrophoderma and cicatricial alopecia. A partial deficiency of a peroxisomal enzyme, DHAPAT, has been identified in some patients.

NEUTRAL LIPID STORAGE DISEASE (CHANARIN–DORFMAN SYNDROME)

This is an autosomal, recessive, multisystem, lipid storage disease which causes an erythrodermic ichthyosis (**374**), hepatitis, myopathy and cataracts with variable other features. It occurs mainly in people of Arabic descent in the Mediterranean region.

A notable feature is the presence of lipid droplets, visible on light microscopy, in basal keratinocytes, circulating polymorphs and monocytes. Leucocyte vacuolation is apparent, if to a lesser extent, in carriers. Biopsies of muscle, liver and skin also contain numerous lipid droplets.

FAMILIAL PEELING SKIN SYNDROME

This is not a true ichthyosis as it causes periodic or continual shedding of large sheets of stratum corneum rather than scaling. Continuous and generalised, non-inflammatory, superficial peeling either starts at birth or in childhood and persists with only slight seasonal variation. The palms and soles are spared. Histology of a lesion shows hyperkeratosis and splitting at the corneal–granular interface. Ultrastructurally, reduced desmosomal plates and an intracellular cytoplasmic split in the lower stratum corneum have been identified.

Hypermelanosis

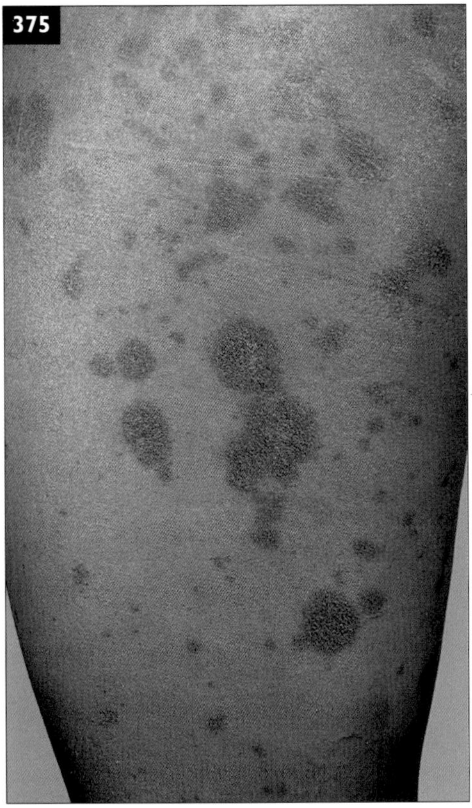

375 Postinflammatory hyperpigmentation.

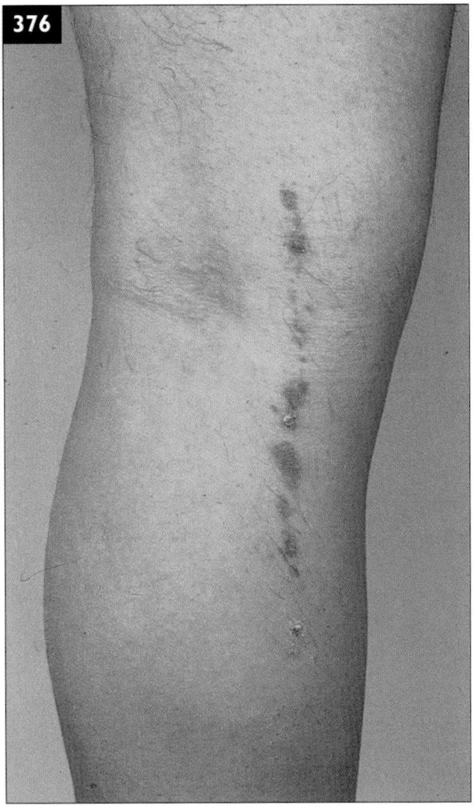

376 Lichen planus.

POSTINFLAMMATORY HYPERPIGMENTATION

Definition and clinical features

A brown or purple-brown discoloration from the accumulation of haem, iron and melanin pigments in the dermis, with or without increased melanin in the epidermis. Postinflammatory hyperpigmentation occurs after trauma, thermal injury or inflammatory dermatoses such as atopic eczema, lichen planus, acne and SLE. The discoloration intensifies and persists after the primary lesions have resolved (**375**). It is particularly likely to occur in dark-skinned individuals.

Differential diagnosis

Other causes of hyperpigmentation including melasma, ochronosis, etc. Exogenous material may stain the skin or be implanted during trauma to produce a dark macule or tattoo. Identification of the cause of postinflammatory hyperpigmentation relies on a history of a pre-existing condition and on examination of coexisting lesions.

Investigations

Histology may be helpful in lichen planus but is often unable to identify the pre-existing inflammatory condition.

LICHEN PLANUS IN DARK SKINS

Definition and clinical features

A form of postinflammatory hyperpigmentation seen especially in Asian skin. A characteristic feature is that resolving plaques often leave hyperpigmented macules that fade only slowly. This hyperpigmentation is marked in dark skins and can be the prominent feature. Linear lesions (**376**) are not unusual.

Hypermelanosis

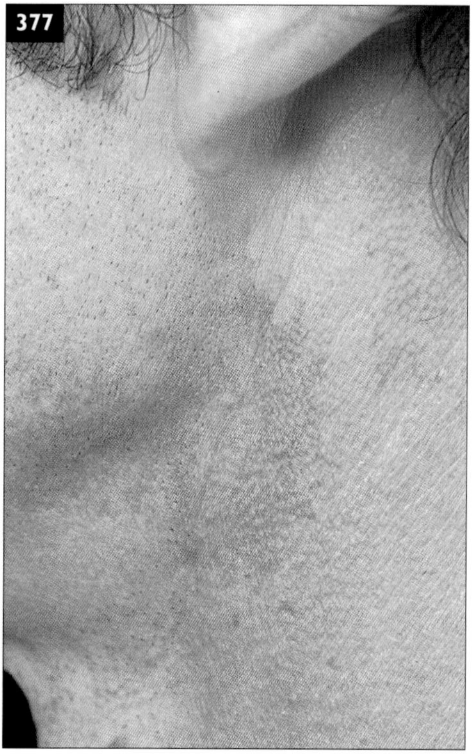

377 Berloque dermatitis.

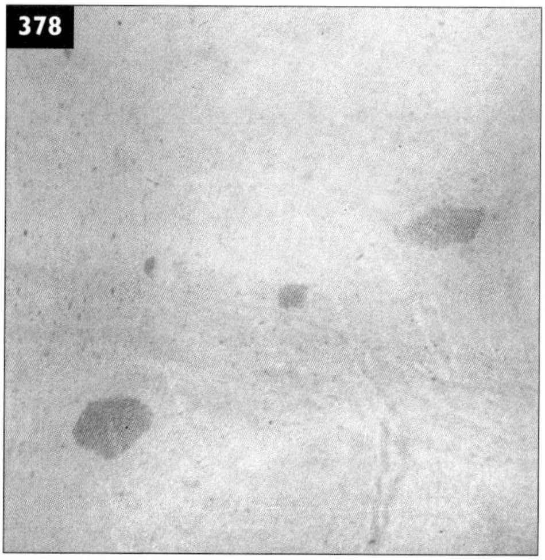

378 Café-au-lait macules.

BERLOQUE DERMATITIS

Definition and clinical features

Berloque (meaning pendent or droplike) dermatitis is a streaky hyperpigmentation resulting from the application of perfumes that contain oil of bergamot, a naturally occurring psoralen. After sun exposure, macular hyperpigmentation with sharp markings and streaking appears on the necks or hands at the site of perfume application (**377**). There is little or no erythema. A more severe reaction, with painful erythema and bullae, may result from exposure to certain concentrated plant juices, such as lime juice, followed by light exposure. The dermatitis usually appears 24 hours after sun exposure, peaking at 48 hours.

CAFÉ-AU-LAIT MACULES

Definition and clinical features

Café-au-lait ('white coffee') macules are hyperpigmented areas occurring on any cutaneous surface, unrelated to UV exposure. Characteristically homogeneous in colour, typically light brown, they vary in size (from 1 mm to many centimetres) and number and may be present at birth or acquired in early childhood. They are sharply demarcated from the surrounding skin by a smooth contour (**378**). The hyperpigmentation is due to increased melanin within epidermal keratinocytes and is enhanced by Wood's light.

Special points

Café-au-lait macules occur as solitary lesions in 10–15% of the normal population, but the presence of six or more café-au-lait macules greater than 1.5 cm in diameter is usually a sign of neurofibromatosis.

ALBRIGHT'S SYNDROME

Definition and clinical features

This genetic syndrome comprises unilateral hyperpigmented macules, fibrous dysplasia of bone and endocrine dysfunction. The full

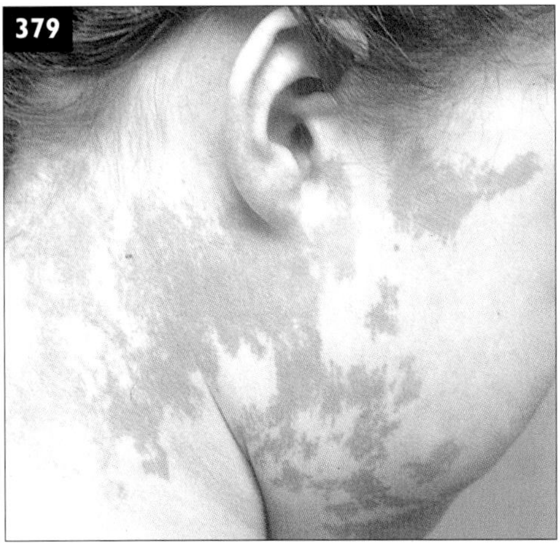

379 Albright's syndrome.

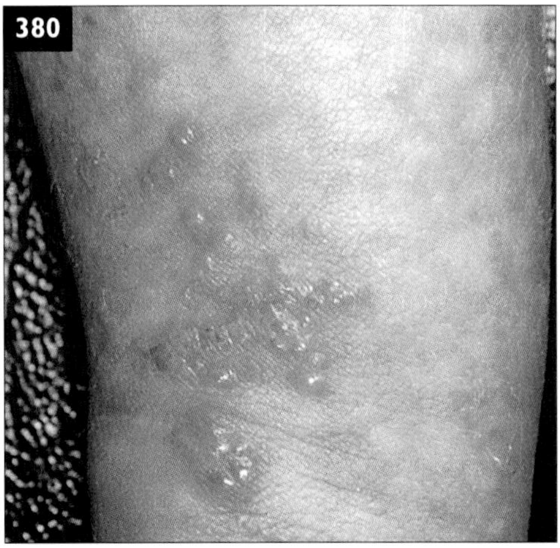

380 Incontinentia pigmenti.

syndrome with precocious puberty occurs only in girls. The dark macules of the syndrome are usually large and few in number, they tend to be unilateral and may be arranged in a linear or segmental pattern (**379**). The hairs within the macules tend to be darker as well, the macules irregular contour helping to distinguish them from café-au-lait macules. The bony lesions tend to be on the same side of the body as the macules. Axillary freckling is not a feature of Albright's (*cf.* neurofibromatosis).

Special points

In girls, precocious puberty occurs below the age of 5 years in about 50% and between 5 and 10 years in 30%. Other developmental abnormalities may be associated.

INCONTINENTIA PIGMENTI

Definition and clinical features

Incontinentia pigmenti is a complex developmental syndrome due to an X-linked dominant trait that is lethal in males; 95% of cases are females. Vesicular, verrucous and pigmented skin lesions are associated with developmental defects of the eye, skeleton and central nervous syndrome. Skin changes are present at or soon after birth.

Three clinical stages are recognised: blisters, warty papules and irregular pigmentation. Linear groups of clear, tense blisters develop on the limbs and/or trunk in recurrent crops (**380**). They are accompanied or followed by smooth red or bluish-purple nodules or plaques. Linear warty lesions may appear on the backs of the fingers or toes. Sometimes pigmentation is the only abnormality. Brown or blue-grey pigmentation may be present from the outset or may develop as the inflammatory lesions are subsiding. A bizarre 'splashed' or 'Chinese figure' distribution is diagnostic (**381**). The pigmentation slowly fades, becoming imperceptible by the third decade.

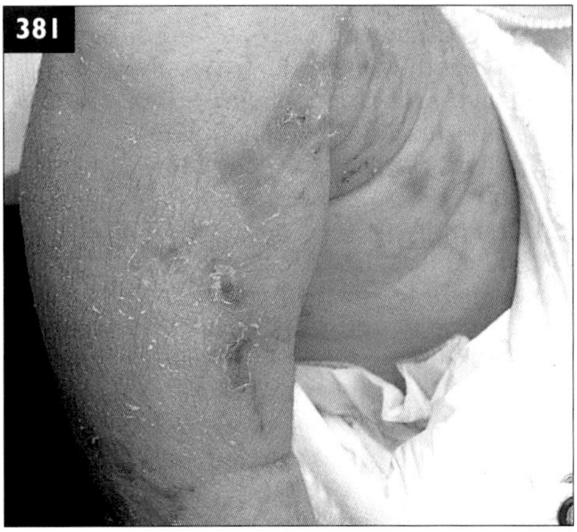

381 'Chinese figure' distribution in incontinentia pigmenti.

Hypomelanosis

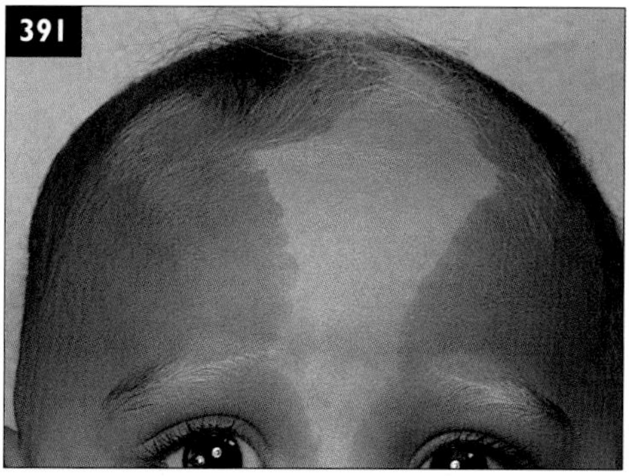

391 Piebaldism.

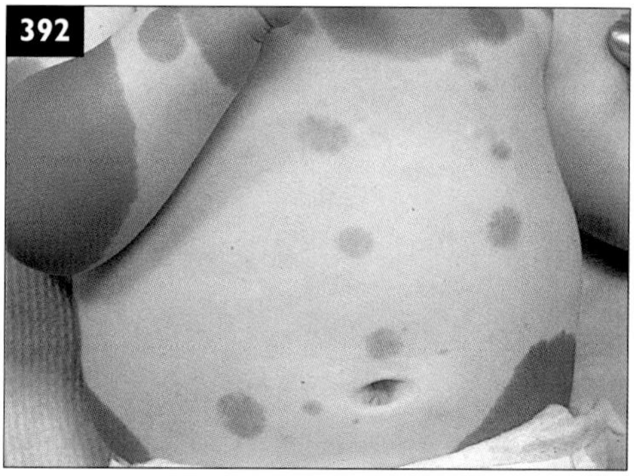

392 Piebaldism.

393 Idiopathic guttate hypomelanosis.

is associated with a forelock of white hair (**391**). Stable white macules are also common on the chest, abdomen and limbs but spare the hands and feet. Islands of normal or hypermelanotic skin occur within the white areas (**392**).

Differential diagnosis
The white forelock and pattern of white macules is quite characteristic. The main differential is Waardenburg's syndrome where, in addition, the interpupillary distance is increased and 20% of patients are deaf. The absence of melanocytes and melanosomes on microscopy differentiates this from naevus depigmentosus.

PITYRIASIS VERSICOLOR
May cause patchy hypo- or hyperpigmentation on the trunk (see p. 72).

PITYRIASIS ALBA
Definition and clinical features
Pityriasis alba is a common, acquired hypomelanosis characterised by poorly circumscribed, fine, scaly macules on the face of children. The aetiology is unknown but may represent a form of low-grade eczema. The term pityriasis alba well describes the pale, scaly and ill-defined patches of hypopigmentation seen most easily in dark-skinned children and affecting usually the face, but sometimes also the trunk and arms.

Differential diagnosis
Vitiligo, tinea and post-inflammatory hypopigmentation.

IDIOPATHIC GUTTATE HYPOMELANOSIS
Definition and clinical features
A common condition of acquired hypomelanosis presenting as small, sharply defined, white macules. It may result from an age-related somatic mutation of melanosomes. The white macules are usually small (2–6 mm in diameter) with sharply defined, angular or irregular borders (**393**). In Caucasian skin they typically occur on sun-exposed areas of the limbs. Sun damage is thought to be an important factor. Non-actinic lesions are seen in Afro-Caribbeans and may be found in unexposed areas on the trunk.

MISCELLANEOUS
Other important causes of hypopigmented skin lesions such as leprosy and sarcoidosis are found elsewhere in this book.

Non-Melanin Pigmentation

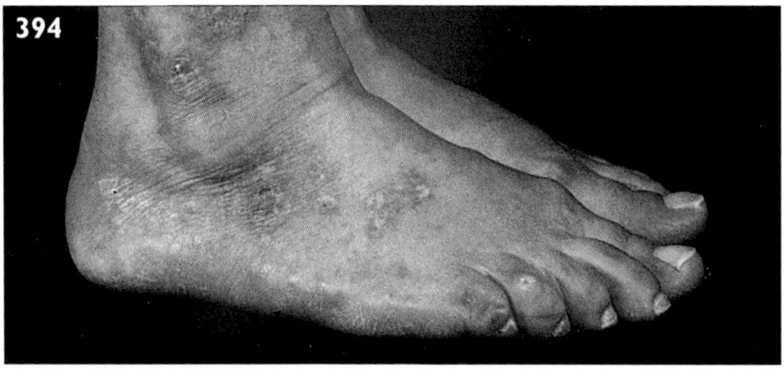

394 Hypostatic haemosiderosis.

HAEMOSIDEROSIS

Definition and clinical features

This is the deposition of the iron-containing pigment haemosiderin within the skin. This commonly results from the local destruction of red blood cells. Haemosiderin deposition stimulates melanogenesis, so that varying degrees of hypermelanosis are usually associated. It is seen most commonly on the lower legs in venous hypertension (hypostatic haemosiderosis); involved areas initially show grouped specks of orange-red pigment (**394**) but, with increasing hypermelanosis, later produce a more uniform deep-brown pigmentation that persists even if the venous hypertension is corrected.

In capillaritis (e.g. Schamberg's disease), cayenne pepper-like haemosiderosis without detectable hypermelanosis is seen especially on the lower legs and thighs (**395**).

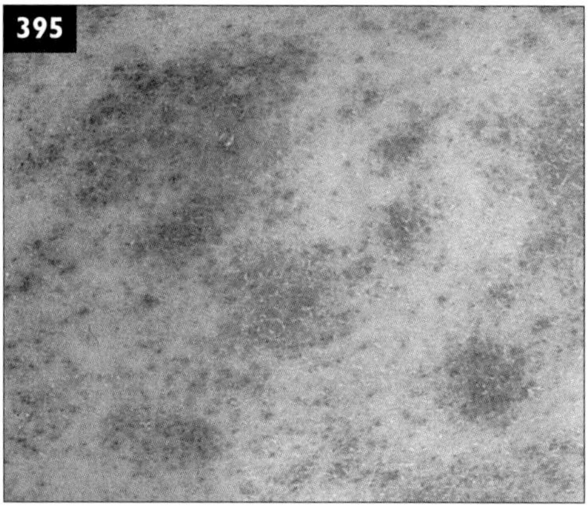

395 Schamberg's disease.

Special points

In haemochromatosis (bronze diabetes), hypermelanosis dominates the clinical picture, giving the distinctive grey-brown pigmentation seen especially on the face, flexural creases and exposed parts.

CAROTENAEMIA

Definition and clinical features

A yellow discoloration of the skin and palate due to excessive blood carotene levels. This yellow discoloration is most marked in areas of hyperkeratosis, especially the palms and the soles (**396**), or where subcutaneous fat is plentiful. It is seen in patients taking β-carotene or in food faddists who eat excessive amounts of carotene-containing foods such as carrots or oranges. Diagnosis is confirmed by measuring blood carotene levels.

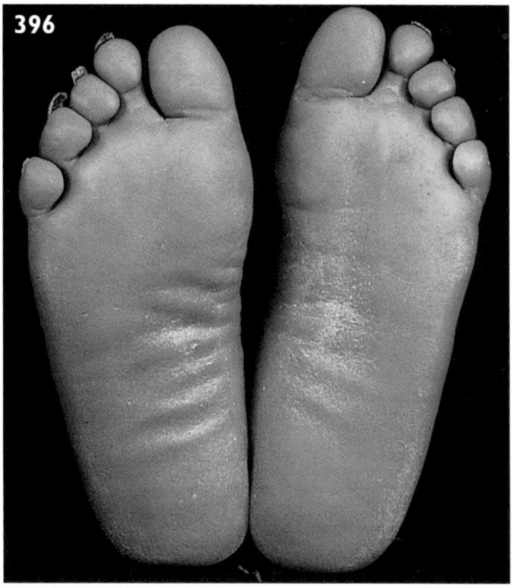

396 Carotenaemia.

Non-Melanin Pigmentation

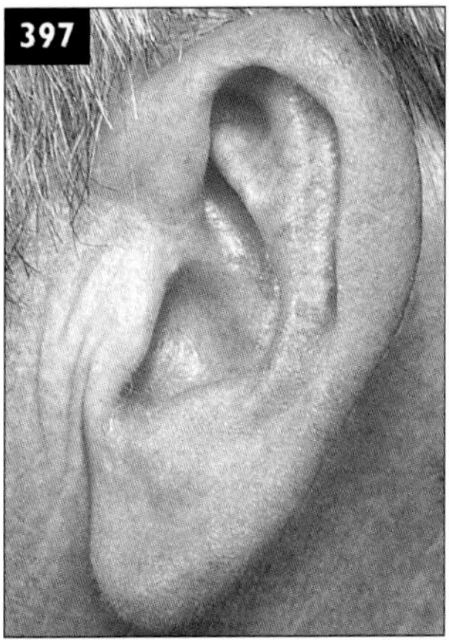

397 Amiodarone pigmentation.

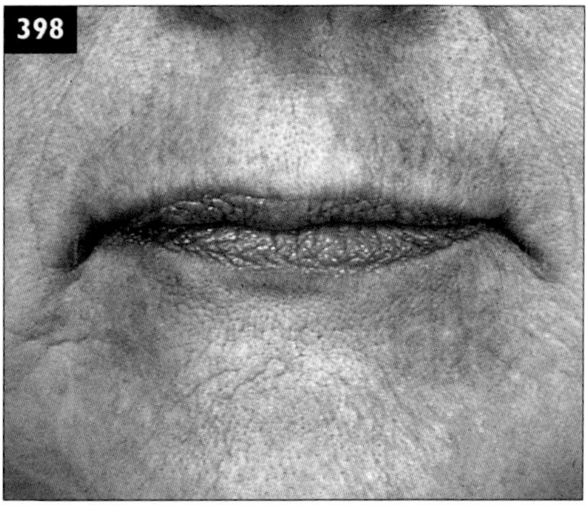

398 Minocycline-induced pigmentation.

Special points

Rarely, carotenaemia is due to an inborn error of metabolism. It may be associated with hyperlipidaemia, diabetes, nephritis or hypothyroidism.

OCHRONOSIS

Definition and clinical features

Ochronosis is the deposition of a melanin-like, brownish-black pigment derived from polymerised homogentisic acid. Part of the rare inherited metabolic disorder alkaptonuria, ochronosis is seen much more commonly in an exogenous or acquired form from the long-term application of hydroquinone-containing skin-lightening creams. A dusky, cutaneous pigmentation is usually most marked over the cheeks and forehead and, in alkaptonuria, the axillae, genitalia, buccal mucosa and larynx.

Differential diagnosis

Alkaptonuria is diagnosed by demonstrating homogentisic acid in the urine. In dark-skinned women, or those receiving treatment for melasma, exogenous ochronosis is important in the differential diagnosis of facial hyperpigmentation.

ARGYRIA

Definition and clinical features

The deposition of silver within the skin, either from industrial exposure or from medication. A slate blue–grey pigmentation slowly accumulates over many years until clinically apparent, especially in sun-exposed areas of skin. Sclerae, nails and mucous membranes may also become pigmented, the pigmentation being permanent.

The diagnosis of argyria is established by skin biopsy. Silver granules are visible within the dermis, particularly in relation to the basal lamina of the eccrine sweat glands.

DRUG-INDUCED PIGMENTATION

Definition and clinical features

A drug-induced alteration in skin colour resulting from a number of mechanisms, including increased melanin synthesis, postinflammatory hyperpigmentation (see Fixed drug eruption, p. 192) and cutaneous deposition of drug-related material.

The clinical picture varies according to the drug in question. The oral contraceptive pill, for instance, may induce melasma. Long-term antimalarial therapy may result in brown or blue-black pigmentation on the shin, face and hard palate. Amiodarone or long-term high dose chlorpromazine can both cause a blue-grey pigmentation of sun-exposed areas (**397**). Lead poisoning may result in a blue-black line at the gingival margin with grey discoloration of the skin.

Minocycline-induced pigmentation is not uncommon following prolonged high dose courses and may present as a diffuse or generalised hyperpigmentation or as a blue-black pigment at sites of previous inflammation such as acne scars (**398**). Skin biopsy shows brown-black granules in the upper dermis that stain for iron.

Tropical Dermatoses

399

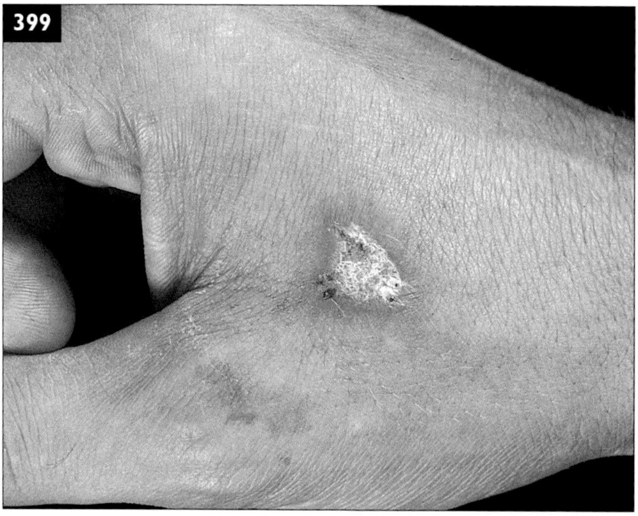

399 Cutaneous leishmaniasis.

400

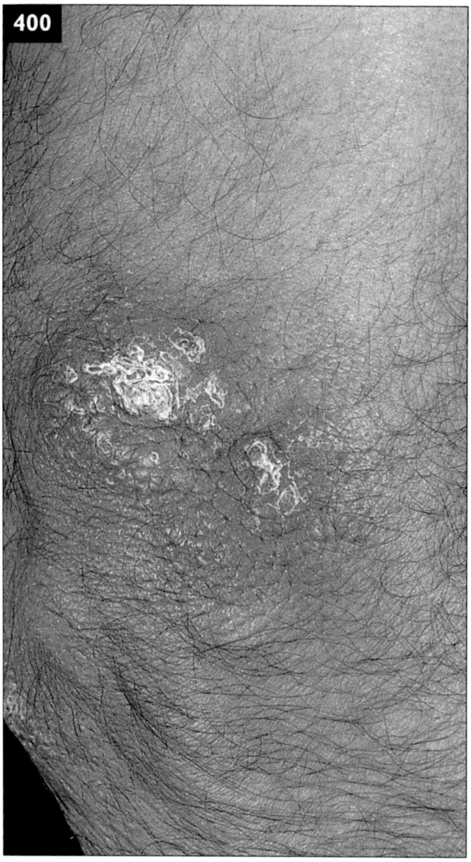

400 Cutaneous leishmaniasis.

CUTANEOUS LEISHMANIASIS (ORIENTAL SORE)

Definition and clinical features

This is a localised cutaneous reaction to infection by *Leishmania* species. Any site exposed to sand flies may be affected.

In the dry urban form, a small, brownish-purple nodule forms after an incubation period of around 2 months. This slowly enlarges to around 1–2 cm, at which time a shallow central ulcer covered by an adherent crust forms (**399**, **400**) which eventually heals by scarring after 8–12 months.

In the wet rural form, the lesions begin earlier after inoculation, and ulceration also

Tropical Dermatoses

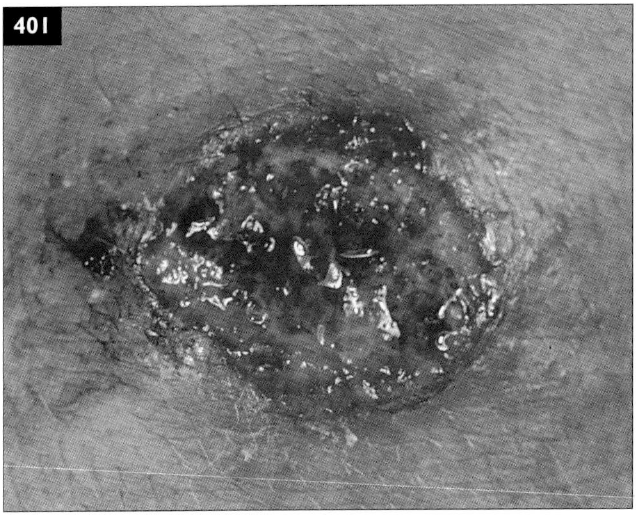

401 Ulcerated cutaneous leishmaniasis.

occurs earlier (**401**). Secondary nodules may occur around lymphatics (**402**) and healing usually takes place in 2–6 months.

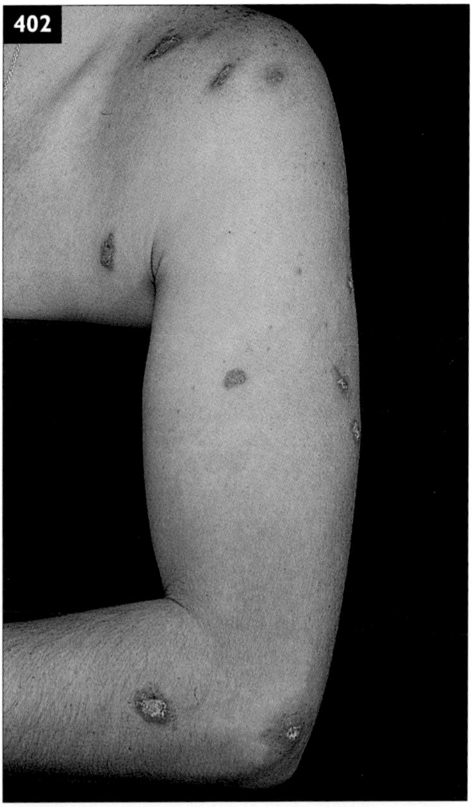

402 Secondary nodules of cutaneous leishmaniasis.

Epidemiology

Many species of Leishmania exist but most cases seen in travellers returning from tropical areas are due to *L. tropica*, *L. major* and *L. aethiopica*. It is a disease of warm countries, occurring around the Mediterranean coast, North Africa, South America, Asia Minor, China and the southern states of the former Soviet Union. The protozoan is transmitted by sandfly bites, commonly *Phlebotomus papatasii*.

Differential diagnosis

Boils are of shorter duration and will grow *Staphylococcus aureus* on culture. Mosquito bites may become secondarily infected with bacteria but reactions are immediate and heal within a few weeks.

Investigations

Skin biopsy or smear for identification of organisms and specialised culture. A cutaneous test (the leishmanin test) is positive in about 90% of cases.

Special points

Small lesions may heal spontaneously. Numerous forms of leishmaniasis can occur including mucocutaneous and visceral forms, all of which can exhibit cutaneous features.

Tropical Dermatoses

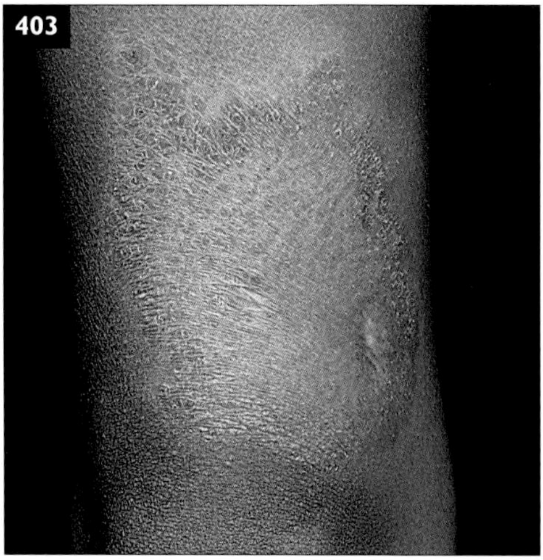

403 Tuberculoid leprosy.

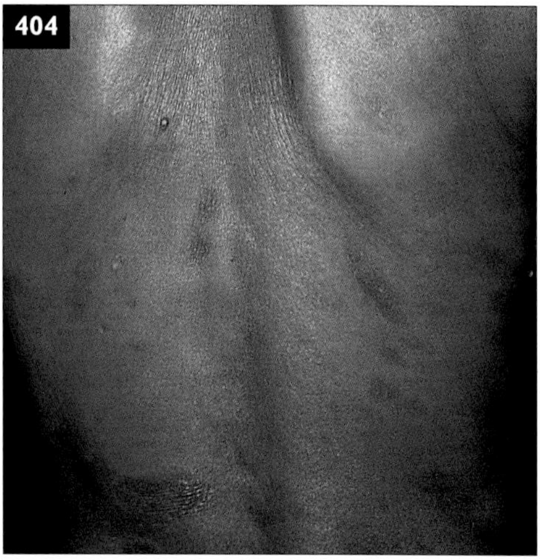

404 Lepromatous leprosy.

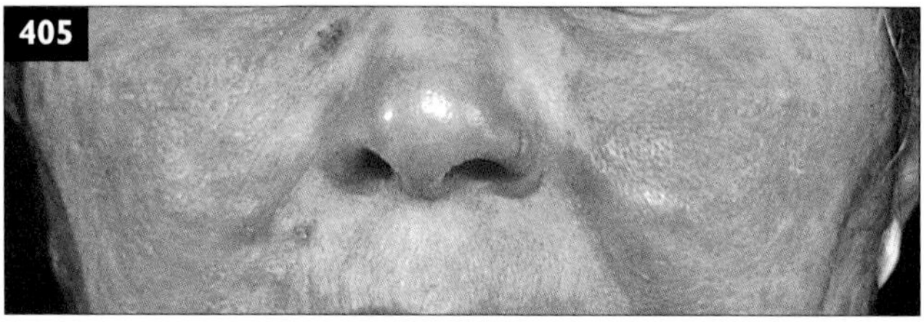

405 Borderline leprosy.

LEPROSY

Definition and clinical features

A chronic mycobacterial infection affecting primarily the peripheral nerves and secondarily involving the skin and other organs. The clinical features depend on the underlying state of immunity of the person.

Tuberculoid leprosy is seen in those with high immunity. Lesions are few, and consist of a well-defined plaque with an erythematous raised border and a hypopigmented, dry, anaesthetic centre (**403**). Thickened peripheral nerves may be palpated.

Lepromatous leprosy occurs in individuals with poor cell-mediated immunity. Lesions are multiple, infiltrating dermal papules, nodules and plaques favouring cooler body sites (**404**).

Various degrees of intermediate forms exist (**405**).

Epidemiology

Leprosy is one of the commonest skin diseases world-wide, affecting around 15 million people in tropical and sub-tropical climates. The young are most susceptible to acquiring infection, and spread occurs mainly via the oronasal route. Nerve involvement typically occurs after an incubation period of 3–5 years.

Differential diagnosis

Occasionally post-inflammatory hypopigmentation may be mistaken for tuberculoid leprosy, but such changes return to normal after a few months. Other granulomatous diseases, such as tuberculosis, leishmaniasis, syphilis, yaws and sarcoidosis, should be ruled out by histology, microbiology and skin testing.

Investigations

Skin smear, skin biopsy, nasal scrape, nerve biopsy and lepromin test.

Special points

Oral corticosteroids are sometimes needed to prevent nerve damage when initiating therapy.

Tropical Dermatoses

406

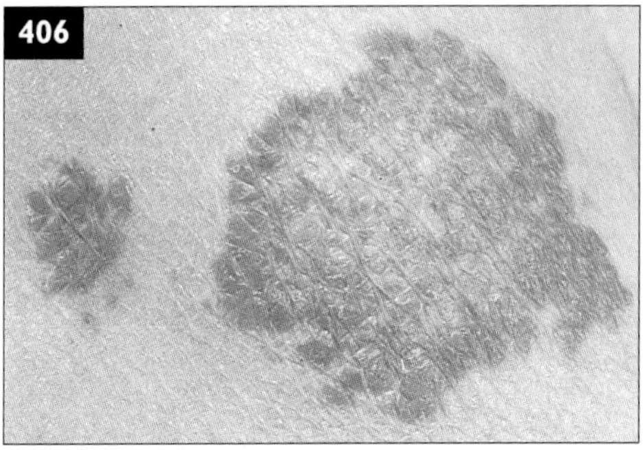

406 Lupus vulgaris.

407

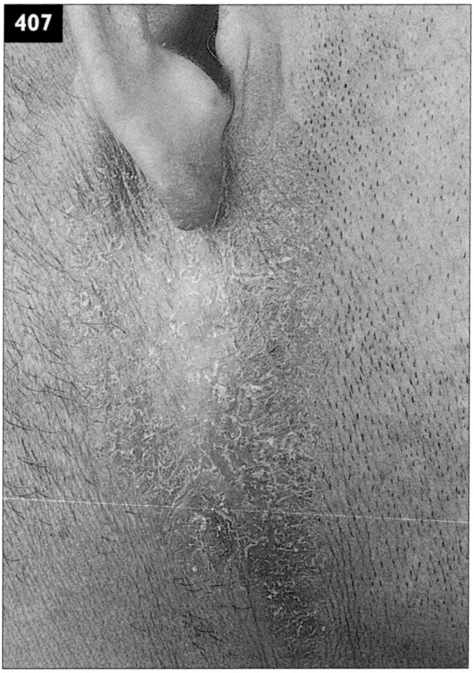

407 Lupus vulgaris.

408

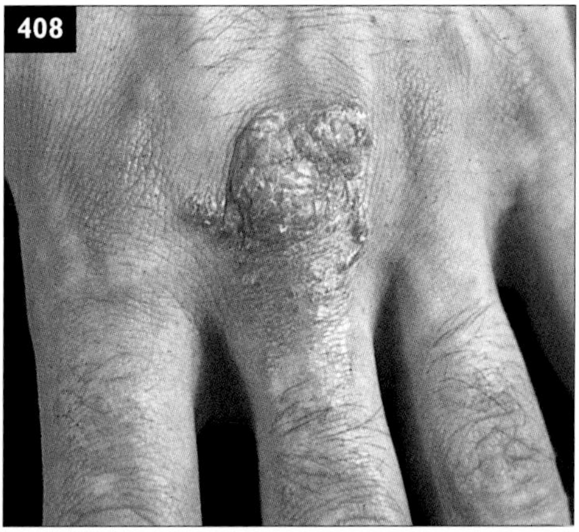

408 Warty TB.

CUTANEOUS TUBERCULOSIS

Definition and clinical features

Invasion of the skin by Mycobacterium tuberculosis. The commonest form is lupus vulgaris, a progressive form in persons with moderate to high immunity. A typical lesion is composed of a solitary, slowly extending, reddish-brown plaque (**406**) located on the head and neck (**407**), which displays an 'apple jelly' appearance when a glass slide is pressed against the surface of the lesion. Cutaneous lesions due to primary inoculation of the skin appear as warty indolent plaques on exposed areas (warty TB) (**408**). Scrofuloderma denotes skin involvement from an underlying tuberculous lymph node.

Epidemiology

Although declining in developed areas, tuberculosis is common in poor countries where various forms of cutaneous involvement are still seen.

Differential diagnosis

Other granulomatous diseases such as leprosy, leishmaniasis, syphilis, and sarcoidosis should be ruled out by histology, microbiology and tuberculin testing.

Investigations

Skin biopsy essential. Material should be sent for culture. Tuberculin test usually strongly positive. Chest radiograph to exclude primary source of infection.

Special points

Untreated lesions may rarely develop into squamous cell carcinoma. Atypical mycobacteria occasionally infect the skin (see p. 67), especially in immunosuppressed individuals. A range of cutaneous reactions to tuberculosis (tuberculides) are recognised.

Tropical Dermatoses

409

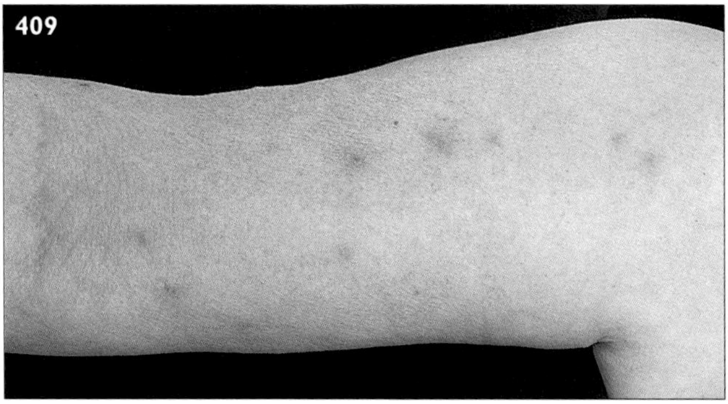

409 Linear insect bite reactions.

410

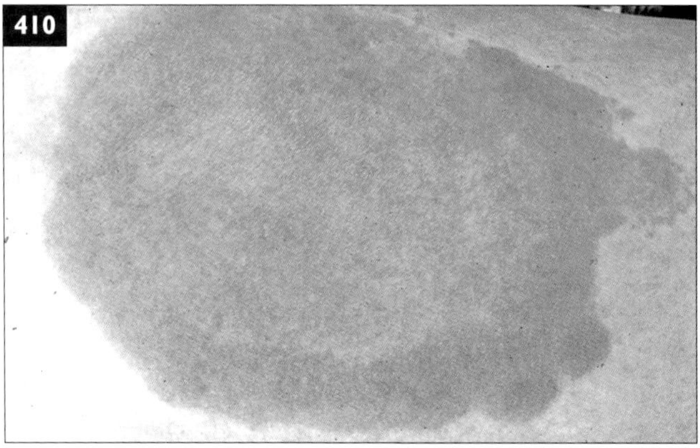

410 Erythema chronicum migrans.

411

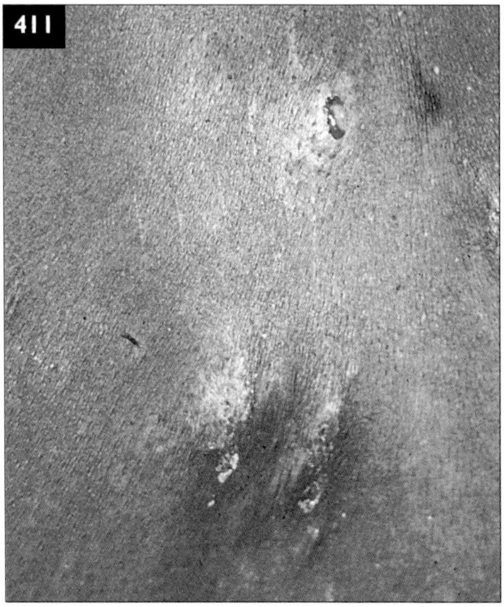

411 Cutaneous myiasis.

INSECT BITES

Definition and clinical features

A localised pruritic reaction of the skin produced by a range of insects, the specific features depending on the offending insect.

Lesions produced by fleas and bed bugs often produce a linear or grouped configuration (**409**). Individual lesions may exhibit a small red punctum corresponding to the puncture wound. Lesions are found on exposed areas. Often a non-specific papular urticaria on exposed limbs is all that is seen. Erythema chronicum migrans (**410**) may follow the tick bite of Lyme disease. Cutaneous myiasis shows furuncle-like lesions (**411**).

Tropical Dermatoses

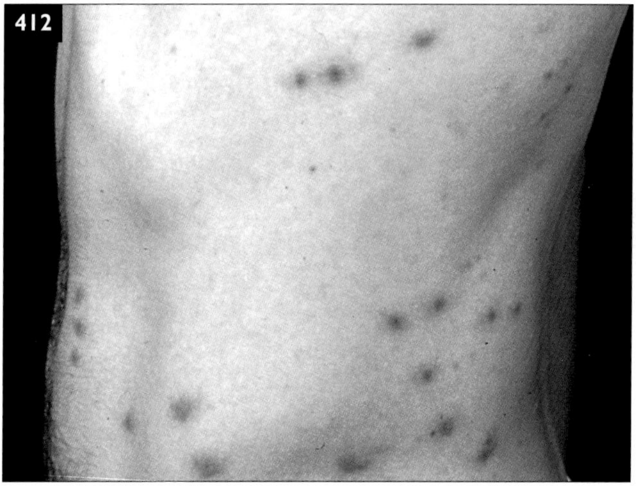

412 Insect bites.

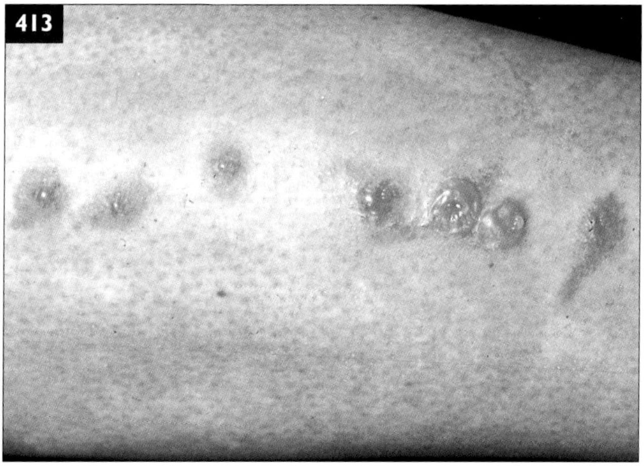

413 Insect bites.

Epidemiology

Insect bites are common and universal throughout the world. In temperate climates, fleas from domestic pets, *Cheyletiella* mites and bed bugs are the commonest causes whereas in tropical regions mosquito and sandfly bites predominate (**412**, **413**). Other infectious diseases such as malaria, filariasis, yellow fever, leishmaniasis and Lyme disease may be transmitted in the process.

Differential diagnosis

The lesions of erythema multiforme may produce groups of annular lesions with a central red area but the symmetrical distribution over extensor areas is characteristic.

Investigations

Examination of pets by a veterinary surgeon if fleas or mites suspected. Biopsy if leishmaniasis suspected. Skin swabs for secondary infection.

Special points

Although often trivialised, insect bites form a considerable burden of skin disease. Intense pruritus may persist for months, and secondary infections with *Staphylococcus aureus* and streptococci can be serious and lead to scarring.

414 Onchocerciasis.

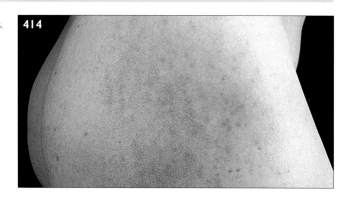

415 Onchocerciasis.

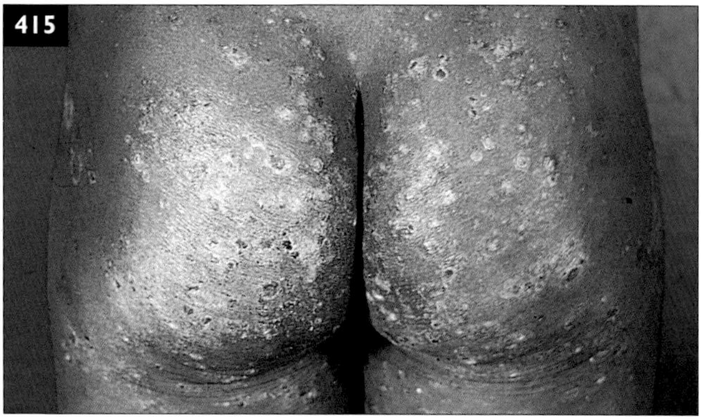

ONCHOCERCIASIS

Definition and clinical features

A filarial disease caused by *Onchocerca volvulus*. The disease usually presents with pruritus followed by a non-specific papular rash. In travellers returning from endemic areas, mild infection is often associated with involvement of the pelvic and buttock area (**414**) and urticarial swellings with unilateral limb swelling may occur. Gross lichenification and small scars eventually develop (**415**) followed by atrophy and loss of skin elasticity. Onchocercomata are painless swellings, sited close to bony prominences, where mature worms may be found.

Epidemiology

Onchocerciasis is found throughout tropical Africa, Arabia, Central America and Mexico. Transmission of larvae occurs through tiny black flies of the Simuliidae family. All ages are affected. Without treatment, symptoms increase in severity until atrophic changes are complete.

Differential diagnosis

General pruritus from other causes such as iron deficiency anaemia should be excluded. Scabies and body lice commonly cause a generalised pruritus but the presence of burrows or lice in clothing seams will help to separate these.

Investigations

Skin snips taken from the legs or buttocks at night are examined in saline for the presence of microfilariae. Nodules can be excised and submitted for histology. A filarial skin test is usually positive. A full blood count may reveal eosinophilia, and a filarial complement fixation test is positive in over 60% of cases.

Special points

Blindness may occur in up to half the adults in hyperendemic areas.

Tropical Dermatoses

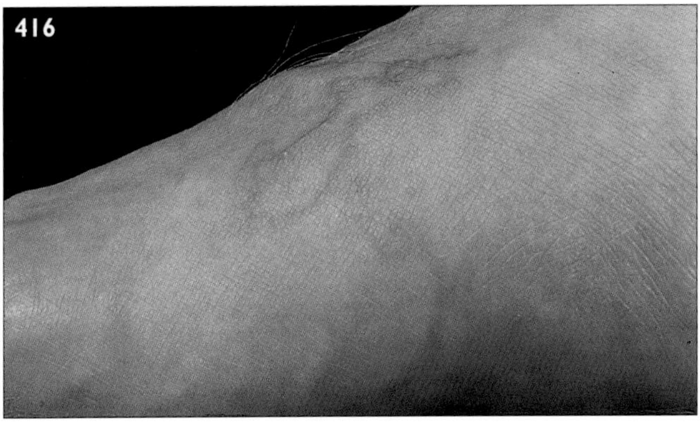

416 Creeping eruption.

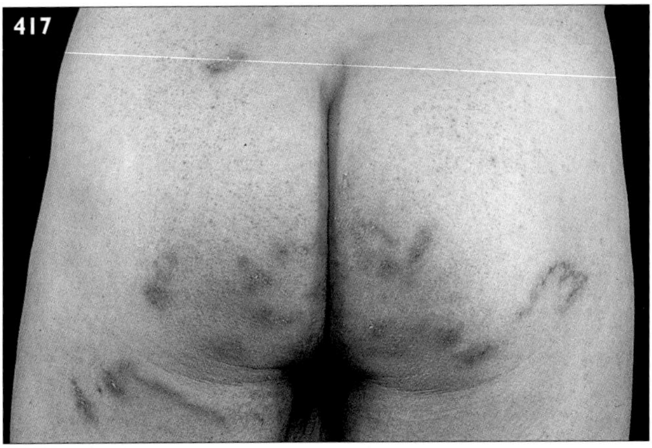

417 Creeping eruption.

CREEPING ERUPTION (CUTANEOUS LARVA MIGRANS)

Definition and clinical features

A self-limiting cutaneous eruption caused by the migration of animal hookworm larvae for whom man is a dead-end host. The eruption is composed of intensely itchy, serpiginous, pink tracks which advance about a centimetre per day (**416**). Large numbers of larvae produce a disorganised collection of tortuous tracks (**417**). Sites exposed to beach sand, such as the feet and buttocks, are the commonest areas to be affected in travellers returning from tropical countries. The larvae wander through the epidermis until they eventually die after around 4 weeks.

Epidemiology

Most creeping eruptions are caused by dog and cat hookworm larvae which penetrate the skin in moist, shaded, sandy areas such as beaches. Although it can occur in temperate climes, most cases are seen in holidaymakers returning from tropical countries.

Differential diagnosis

Lesions of *Strongyloides stercoralis* advance faster, are frequently perianal, and are associated with intestinal involvement. Migratory myiasis produces shorter tracks with a terminal vesicle which often breaks down.

Investigations

None usually required.

Special points

The lesions can be intensely itchy but respond quickly to treatment with a single dose of 400 mg of oral albendazole.

Drug Eruptions

Drug eruptions are probably the most frequent manifestation of drug sensitivity. Their true incidence is difficult to determine because mild and transitory eruptions are often not recorded and because skin disorders may be falsely attributed to drugs. Certain patient groups are at increased risk of developing an adverse drug reaction. The ampicillin rash seen in patients with infectious mononucleosis is a classical example (**418**). Elderly patients and patients with acquired immunodeficiency syndrome (AIDS) appear predisposed to adverse drug reactions. A 5-year survey of in-patients, published in 1989, incriminated antimicrobial agents most frequently (42%), then antipyretic/anti-inflammatory analgesics (27%), with 10% of reactions due to drugs acting on the CNS. More recent surveys have found an increased proportion of cardiac drugs especially ACE inhibitors, calcium channel-blockers and amiodarone.

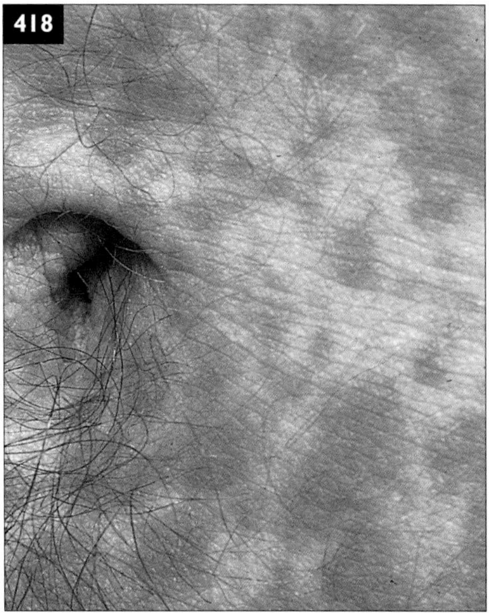

418 Ampicillin rash.

EXANTHEMATIC (MACULOPAPULAR) REACTIONS

Definition and clinical features

The commonest of all cutaneous drug eruptions, occurring in 2–3% of patients, and seen with almost any drug at any time up to 3 weeks after administration.

Typically, there is a fine erythematous morbilliform maculopapular eruption of the trunk and extremities that may become confluent (**419**). Exanthematic drug reactions often start in areas of trauma or pressure and can be very variable, with either predominantly small papules, or large macules, a reticular eruption, or polycyclic or sheet-like erythema. Intertriginous areas may be favoured, palmar and plantar involvement can occur and the face is often spared. Purpuric lesions are common on the legs and erosive stomatitis may develop. Drug exanthem may be accompanied by fever, pruritus and eosinophilia. These eruptions usually fade with desquamation, sometimes with postinflammatory hyperpigmentation.

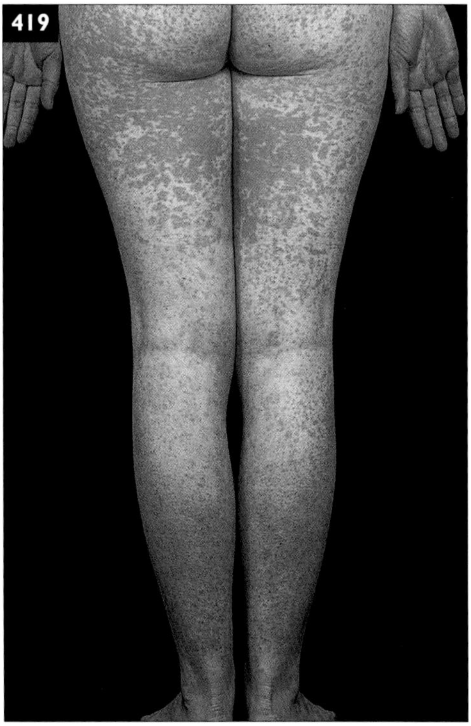

419 Exanthematic drug reaction.

Drug associations

Drugs commonly causing exanthematic reactions include: ampicillin and penicillin, sulfonamides, phenylbutazone, phenytoin, carbamazepine, gold and gentamicin.

Drug Eruptions

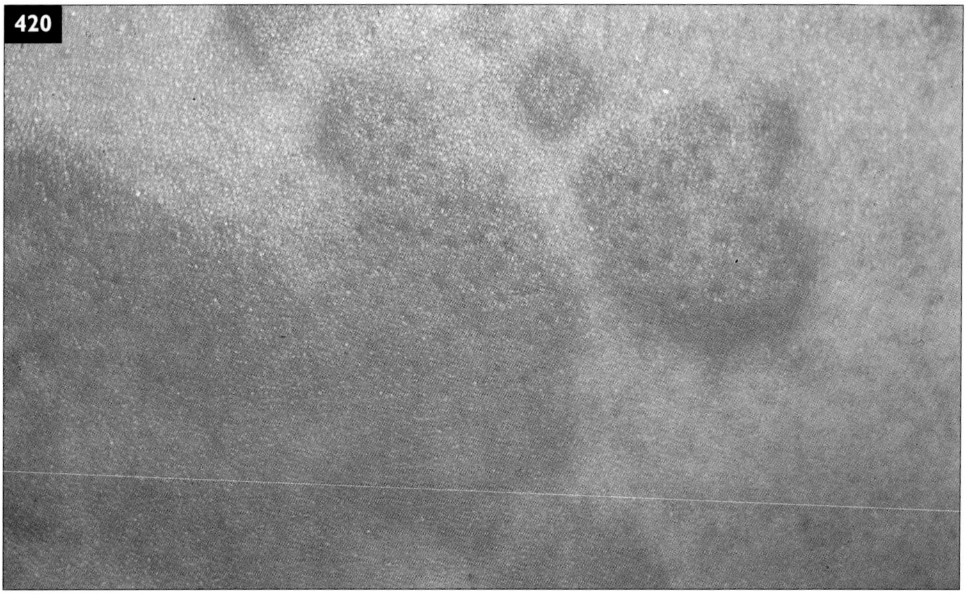

420 Urticarial drug reaction.

BULLOUS DRUG ERUPTIONS

Definition, clinical features and drug associations

This is a heterogeneous group involving many different clinical reactions and mechanisms. Pemphigus and pemphigoid may be drug induced (see pp. 134 and 136), as may acquired epidermolysis bullosa (EBA) and cutaneous porphyria. Penicillamine-induced pemphigus is usually of the foliaceus type, while captopril causes a pemphigus vulgaris-type eruption. Cicatricial pemphigoid has been described with clonidine and previously with practolol. Fixed eruptions and drug-induced vasculitis may have a bullous component, while toxic epidermal necrolysis (TEN; see below) has widespread blistering. A number of drugs may induce phototoxic bullae (see below). Bullae, often at pressure points, can be present in patients comatose after overdosage with barbiturates, methadone, tricyclic antidepressants and benzodiazepines.

URTICARIA

Definition and clinical features

Urticaria is the second most common allergic cutaneous reaction to drugs. Allergic urticaria is the cutaneous manifestation of a Type 1 (IgE antibody mediated) or Type 3 (immune complex mediated) hypersensitivity reaction. Some drugs, e.g. morphine and codeine, can act as direct histamine liberators. Urticaria may accompany serum sickness reactions or systemic anaphylaxis.

Urticaria appears as firm, erythematous, oedematous plaques with normal overlying epidermis and no scaling (**420**). Lesions characteristically last for less that 24 hours and are replaced by new lesions in different sites. Giant, papular, arcuate and annular lesions may be seen (**421**). Angio-oedema may be associated. Pruritus is prominent and bronchospasm, hypotension and eosinophilia may occur. Urticaria usually resolves quickly when the offending drug is withdrawn but, not uncommonly, episodes of urticaria may persist for several weeks after drug discontinuation.

Drug associations

Penicillin and salicylates are common provokers. Other commonly implicated agents include blood products, vaccines, radiocontrast agents, NSAIDs, opiates, cephalosporins and ACE inhibitors.

Drug Eruptions

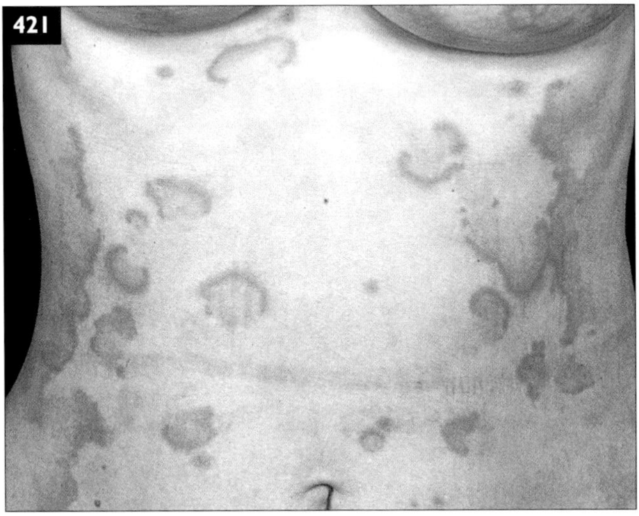

421 Urticarial drug reaction.

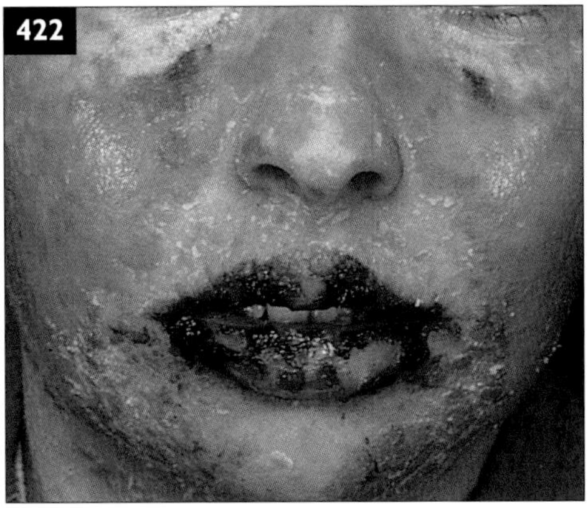

422 Stevens–Johnson syndrome.

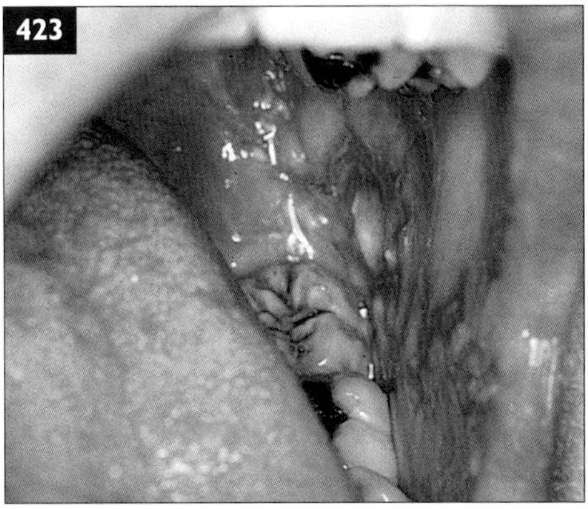

423 Stevens–Johnson syndrome.

STEVENS–JOHNSON SYNDROME

Definition and clinical features

Stevens–Johnson syndrome is a severe variant of erythema multiforme (EM) characterised by widespread involvement of mucosal surfaces.

A prodrome of fever, malaise and prostration is followed by eruption of mucosal bullae, with or without the widespread cutaneous target lesions of EM. Mucosal surfaces, commonly the oral mucosa, respiratory tract and conjunctivae may be extensively involved and secondary infection is common (**422**, **423**). Morbidity is significant, with pain, ocular complications, respiratory compromise, dysuria and difficulty maintaining adequate oral fluid intake.

Drug associations

Erythema multiforme (see p. 159) is more commonly precipitated by various infections, but both EM and Stevens–Johnson syndrome can be drug induced. Commonly incriminated are sulfonamides/co-trimoxazole, barbiturates, phenylbutazone, phenytoin, carbamazepine, phenothiazines, chlorpropamide, thiazide diuretics and malaria prophylaxis.

Drug Eruptions

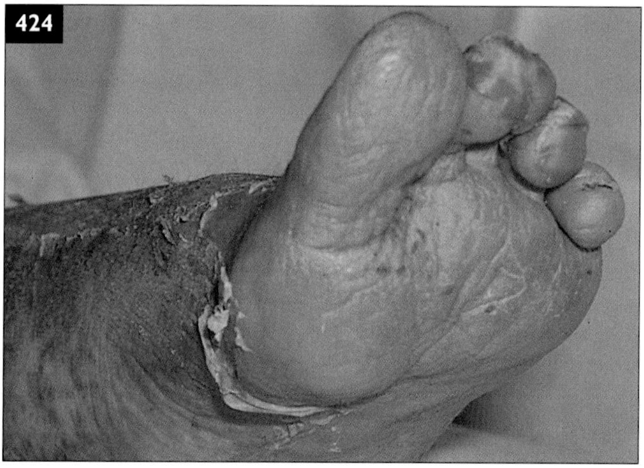

424 Toxic epidermal necrolysis.

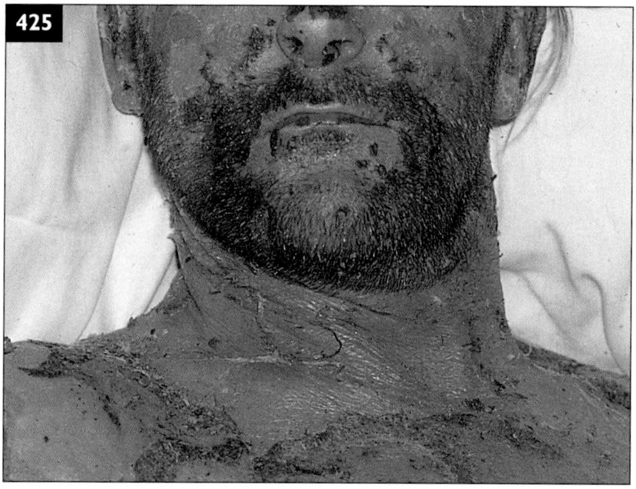

425 Toxic epidermal necrolysis.

TOXIC EPIDERMAL NECROLYSIS (TEN)

Definition and clinical features

This dermatological emergency is characterised by generalised erythema that rapidly develops full thickness epidermal necrolysis and exfoliation, associated with mucosal involvement and serious secondary complications. There is an appreciable mortality.

Often a prodrome of 1–2 days precedes a morbilliform or generalised erythema of the face and extremities. The widespread erythema is rapidly followed by blister formation with confluence into large, flaccid bullae that are easily ruptured, resulting in sloughing of large sheets of epidermis (**424**, **425**). Mucous membranes are usually severely affected, including the oral mucosa (**426**), conjunctivae, trachea, bronchi and anogenital region. Nail shedding may also occur.

Systemic involvement is reflected by fever, leucocytosis, electrolyte imbalance and elevated hepatic enzymes. Pigmentary changes and a sicca syndrome are frequent sequelae.

Drug associations

A drug aetiology is identified in up to 75% of cases. Many drugs have been associated but most frequently implicated are sulfonamides,

Drug Eruptions

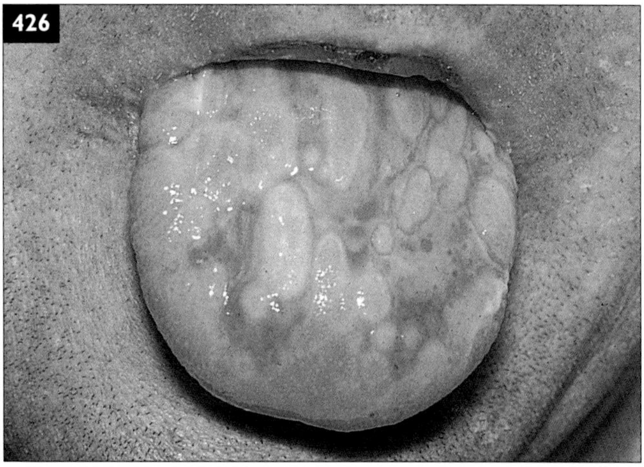

426 Toxic epidermal necrolysis.

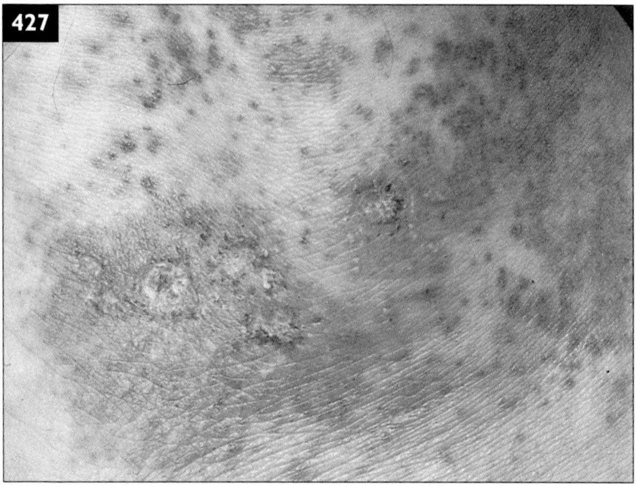

427 Drug-induced vasculitis.

NSAIDs, phenytoin, penicillins, allopurinol, carbamazepine and barbiturates.

VASCULITIS

Definition and clinical features

Vasculitis is a manifestation of immune complex disease with inflammation and necrosis of blood vessels (see pp. 155–158). Drug-induced vasculitis may involve the skin and/or internal organs. The pattern of the cutaneous eruption may indicate the calibre of the involved vessel. Capillaritis is characterised by cayenne pepper spots of pigmentation, venulitis by palpable purpura (**427**) and arteritis by painful nodules. All arise most commonly on the lower extremities. The distinctive patterns of Henoch–Schönlein vasculitis, polyarteritis nodosa and hypocomplementaemic vasculitis are not commonly caused by drugs.

Drug associations

Many groups of drugs have been associated with vasculitis, including thiazides, sulfonamides, penicillin, fluoroquinolone antibiotics, ACE inhibitors, cimetidine, allopurinol, hydralazine, quinidine and phenylbutazone. Serum products, food additives, BCG vaccination and radiographic contrast media are other causes.

Drug Eruptions

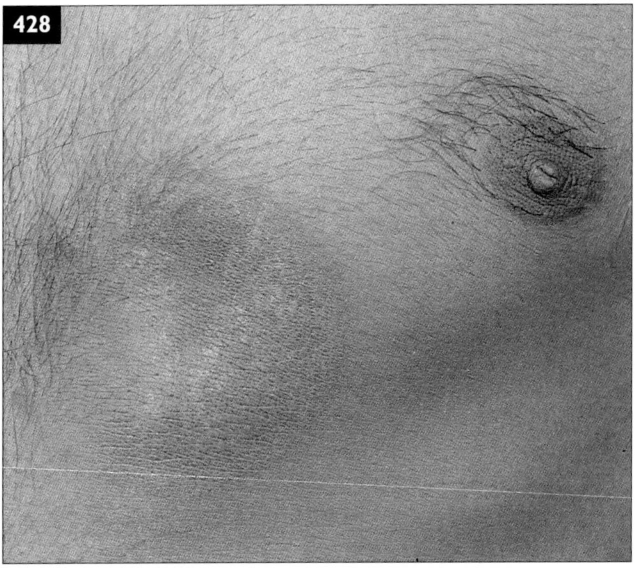

428 Fixed drug eruption.

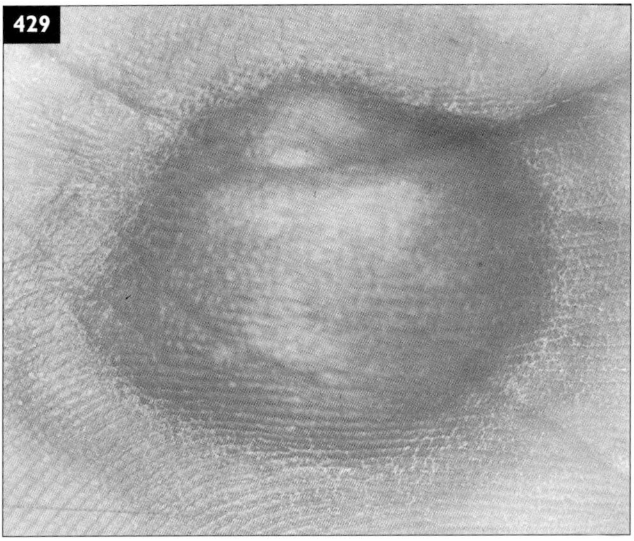

429 Fixed drug eruption.

FIXED DRUG ERUPTION

Definition and clinical features

A cutaneous reaction that characteristically recurs in the same site(s) each time the drug is administered. Usually just one drug is involved but cross-sensitivity to related drugs may occur. Typical lesions are well-demarcated, round or oval, erythematous, dusky plaques (**428**) with subsequent postinflammatory hyperpigmentation. Bullae are quite common (**429**). Lesions arise within 8 hours of drug administration and are commoner on the extremities, genitalia and perianal areas. Mucous membranes may be involved.

Drug Eruptions

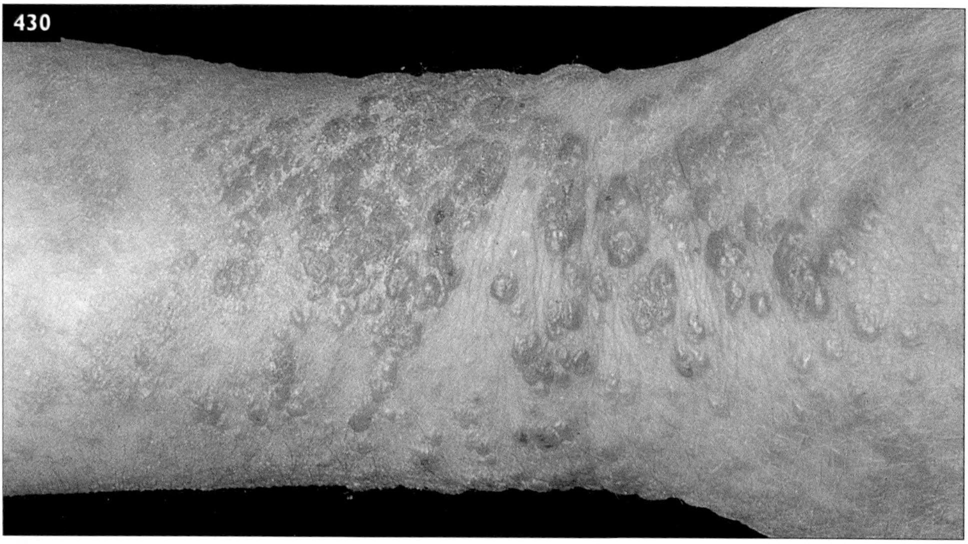

430 Lichenoid drug eruption.

431 Lichenoid drug eruption.

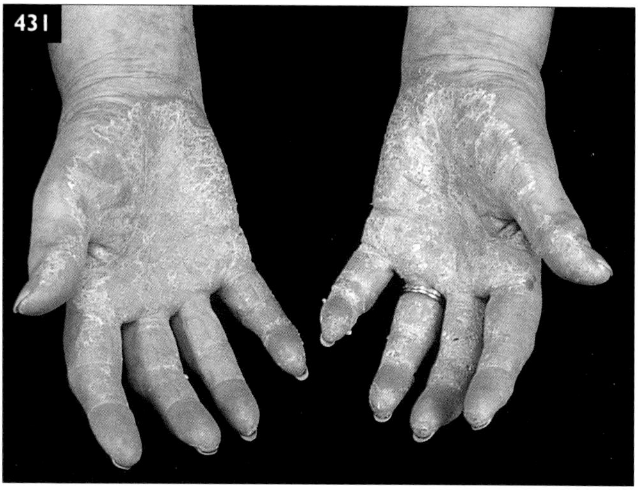

Drug associations

A large number of drugs have been reported, but especially tetracyclines, sulphonamides, phenolphthalein and oxyphenbutazone.

LICHENOID ERUPTIONS

Definition and clinical features

A drug eruption that may closely mimic idiopathic lichen planus (see Chapters 2 and 6). Histologically, there is additional focal parakeratosis and eosinophils. Typical lesions are violaceous, flat-topped, shiny papules. Lichenoid drug eruptions tend to be extensive (**430**) and may be linked with or develop into an exfoliative dermatitis (**431**). The eruption may develop weeks or months after initiation of therapy and usually only resolves slowly with withdrawal of the inciting agent. With

Drug Eruptions

432

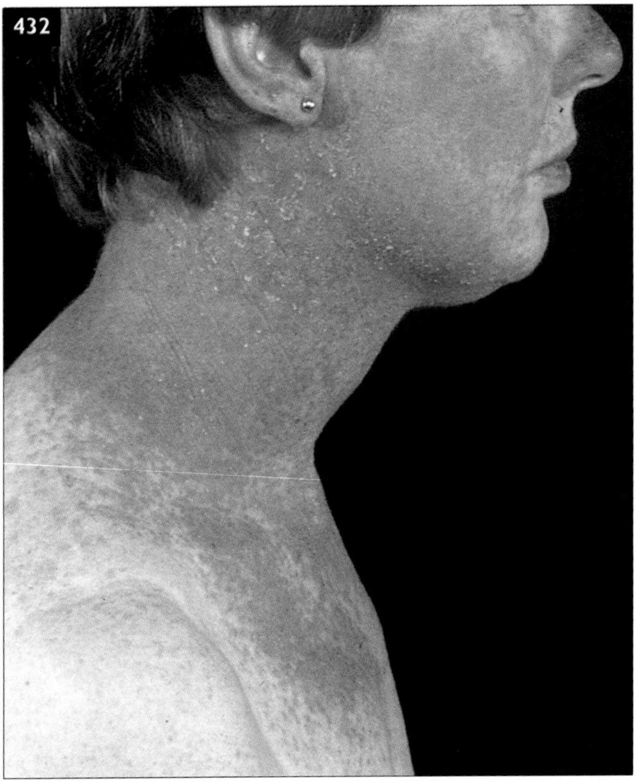

432 Photosensitive drug reaction.

thiazides and pyritinol, lesions may be preferentially distributed in light-exposed sites. An LP-like eruption occurs as a contact reaction after exposure to colour film developers.

Drug associations

Lichenoid drug reactions are especially seen with gold, penicillamine, β-blockers, captopril, thiazide diuretics, tetracyclines, antimalarials and anti-tuberculous agents.

PHOTOSENSITIVITY

Definition and clinical features

Drug–light reactions may be phototoxic or photoallergic. Clinically, it may not be possible to distinguish between the two and some drugs may produce both. Phototoxic reactions are much more common and will occur in almost all individuals, given adequate amounts of the drug and adequate light exposure. Photoallergic drug reactions require the interaction of the drug, UV light and the immune system.

Phototoxic reactions present as exaggerated sunburn with erythema, oedema, blistering, weeping, desquamation and subsequent hyperpigmentation on exposed areas. There may be photo-onycholysis. Phototoxic eruptions appear within 24 hours of drug exposure and resolve within 1 week; photoallergic eruptions may take weeks or months to resolve. With photoallergic reactions the eruption is variable. Erythematous plaques, eczema, vesicles and bullae all occur. The distribution is characteristically in sun-exposed areas, including the face, V of the neck and the backs of the hands and forearms (**432**).

Drug associations

Common associations with photosensitivity include NSAIDs, tetracyclines, sulfonamides, thiazide diuretics and cardiac drugs, especially

Drug Eruptions

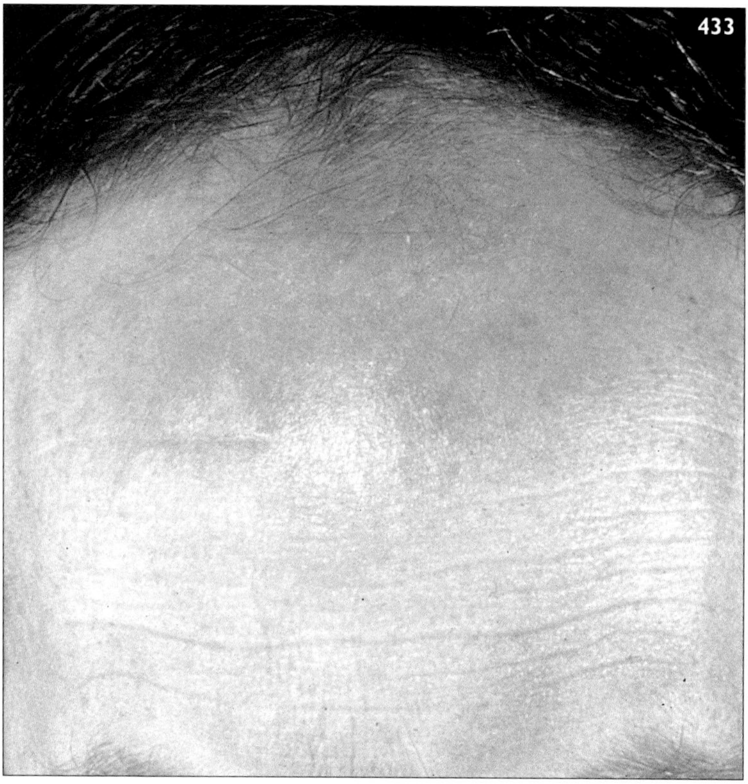

433 Amiodarone pigmentation.

ACE inhibitors and amiodarone. Patients with amiodarone photosensitivity often develop a blue-grey discoloration in sun-exposed areas (**433**).

GINGIVAL HYPERPLASIA

Definition and clinical features

Drugs cause gingival hyperplasia by inducing neutropenia and immunosuppression or by altering fibroblast proliferation and metabolism. Cyclosporin affects both the immune system and the fibroblast.

Gingival hyperplasia related to cyclosporin is usually confined to the free gingival margin and the interdental papilla. Associated bleeding is common. Calcium-channel blockers (especially nifedipine) may cause a nodular or a diffuse gingival hyperplasia. Proliferation of fibroblasts containing sulfated mucopolysaccharides is found in phenytoin-induced hyperplasia.

Drug associations

Cyclosporin, nifedipine and phenytoin.

IODODERMA

Definition and clinical features

Prolonged administration of small doses of iodide or bromide may provoke eruptions with or without mucosal or systemic symptoms. Acneiform or vegetating masses are the most distinctive.

A number of eruptions can be caused by iodine including urticaria, acneiform papules and pustules, tense haemorrhagic bullae arising on plaques of erythema, and hypertrophic vegetating masses. In bromism, acneiform and vegetating lesions occur more, and bullae less, frequently than with iodism. Vegetating iododermas/bromodermas may be very florid, with heaped-up masses of hypertrophic epithelium with many pustules simulating pemphigus vegetans or a granulomatous infection. Serious and even fatal reactions have been caused by radiographic contrast media in sensitised individuals.

Hair Disorders

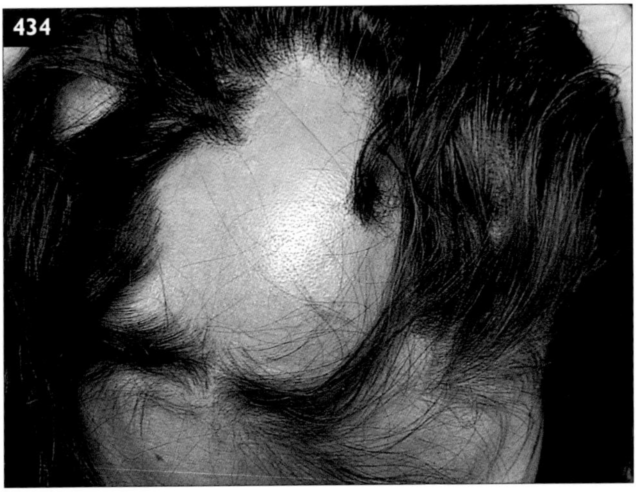

434 Alopecia areata.

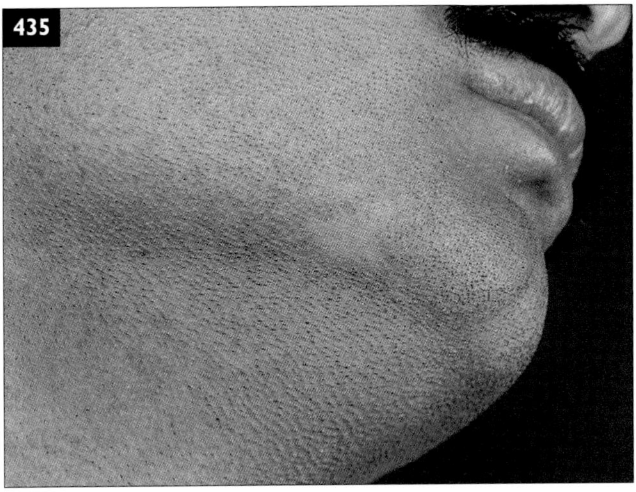

435 Facial alopecia areata.

ALOPECIA AREATA

Definition and clinical features

A non-scarring autoimmune disorder affecting any hair-bearing area. Typically, there is a sudden onset of solitary or multiple circular or oval bald areas, usually affecting the scalp (**434**) but any hair-bearing area may be affected. The residual hair follicles are visible confirming a lack of scarring. Diagnostic exclamation mark hairs may be visible at the margins of the lesion. The affected scalp is usually normal in colour but may be erythematous. Hairs at the edge of the patch may be easily removed on slight traction. Spontaneous regrowth frequently occurs, but the areas may spread peripherally and may eventually involve the whole scalp (alopecia totalis) and even facial (**435**) and body hair (alopecia universalis).

Rarely, a diffuse alopecia may be seen without discrete bald patches. This may occasionally preferentially affect dark hairs leaving pre-existing white hairs in place. Regrowth is frequently pure white. Nail changes may also occur, particularly in extensive disease, as fine regular pitting or a roughened, sandpaper appearance (trachyonychia) (**436**).

Hair Disorders

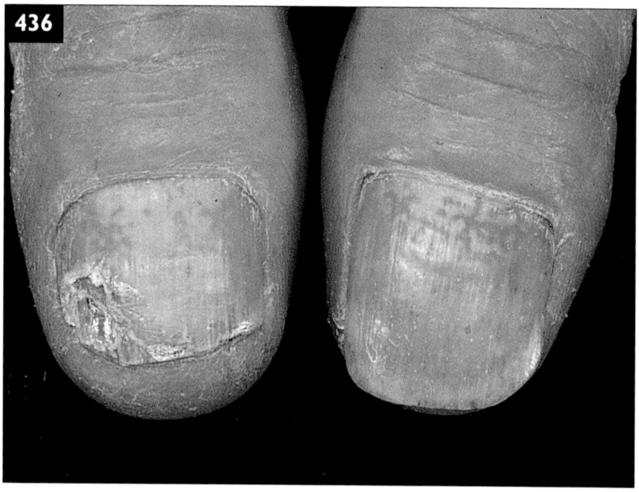

436 The nails in alopecia areata.

Epidemiology
A common disorder affecting all races and either sex equally. It occurs at any age, with the highest incidence between 10 and 30 years.

Differential diagnosis
Scalp fungal infections in children may be confirmed on mycological examination and Wood's light. Trichotillomania shows broken hairs of varying lengths. In older patients, scarring alopecia due to lichen planus or discoid lupus erythematosus may also cause patchy alopecia. Telogen effluvium also causes diffuse non-scarring alopecia.

Investigations
An autoimmune basis is suggested. Organ-specific autoantibodies may be demonstrated. A family history of alopecia areata occurs in 20–50% of patients. Scalp biopsy is supportive.

Special points
Spontaneous regrowth usually occurs in localised disease. Topical, intralesional and systemic corticosteroids can produce temporary regrowth. Contact sensitisation therapy using irritants (dithranol) or allergens (diphencyprone) and PUVA are also used. The more extensive the hair loss, the less likely the prospect of regrowth. Extensive involvement, atopy, other autoimmune diseases, nail involvement and onset in childhood are poor prognostic factors.

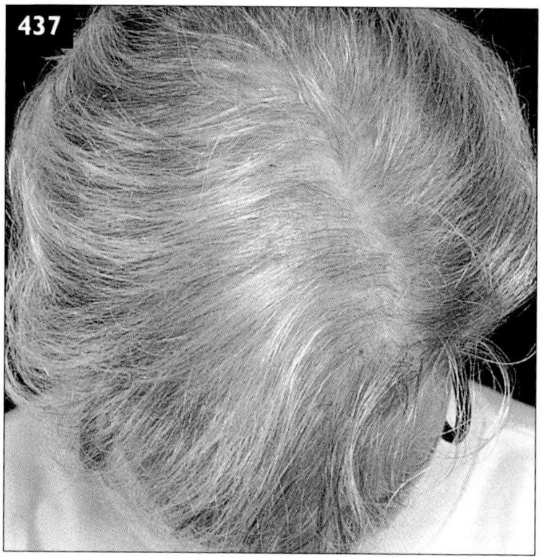

437 Diffuse alopecia in telogen effluvium.

TELOGEN EFFLUVIUM
Definition and clinical features
Sudden extensive hair loss occurring 4–8 weeks following the precipitating event. Several hundred hairs may be lost per day, producing an alopecia diffusely affecting the entire scalp (**437**). Other hair-bearing areas may also be involved. Pre-existing androgenetic alopecia may become more evident, the scalp appears normal and duration is variable (but recovery is usually complete within 6 months).

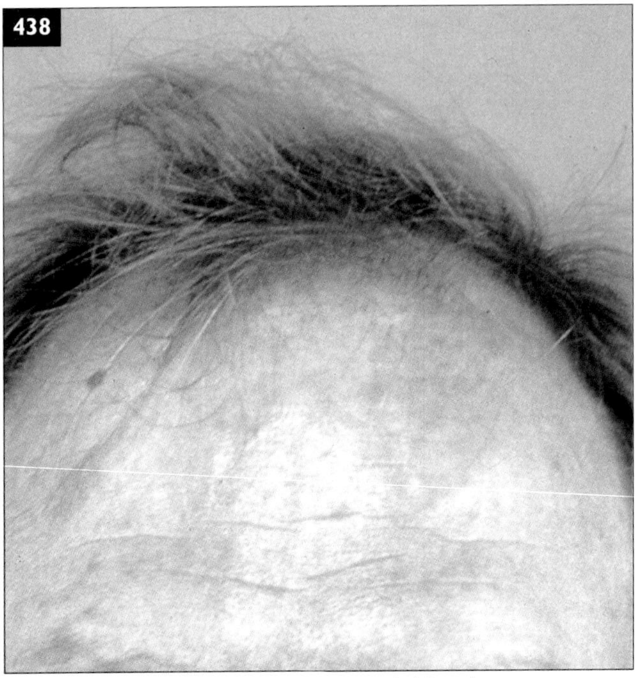

438 Androgenetic alopecia (male pattern baldness).

Epidemiology
Occurs at any age but most frequently in young adults. More commonly affecting females in the ratio 2:1.

Differential diagnosis
Diffuse scalp alopecia may also occur with alopecia areata, hypothyroidism, iron deficiency, anaemia and may be caused by drugs. Anagen effluvium occurs within 1–2 weeks of the precipitating drug or event.

Investigations
Trichogram (plucked scalp hairs) will show an increase in the number of telogen hairs and reduction in anagen hairs.

Special points
Acute precipitating factors include childbirth, pyrexia, haemorrhage, commencing, changing or discontinuing hormonal therapy (including oral contraceptive pill), eating disorders, strict dieting and nutritional deficiencies. More than the usual 10% of hairs on the scalp in telogen are precipitated into the resting phase of the hair cycle.

ANDROGENETIC ALOPECIA (MALE PATTERN BALDNESS)

Definition and clinical features
Miniaturisation of the hair follicles through successive cycles affecting the fronto-vertex and crown of the scalp, producing a gradual conversion of terminal to vellus hairs. The scalp hair loss begins with recession at the temples and the frontal hairline in men (Hamilton pattern) (**438**) and thinning over the crown and vertex. This progresses slowly over several years; in severe cases hair remains at the occiput and sides of the scalp alone. Vellus hairs may remain on the vertex. In women (Ludwig pattern) the frontal hairline is frequently kept but a diffuse thinning occurs over the top of the scalp. Although increased shedding may occur initially, the history is usually one of gradual thinning. In women, associated hirsutism, acne vulgaris, obesity and irregular menses may suggest an underlying polycystic ovarian syndrome.

Hair Disorders

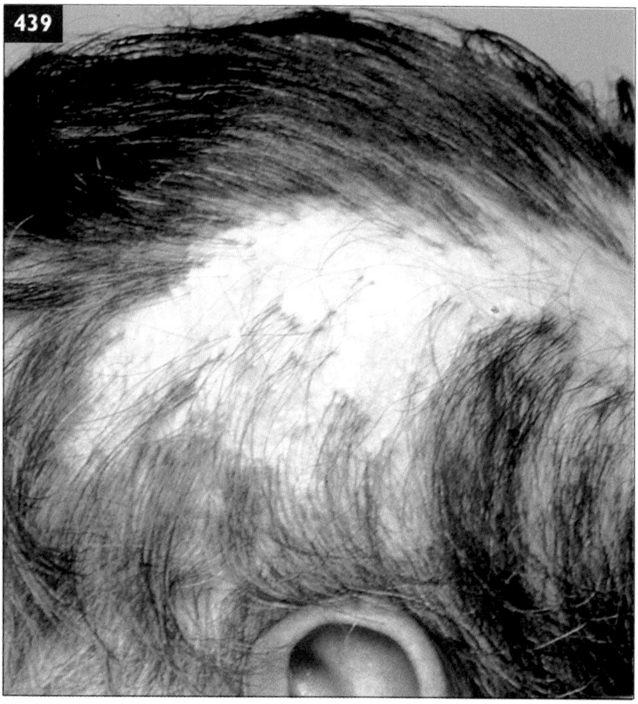

439 Scarring alopecia.

Epidemiology
Affects all races world-wide, occurring physiologically from the late teens to the 50s. Usually occurs in women post-menopausally. The condition requires genetic predisposition (dominant gene) and normal amounts of circulating plasma androgens.

Differential diagnosis
Telogen effluvium may produce diffuse alopecia but usually affects the back and sides of the scalp as well as the fronto-vertex. Hairstyles producing traction may cause recession of the anterior hair margin.

Investigations
In women, hormone profile and ovarian ultrasound scan may confirm underlying polycystic ovarian syndrome.

Special points
Treatment includes topical measures such as minoxidil lotion, systemic anti-androgens in women or scalp surgery (transplantation and scalp reduction).

SCARRING ALOPECIA

Definition and clinical features
Permanent destruction of hair follicles secondary to inflammatory and scarring cutaneous disorders. Scarred patches of alopecia without visible hair follicles occur irregularly throughout the scalp (**439**) or other hair-bearing area. The skin is usually scarred and atrophic. There may be signs of active cutaneous disease, such as lichen planus causing follicular plugging and pale atrophic areas, or discoid lupus erythematosus with erythematous indurated scaling plaques and follicular plugging.

Pseudopelade is a non-inflammatory form of scarring alopecia characterised by pale, waxy, patchy areas of skin atrophy. Other disorders causing scarring include burns, X-ray therapy, trauma, staphylococcal infection, fungal infections and neoplasms.

Differential diagnosis
Patchy alopecia may be produced by alopecia areata, which is non-scarring.

Hair Disorders

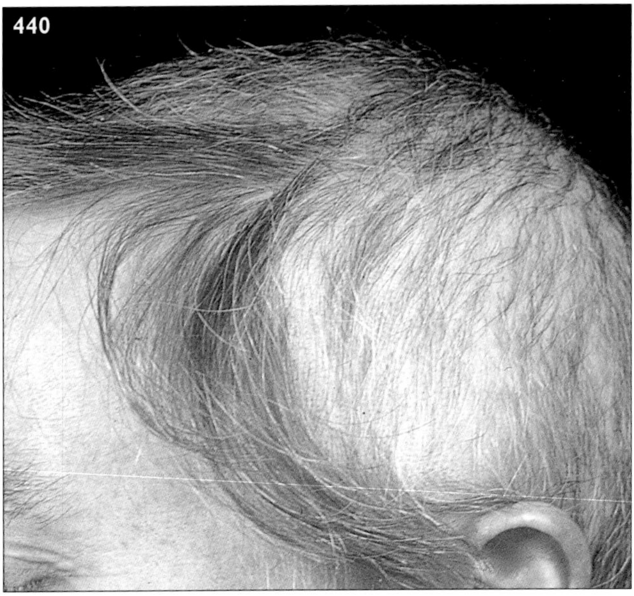

440 Trichotillomania (traumatic alopecia).

Investigations
Scalp biopsy will confirm the presence of scarring, with destruction of hair follicles and sebaceous glands, and may provide evidence of the underlying inflammatory disorder.

Special points
In scarring alopecia there is no potential for regrowth: the hair loss is permanent. Therapy includes treating any underlying disorder and long-term therapy with corticosteroids or antimalarial drugs may be required. Plastic cosmetic procedures may be useful at a later stage.

TRICHOTILLOMANIA
Definition and clinical features
Self-induced alopecia produced by deliberate trauma to the hair. A diffuse area of thinned hair with a poorly defined margin (**440**). Scalp skin is normal. Affected hairs show breakage of varying lengths. The area may be solitary or multiple. A normal, tonsural, long-haired margin often remains. Patients may exhibit other evidence of self mutilation (see dermatitis artefacta, p. 29). The scalp is usually affected but hair loss may also occur in the eyebrows, eyelashes, or body hair.

Epidemiology
Trichotillomania occurs more frequently in females than males (a ratio of 3:1) but may occur at any age. Most frequently it occurs between the ages of 5 and 10 years developing as a habit tic. In older women it may be a sign of underlying psychiatric disorder. Anxiety and emotional stress are precipitating factors.

Differential diagnosis
Alopecia areata produces more discrete, completely bald areas of alopecia. Tinea capitis can produce broken hairs, and scaling and inflammation may be present. Mycological examination confirms the diagnosis.

Investigations
Hair microscopy will reveal broken hairs of various lengths.

Special points
Occlusion of the area often allows recovery. Children frequently outgrow the habit tic, whilst in adults psychiatric therapy may be required.

Genital and Perianal Dermatoses

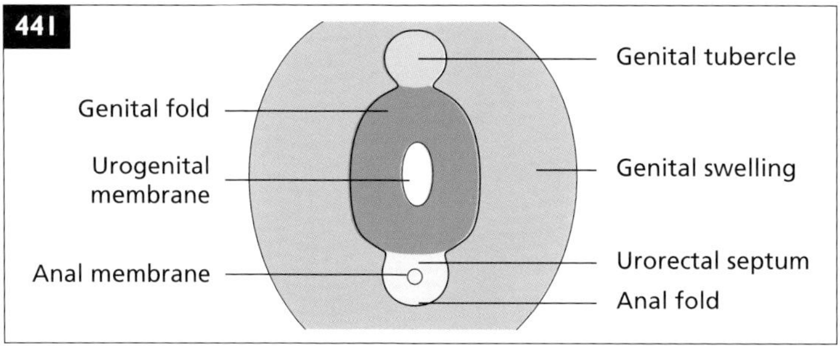

441 Primitive perineum (simplified) at 7 weeks.

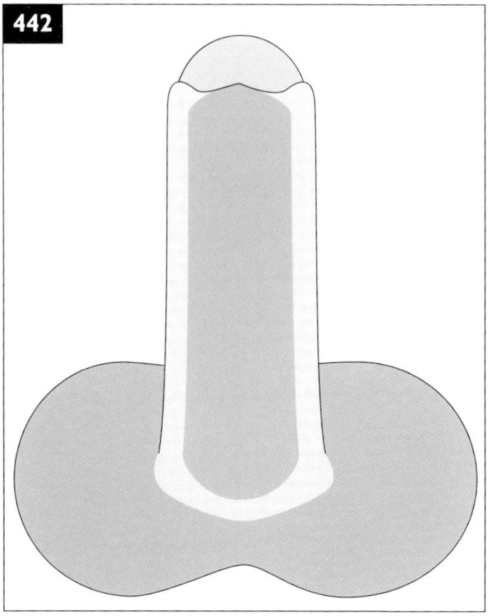

442 Adult male external genitalia (simplified).

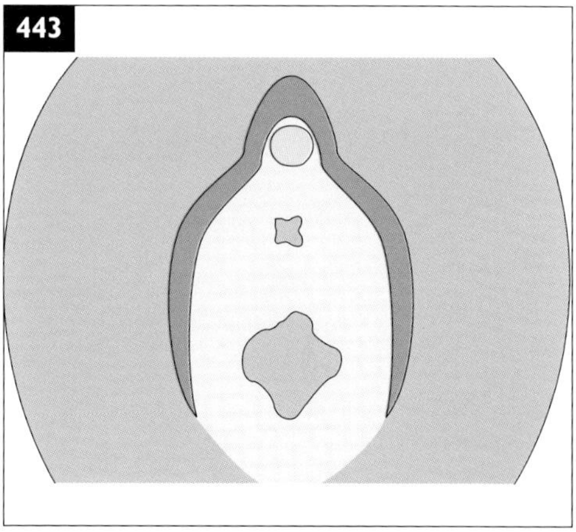

443 Adult female external genitalia (simplified).

The genital and perianal skin can be affected by many of the dermatoses that characteristically occur at other sites, but some conditions have a predilection for this anatomical region. Difficulties arise in diagnosis as the classical morphology is altered due to the occlusive effect of these flexural sites.

A brief review of the embryology and anatomy of this area is important in understanding the nature and distribution of the dermatoses that do occur.

EMBRYOLOGY AND ANATOMY

The external genitalia begin to form at about 4 weeks, shortly after the cloaca has developed, but sexual differentiation is not apparent until 12 weeks. At 7 weeks, the primitive perineum is formed (**441**) when the urorectal septum has reached the cloacal membrane, dividing it into the anterior urogenital membrane and posterior anal membrane. Subsequent masculinisation (**442**) or feminisation (**443**) is a consequence of tissue response to the presence or absence of androgens.

LICHEN SCLEROSUS

Definition and clinical features

A chronic, scarring, inflammatory dermatosis that can occur at any site but has a predilection for the genital and perianal skin. Typically, at

Genital and Perianal Dermatoses

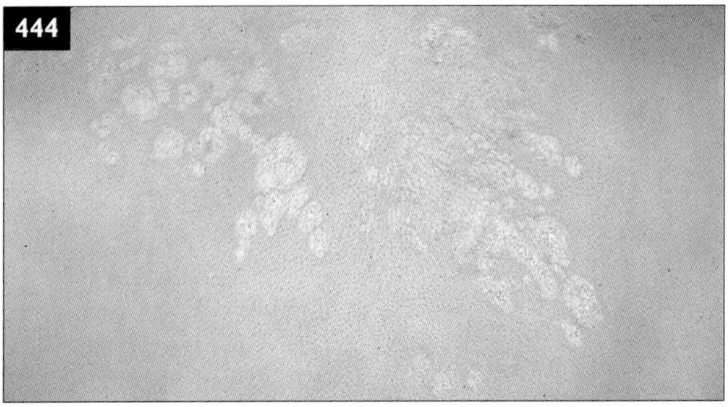

444 Lichen sclerosus.

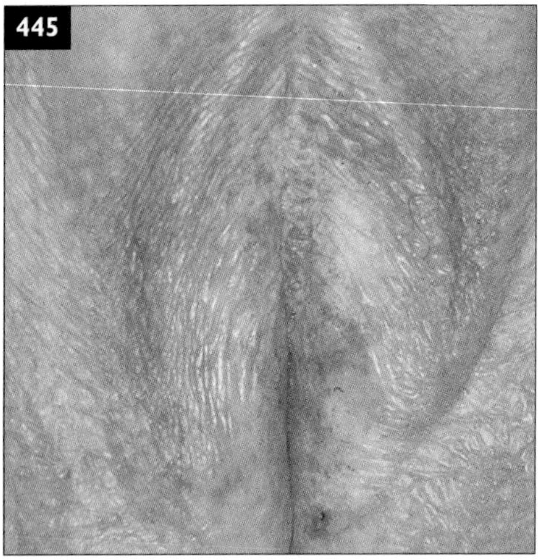

445 Lichen sclerosus.

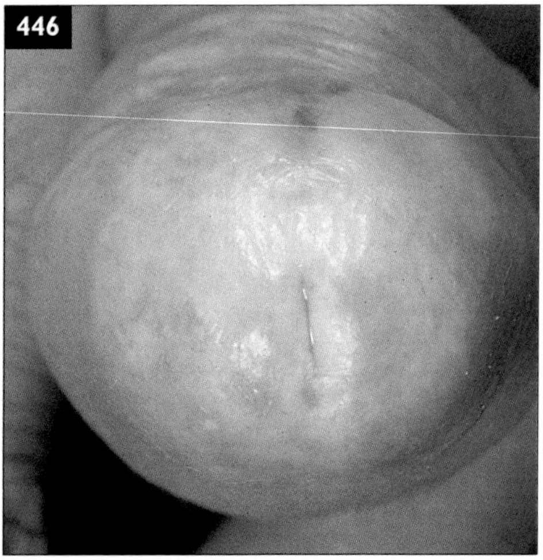

446 Balanitis.

extragenital sites, the lesions are porcelain white papules and plaques (**444**). Follicular delling may sometimes be marked. The individual lesions may coalesce to form sheets of atrophic skin, often with extensive areas of purpura. Bullous lesions can occur. In the anogenital area there are usually confluent, white, atrophic patches (**445**), occurring in a figure-of-eight pattern. There is usually architectural distortion, with either partial or complete loss of the labia minora, burying of the clitoris and introital narrowing in females, and partial or complete phimosis and meatal stenosis in males (**446**).

Epidemiology

The incidence and aetiology are unknown. It is commoner in women than men. Female patients appear to present most frequently in childhood or around the menopause. It is even more difficult to assess the incidence in boys, as, very often, they are circumcised for phimosis but the tissue is not routinely examined histologically, so may go undiagnosed.

Differential diagnosis

Other dermatoses that can produce atrophy and scarring, i.e. lichen planus, cicatricial pemphigoid and pemphigus.

Genital and Perianal Dermatoses

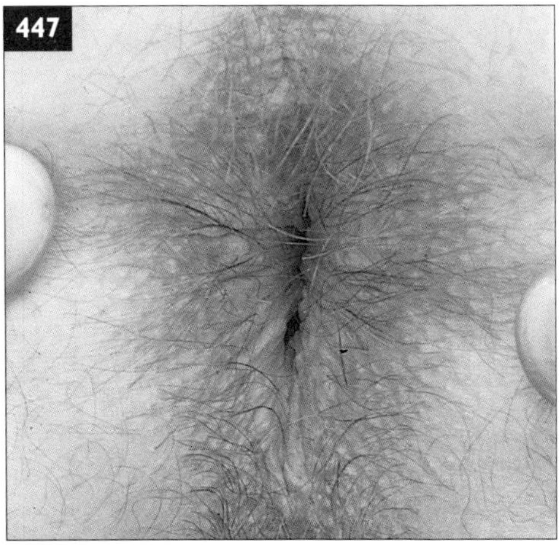

447 Lichen planus.

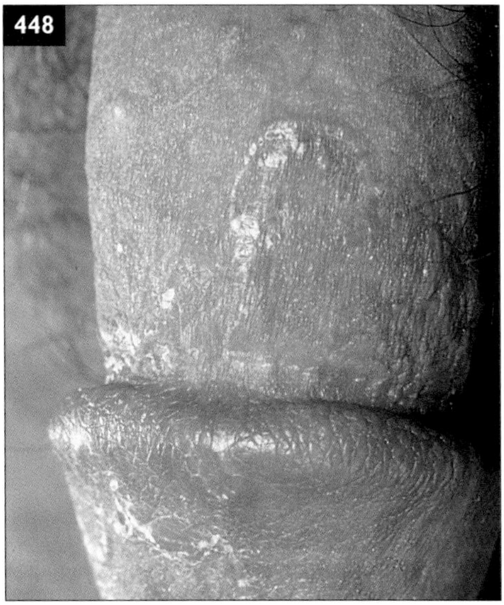

448 Annular lichen planus.

Investigations

A skin biopsy will show epidermal atrophy with hyalinisation of the underlying papillary dermis, and a lymphocytic inflammatory infiltrate beneath this. Other autoimmune diseases may be associated with lichen sclerosus, in particular thyroid disease, so if clinically indicated thyroid function should be assessed.

Special points

Squamous cell carcinoma may develop on a background of lichen sclerosus. It occurs in 6% or less of patients with known lichen sclerosus. Surgical excision is inappropriate in the treatment of uncomplicated lichen sclerosus.

LICHEN PLANUS

Definition and clinical features

A lymphocyte-mediated, inflammatory, mucocutaneous disease with characteristic lesions on the skin and mucous membranes of the mouth and genitalia (see pp. 55–57).

Lichen planus can present in the anogenital area with the classical lesions of flat-topped, shiny, violaceous papules and Wickham's striae (**447**). Annular lesions may occur, particularly on the penis (**448**). However, lichen planus may present either as erosive disease (**449**) or with hypertrophic, hyperkeratotic plaques. In either of these variants there may be associated atrophy and

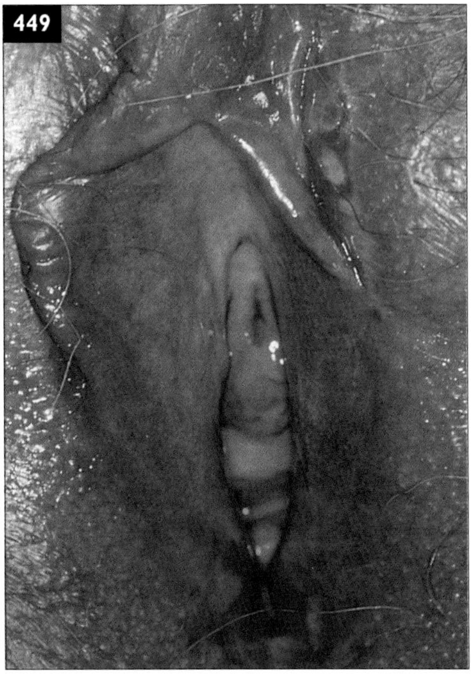

449 Erosive lichen planus.

Genital and Perianal Dermatoses

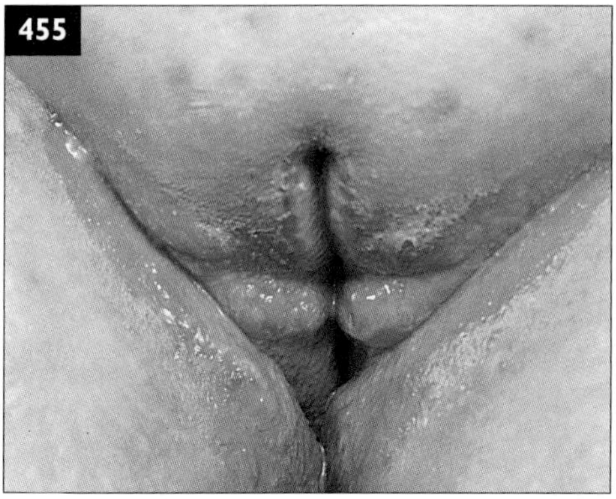

455 Cutaneous Crohn's disease.

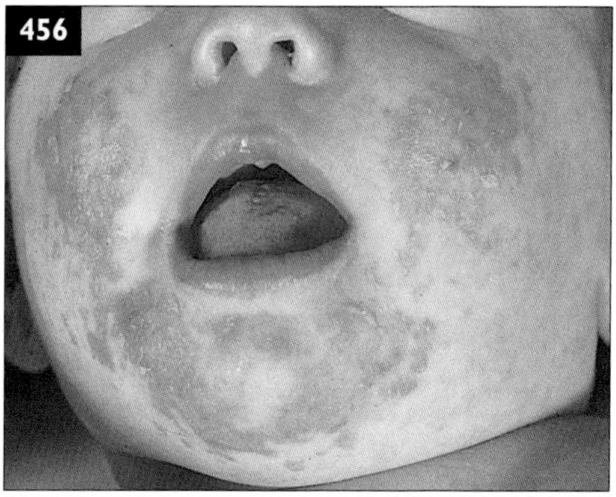

456 Acrodermatitis enteropathica.

CUTANEOUS CROHN'S DISEASE

Definition and clinical features

Chronic inflammatory changes of flexural skin, characterised by lymphoedema or ulcerative necrosis, occurring in association with either active or inactive Crohn's disease of the intestine.

The commonest site to be involved is the perianal area, where chronic sinuses and ulcers develop which can lead to fistulas and ischiorectal abscesses. There is also marked oedema and tag formation. Vulval involvement usually presents with severe, generalised oedema of the labia majora and minora, but it may be unilateral. There is often intense erythema and oedema. There may be deep, linear fissuring along the skin folds (**455**).

Epidemiology

Cutaneous Crohn's usually occurs simultaneously or after the onset of intestinal disease. However, in some cases it may precede the onset of intestinal symptoms by many years.

Differential diagnosis

Apocrine acne (hidradenitis suppurativa), deep fungal infection, lymphogranuloma venereum, amoebiasis, Behçet's syndrome and sarcoidosis.

Investigations

Skin biopsy may show characteristic granulomatous inflammation or lymphangiectasia. If relevant, investigation of gastrointestinal function.

Special points

There is not always a strong correlation between active bowel disease and degree of skin involvement.

ACRODERMATITIS ENTEROPATHICA

Definition and clinical features

A rare condition of abnormal zinc metabolism, characterised by dermatitis, diarrhoea, failure to thrive and alopecia. Typically, the infant develops symptoms and signs at about 6 weeks after weaning (**456**, **457**) or earlier if not breast fed. Erythematous, scaly areas develop periorificially, around the eyes, mouth and nappy area. Lesions also develop on the hands and feet. There may be vesicobullous areas. The scalp hair becomes sparse and is lost.

Epidemiology

This is thought to be inherited as an autosomal recessive trait. The reason for the zinc malabsorption is unknown but it improves with age.

Differential diagnosis

Eczema, psoriasis and candidiasis.

Investigations

Measurement of plasma or serum zinc level. However, blood levels vary rapidly with infection or injury and may not always reflect the true zinc status.

Special points

Oral zinc clears the clinical lesions within 2 weeks but must be continued indefinitely.

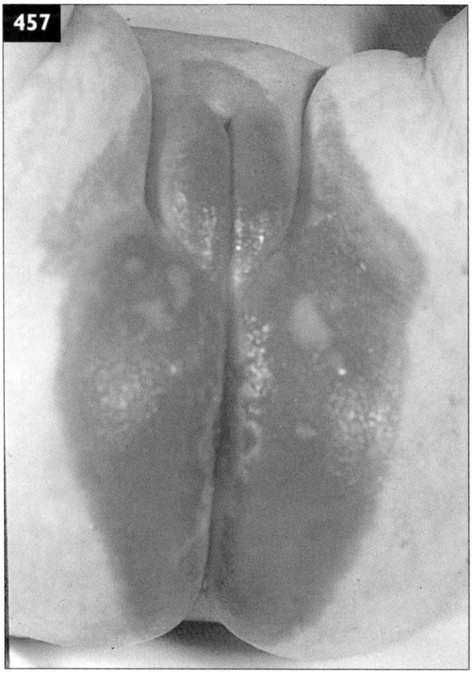

457 Acrodermatitis enteropathica.

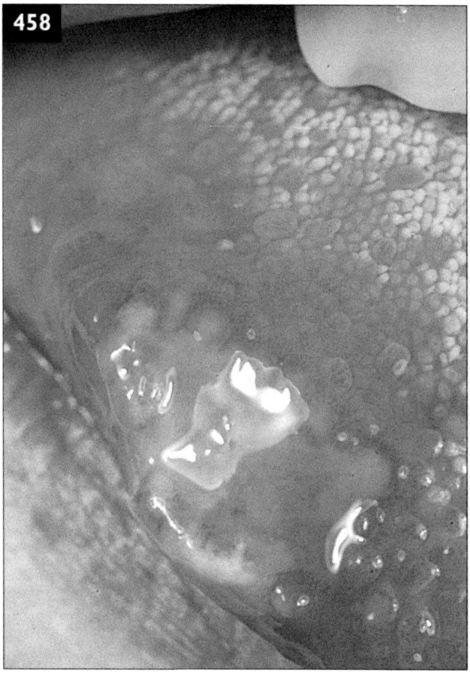

458 Behçet's syndrome.

BEHÇET'S SYNDROME

Definition and clinical features

Behçet's syndrome is the association of orogenital ulceration with eye disease. In addition, there may be other cutaneous and systemic manifestations that are included in the diagnostic criteria.

The oral and genital ulcers are usually large and classified as major aphthae. They are painful and recurrent. Over 90% of patients have eye involvement, including iridocyclitis, anterior and posterior uveitis, retinal vasculitis and optic atrophy (**458**, **459**). An associated arthralgia and occasionally erythema nodusum may occur. There may also be profound, systemic symptoms; neurological involvement is a serious complication.

Epidemiology

The majority of the patients are male and of Mediterranean or Eastern origin. There are familial cases and an association with certain HLA types. Various abnormalities of cell-mediated immunity have been described but these are not always a universal finding.

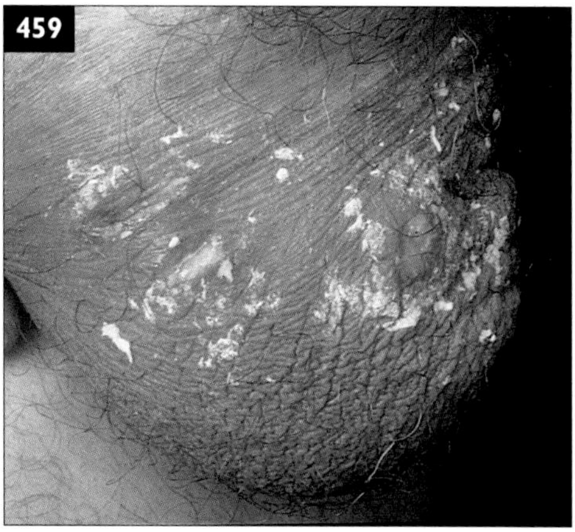

459 Behçet's syndrome.

Differential diagnosis

Aphthous ulceration, cytomegalovirus infection, secondary syphilis, Crohn's, Stevens–Johnson syndrome or erythema multiforme.

Genital and Perianal Dermatoses

460

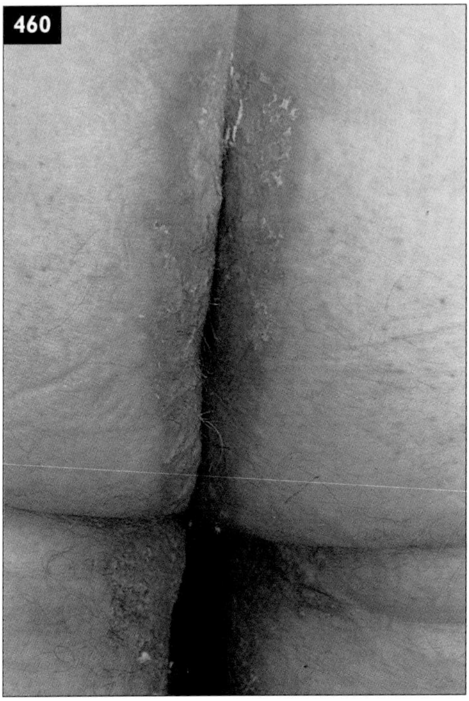

460 Hailey–Hailey disease.

Investigations
There is no diagnostic test and it is a diagnosis of exclusion. Therefore, investigations must be directed to exclude other causes of genital ulceration.

Special points
Pathergy, the tendency to pustulate at a site of trauma, is a characteristic feature.

HAILEY–HAILEY DISEASE (BENIGN FAMILIAL CHRONIC PEMPHIGUS)
Definition and clinical features
A chronic, vesicobullous, genodermatosis affecting the flexural zones (see p. 135). It is unrelated to pemphigus. Clusters of small vesicles develop on normal or erythematous skin, usually in flexural zones where heat and friction appear to play a role (**460**). The neck, scalp and extremities may rarely be involved. Oral lesions have been described. The vesicles are easily ruptured leaving erosions and crusts. The lesions extend out peripherally sometimes with central clearing. Cold weather promotes spontaneous remissions.

Epidemiology
Males and females are equally affected. Heat, friction and infection cause exacerbations. Onset is usually in adolescence and early adult life.

Differential diagnosis
Pemphigus, Darier's disease, bacterial or candidal intertrigo.

Investigations
Skin biopsy for histological and immunofluorescence studies. Histologically, there is suprabasal clefting with acantholysis. Immunofluorescence is negative. Skin swabs for microbiological assessment.

Special points
In severe cases, skin grafting may help.

INTRAEPITHELIAL NEOPLASIA
Definition and clinical features
The grading of genital and perianal epidermal neoplasia has been based on that used for cervical intraepithelial neoplasia (CIN), CIN III representing two-thirds to full-thickness epidermal atypia. Vulval, penile and perianal lesions with this degree of atypia are referred to as VIN III, PIN III, and PAIN III, respectively. This terminology is now being introduced to replace the older clinical terms Bowen's disease, Bowenoid papulosis and erythroplasia of Queyrat (see pp. 117–118).

Morphologically, there is great variation in these lesions. Solitary lesions may arise, which clinically can appear as erythematous scaly plaques, erosions or white patches (**461**). Multifocal disease may demonstrate a variety of lesions with different morphological features in the same patient. These range from pigmented papules and plaques, resembling seborrhoeic keratoses, to typical warts (**462**). These pigmented lesions are characteristic of multifocal VIN III, previously termed Bowenoid papulosis.

Epidemiology
The multifocal lesions tend to occur in young adults and the majority remit spontaneously. They are usually associated with human papilloma viruses Types 16 and 18. Two-thirds of the women will have evidence of CIN. The association with HPV in older patients is not so clearly established.

Genital and Perianal Dermatoses

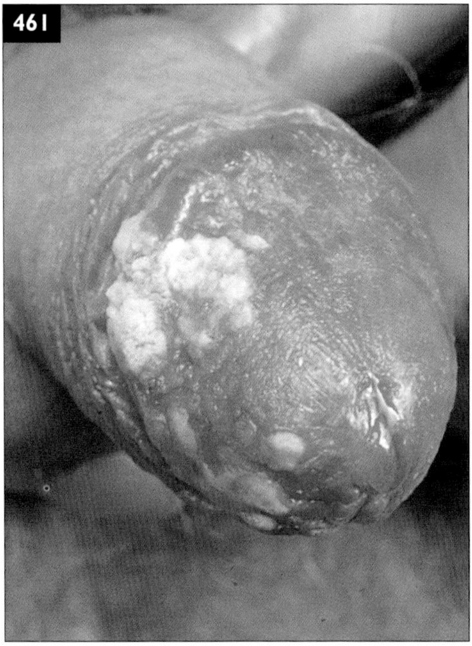

461 Intraepithelial neoplasia.

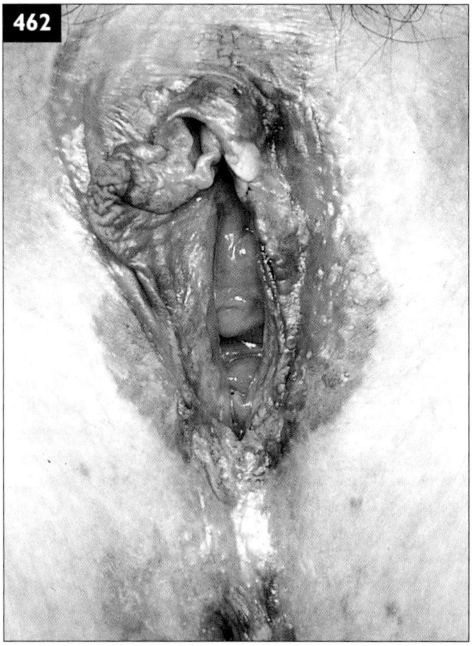

462 Multifocal VIN III.

Differential diagnosis
Lichen planus, lichen sclerosus, squamous cell carcinoma and viral warts.

Investigations
Skin biopsy will show full thickness atypia. Screening for other sexually transmitted diseases including VDRL. Cervical screening for affected women, and all those whose sexual partners have lesions.

Special points
Conservative management and careful follow up.

HERPES SIMPLEX VIRUS INFECTION
Definition and clinical features
There are two closely related herpes simplex viruses (HSV) Type I and Type II. Either can produce primary and recurrent mucocutaneous infections (see pp. 69–70).

Primary infection is the first infection and results in multiple turbid vesicles that are usually bilateral and coalesce to produce eroded areas which are very painful (**463**). There may be marked oedema and secondary urinary retention. Recurrent disease

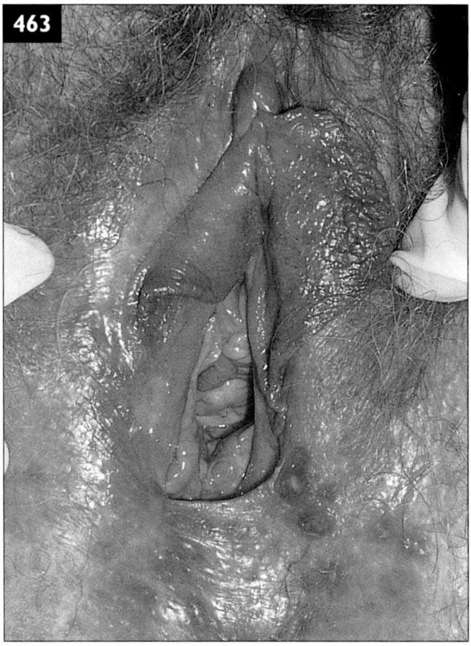

463 Vulval herpes simplex.

Genital and Perianal Dermatoses

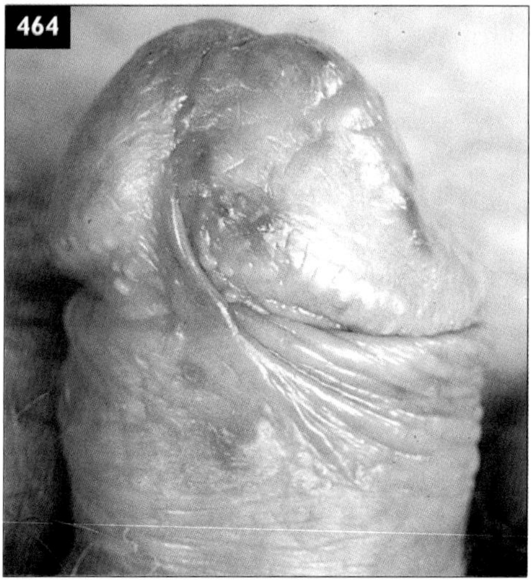

464 Recurrent penile herpes simplex.

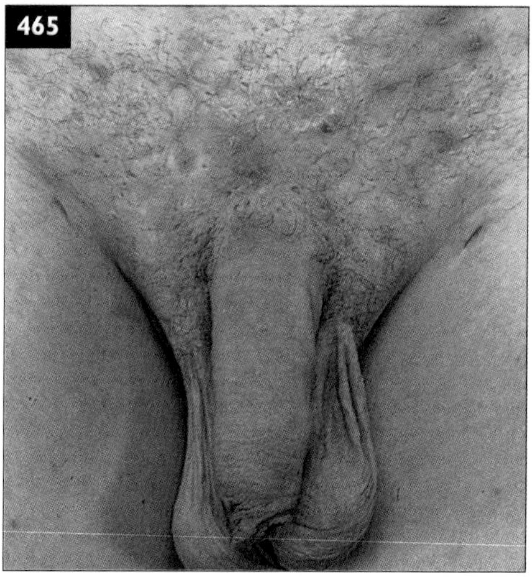

465 Hidradenitis suppurativa.

is due to reactivation of the virus, which is dormant in the dorsal root ganglion (**464**).

Epidemiology

The majority of infections are sexually acquired and, depending on geographical location, 50–90% of genital infections are HSV Type II. HSV Type II is more likely to be associated with recurrent disease.

Differential diagnosis

Impetigo, herpes zoster

Investigations

A Tzanck smear from a blister base will show multinucleated giant cells. Swabs from deroofed blister taken for culture. Smears for electron microscopy. Screening for other sexually transmitted disease. Currently serology tests are unreliable. PCR may be helpful.

Special points

Herpes simplex infection is one of the commonest triggers of erythema multiforme.

HIDRADENITIS SUPPURATIVA (APOCRINE ACNE)

Definition and clinical features

A chronic inflammatory and suppurative condition of the skin at sites where apocrine sweat glands are present. Tender, inflamed, papules, pustules and cysts arise in the axillae, inguinal areas, perianally and on the perineum (**465**). The inframammary zones and breasts may be involved in women. The initial lesions may go on to form sinuses and fistulous tracts with considerable scarring (**466**). Double-pored or polyporous comedones are often present in the affected areas. Hidradenitis suppurativa usually occurs alone but may be associated with acne conglobata and dissecting cellulitis of the scalp, the so-called follicular triad. There have also been reports of an association with Crohn's disease.

Aetiology

This is unknown and it is generally not considered to be a primary problem of the apocrine gland, although this is involved in the process. It occurs after puberty when the apocrine glands are fully developed. It is commoner in women than men.

Differential diagnosis

Furunculosis, Crohn's disease and lymphogranuloma venereum.

Investigations

Specimens should be taken for microbiological assessment to determine the appropriate

Genital and Perianal Dermatoses

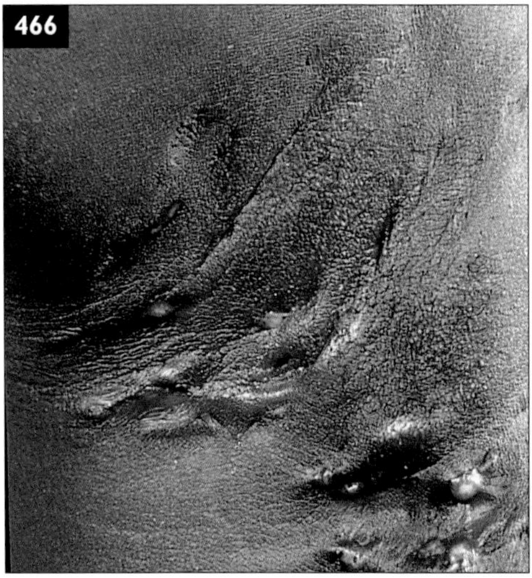

466 Hidradenitis suppurativa.

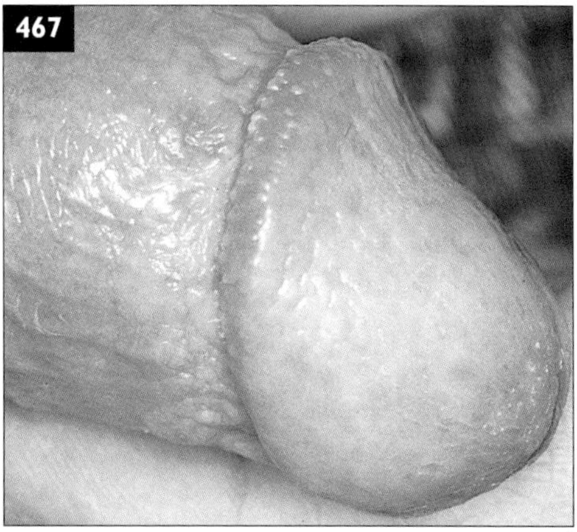

467 Penile pearly papules.

antibiotic treatment. Skin biopsy of chronic ulcers on long-standing disease to exclude malignancy.

Special points
Acute cellulitis may be a complication giving rise to sudden fever and toxicity.

PAPILLOMATOSIS
Definition and clinical features
Benign papillary projections of the epithelium. These occur as shiny, opalescent micropapules encircling the coronal sulcus in men and are known as penile pearly papules (**467**). They also occur in women, sited symmetrically on the inner aspects of the labia minora or the vulval vestibule (**468**). They may be very tiny projections giving the affected epithelium a granular appearance but occasionally they may be long and filiform. The lesions are normally asymptomatic.

Aetiology
The incidence and aetiology is unknown but is considered to be a variant of the normal. There is no evidence that human papilloma virus is responsible for these lesions.

Differential diagnosis
Viral warts.

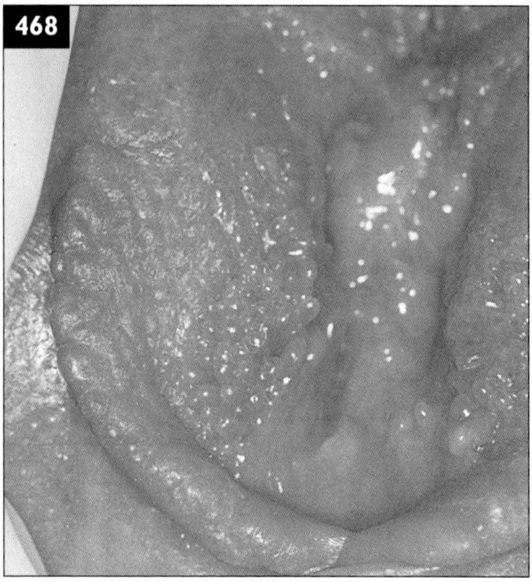

468 Vestibular papillomatosis.

Investigations
This is not usually necessary. However, a biopsy will show epithelial projections with a core of normal connective tissue and a dense vascular network, histologically identical to angiofibromas.

Special points
No treatment is necessary other than reassurance.

Genital and Perianal Dermatoses

469

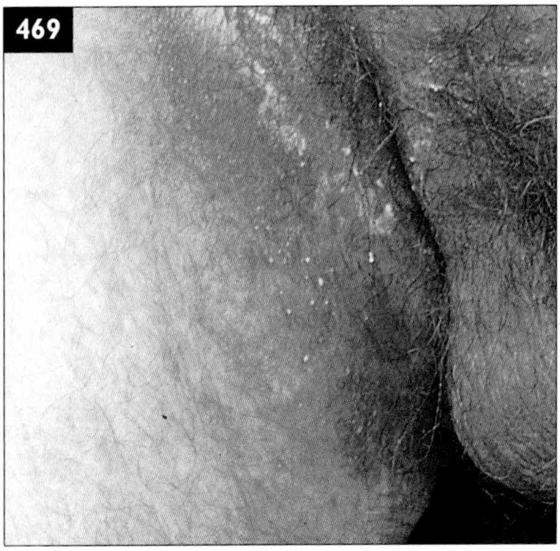

469 Vulval candidiasis.

470

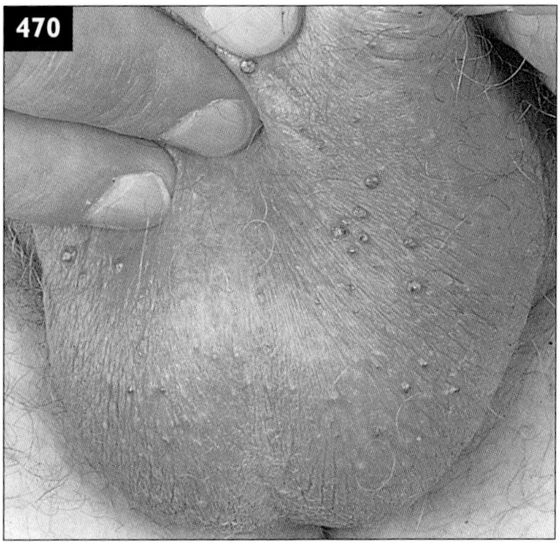

470 Angiokeratomas of Fordyce.

CANDIDIASIS

Definition and clinical features

An opportunistic infection with yeasts of the *Candida* genus that can occur on any epithelium but has a predilection for mucosal surfaces (see pp. 72–73). Various sites in the anogenital area may be affected in isolation or together.

Vulval candidiasis is usually associated with vaginal infection and a curdy, white vaginal discharge. The vulval skin is red, oedematous and sometimes studded with subcorneal pustules (**469**).

In men, balanitis is characterised by micropapules or pustules which rupture, leaving very superficial erosions on the glans. Flexural candidiasis affects the genitocrural folds, perianal area and natal cleft. The classical features of this intertrigo are erythema and maceration which spread on to the surrounding skin where the typical subcorneal pustules develop.

Epidemiology

Over 70% of infections are caused by *Candida albicans*. It is the cause of balanitis in males, vulvovaginitis in females and anorectal infection in both. *Candida albicans* has both yeast and mycelial forms and can be a normal commensal in the mouth, vagina and perianal skin. Infection occurs with an overgrowth of the fungus. There are usually predisposing factors, i.e. pregnancy, high-dose oral contraceptive, diabetes, oral antibiotics, inflamed macerated dermatoses and immunosuppression due to disease or drugs.

Differential diagnosis

Bacterial or tinea intertrigo, trichomonas, Hailey–Hailey disease, psoriasis, seborrhoeic eczema, pemphigus and contact eczema.

Investigations

Direct microscopy of smears with 10% potassium hydroxide (KOH). Culture of swabs. Exclude diabetes mellitus.

Special points

Herpes simplex infection needs to be excluded in men with vesicopustular balanitis.

ANGIOKERATOMAS OF FORDYCE

Definition and clinical features

Acquired, ectatic, thin-walled vessels covered by hyperkeratotic epithelium, affecting the scrotum or labia majora. Bright red papules develop on the scrotum (**470**) and labia majora (**471**), which darken with age. They develop most commonly in middle age and are usually asymptomatic. Some patients complain of itch or soreness. Rarely, they may be extensive, affecting the penis and upper thighs.

Epidemiology

Angiokeratomas are considered to be a degenerative phenomenon as their incidence becomes more frequent with age. However, they may be seen from the late teens onwards. Local venous tension may be a contributory factor.

Genital and Perianal Dermatoses

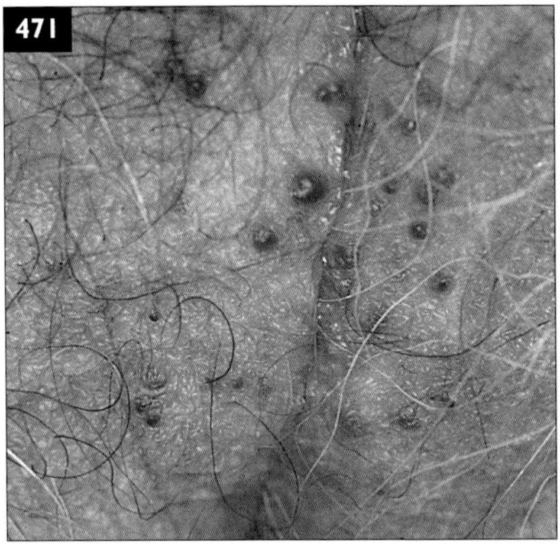

471 Angiokeratomas of Fordyce.

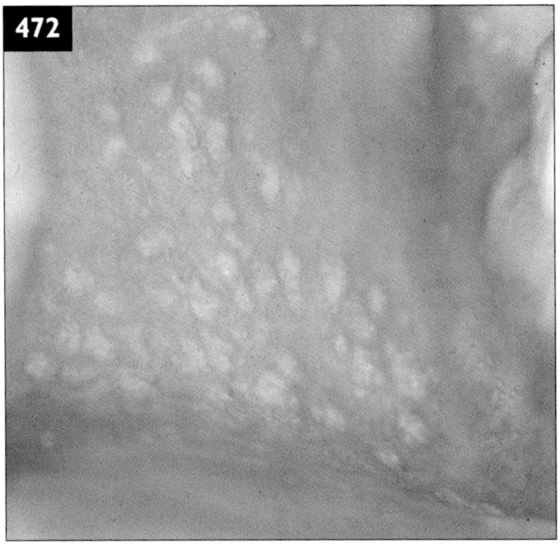

472 Fordyce spots.

Differential diagnosis

Angiokeratoma corporis diffusum (Fabry's disease) (see pp. 146–148).

Investigations

Histological features include ectatic blood vessels within the papillary dermis with acanthosis and hyperkeratosis of the overlying epithelium.

Special points

The histopathology may help to differentiate between these angiokeratomas and those seen in Fabry's disease, as vacuoles may be seen in the endothelial and smooth muscle cells in the latter.

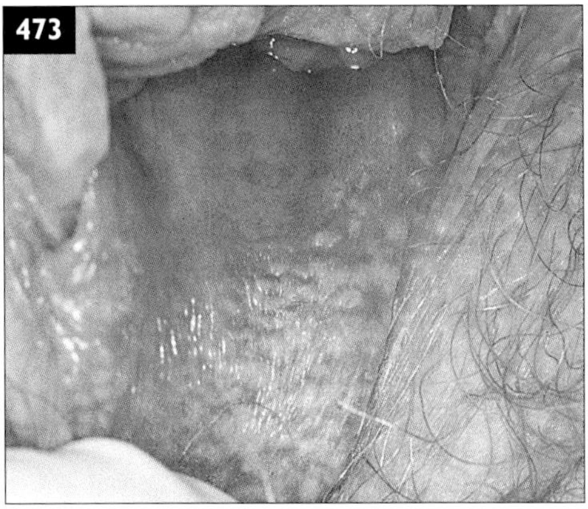

473 Fordyce spots.

FORDYCE SPOTS

Definition and clinical features

Fordyce spots are free sebaceous glands without an associated hair follicle. The sebaceous glands are distributed symmetrically as individual creamy-white or yellow papules (**472**). Sometimes they are so numerous that they appear as confluent patches (**473**). They are found on the labia minora, interlabial sulci, penile shaft and buccal mucosae.

Epidemiology

Fordyce spots are common and are now considered a variant of the normal. They are not seen in children as they only become visible after puberty.

Differential diagnosis

Epidermoid cysts, milia (see pp. 111–112).

Investigations

Histopathologically, lobules of mature sebaceous glands are associated with a sebaceous duct which opens directly on to the surface epithelium.

Special points

They are usually asymptomatic but in some female patients they may be associated with pruritus.

Genital and Perianal Dermatoses

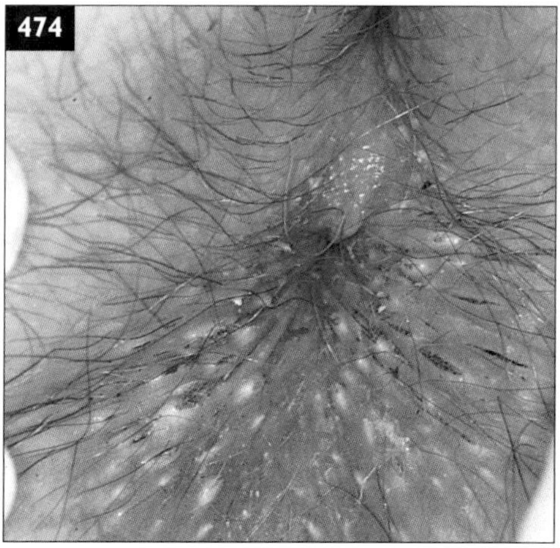

474 Epidermoid cysts.

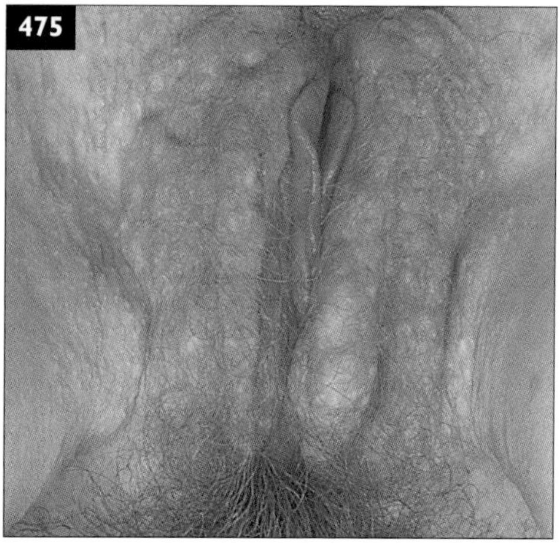

475 Epidermoid cysts.

EPIDERMOID CYSTS

Definition and clinical features

A dermal cyst lined with stratified squamous epithelium and filled with keratin and its breakdown products (see pp. 111–112).

Epidermoid cysts usually arise on the cornified squamous epithelium of the anogenital skin and are not seen on the glans penis or vulval vestibule (**474, 475, 476**). They are more often multiple than solitary lesions, arise as dome-shaped papules and are yellow or white. A central punctum can sometimes be seen. The cysts enlarge slowly and occasionally can become inflamed and tender.

Epidemiology

These cysts are common, occurring in adolescents and mid life. They are often associated with acne and many are the result of inflammation around a pilosebaceous follicle.

Differential diagnosis

Steatocystoma multiplex, eccrine gland tumours (see p. 116).

Investigations

Histological features include a layered, lining wall with lamellated and birefringent keratin filling the cavity. A hair may be present within the cyst. Some cysts have an associated chronic inflammatory or foreign body reaction around them.

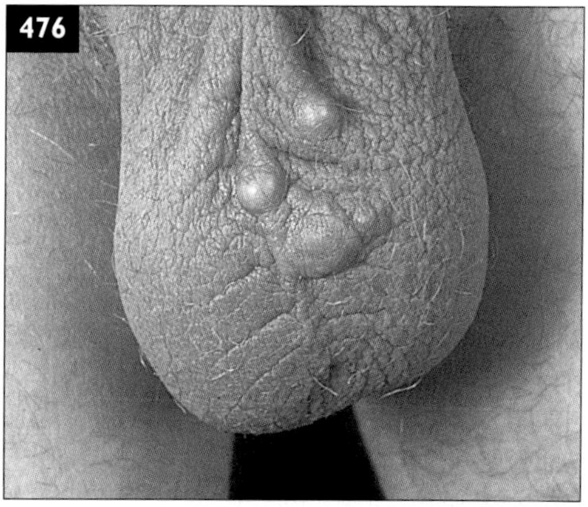

476 Epidermoid cysts.

Special points

Sometimes these cysts are erroneously referred to as sebaceous cysts but a sebaceous cyst has a lining wall resembling the external hair root sheath, i.e. the cells do not flatten and form a granular layer as they differentiate and the cyst contents are not birefringent lamellae. They are more likely to calcify.

SYPHILIS

Definition and clinical features

Syphilis is a contagious, sexually acquired infection, which, if untreated is characterised by a variety of cutaneous and systemic signs and symptoms.

Genital and Perianal Dermatoses

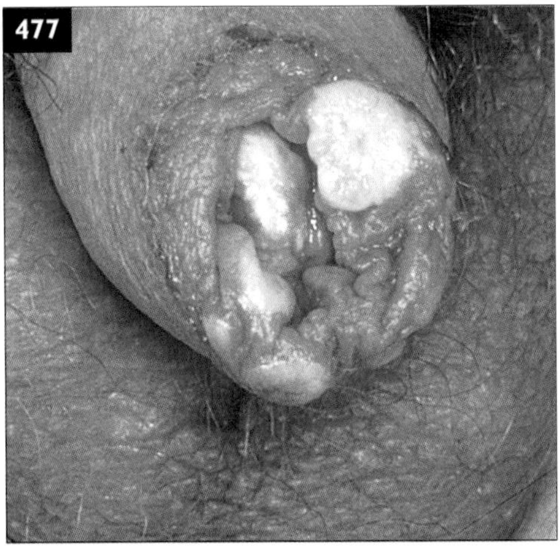

477 Primary syphilis.

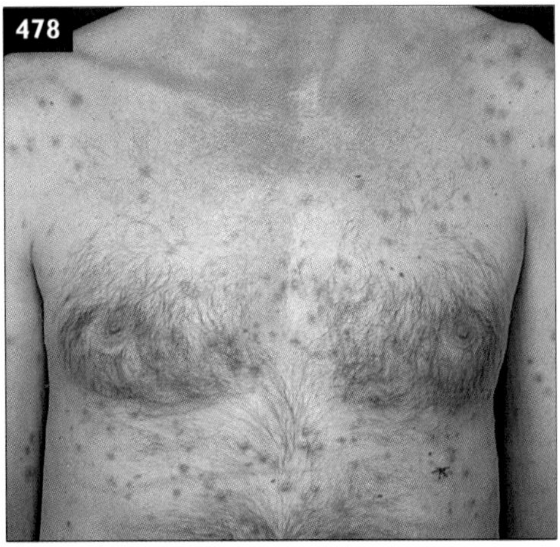

478 Secondary syphilis.

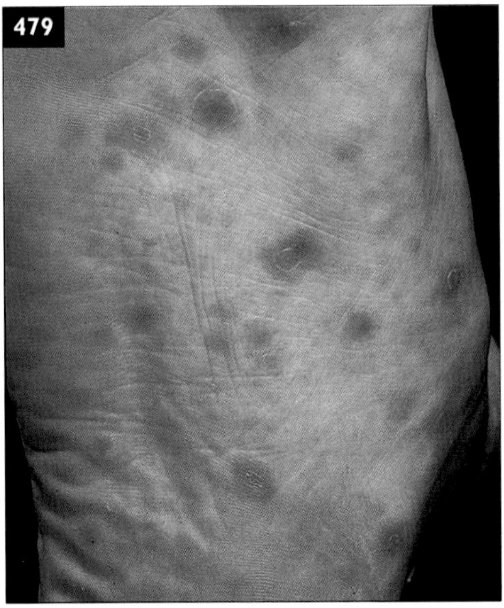

479 Secondary syphilis.

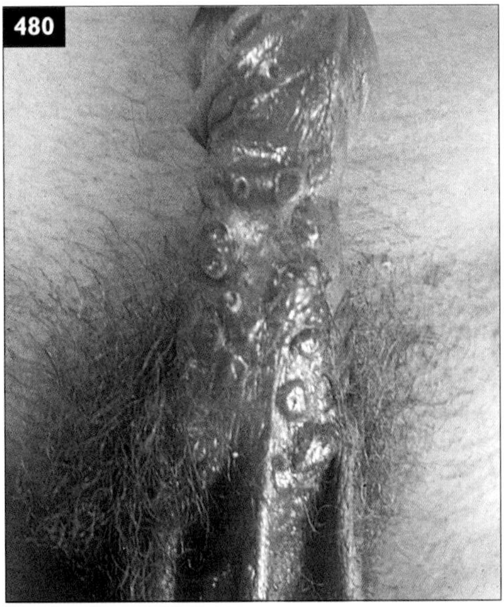

480 Condylomata lata.

Primary syphilis (**477**) is characterised by a chancre which is a well-defined, painless ulcer at the site of contact, most frequently in the anogenital area. It is usually solitary but there may be multiple lesions.

With secondary syphilis (**478**), in the untreated patient, a maculopapular eruption occurs on the face, trunk and limbs which has a psoriasiform appearance with distinctive lesions on the palms and soles (**479**). In flexural sites of the anogenital area, clusters of papules develop which vary from being smooth and shiny to wart-like and are known as condylomata lata (**480**).

Genital and Perianal Dermatoses

Epidemiology
Treponema pallidum is the causative organism and there is a steady increase in the incidence of syphilis in men, with a high prevalence in homosexuals. Changes in sexual practices with the advent of HIV infection has led to a slight decline in incidence.

Differential diagnosis
Primary chancre – any ulcer, e.g. Behçet's, Sutton's, aphthous. Secondary – psoriasis, pityriasis rosea. Condylomata lata – viral warts.

Investigations
Smears of primary and secondary lesions with dark field microscopy. Serology for antibody detection. Histopathology.

Special points
Congenital syphilis is now very rare due to routine screening for syphilis in pregnancy.

HUMAN IMMUNODEFICIENCY VIRUS (HIV) INFECTION

Definition and clinical features
HIV is the viral agent responsible for the acquired immunodeficiency syndrome (AIDS).

The specific cutaneous manifestations in the anogenital region are few and include Kaposi's sarcoma and chronic cytomegalovirus or herpes simplex infection. There is an increased incidence of syphilis and as there is impaired cell mediated immunity, more problems with recurrent candidiasis, fungal infections, herpes virus, human papilloma virus infection and molluscum contagiosum. Generalised drug eruptions are also a problem and, in particular, fixed drug eruptions characteristically occur in the anogenital area and this has been well documented with penile erosions in patients receiving pentamidine. There are also well documented case reports of intraepithelial neoplasia and invasive carcinomas of the anogenital region in patients with HIV infection.

Epidemiology
The main routes of transmission are via sexual intercourse, transplacentally to the foetus and the use of contaminated syringes and needles. Transfusion of contaminated blood and blood products is no longer a risk in the UK since the introduction of routine screening in 1984. In Africa, spread is mainly through heterosexual intercourse and transplacentally. Transmission in the industrialised countries is predominantly through homosexual or bisexual men, and intravenous drug abusers.

Diagnosis
Serology for antibodies and antigen.

Index

Index

Index

Index